The Concise Book of Acupoints

John R. Cross

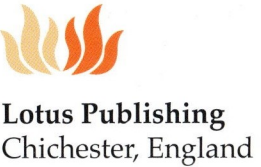

Lotus Publishing
Chichester, England

First published in 2010 by
Lotus Publishing
Apple Tree Cottage, Inlands Road, Nutbourne, Chichester, PO18 8RJ, UK

Illustrations Amanda Williams, John Tyropolis, Michael Evdemon and Ilaira Bouratinos
Text Design Wendy Craig
Cover Design Jim Wilkie
Printed and Bound in the UK by Scotprint

British Library Cataloguing in Publication Data
A CIP record for this book is available from the British Library
ISBN 978 1 905367 19 1

Contents

Introduction

What Is an Acupoint? Traditional and Modern Concepts

Traditional Concepts

Traditional Chinese Medicine (TCM) has been practiced for over 5000 years as a way of maintaining health, not necessarily to ease symptoms. It is believed that acupuncture originated in India and was later spread to China, Egypt and Asia by Buddhist monks. It then transferred to Japan and other Far Eastern countries. It has only been popular in the West since the middle of the twentieth century. It was quaintly thought that warriors returning from war exhibiting spear and arrow wounds would slowly be healed of other conditions as their wounds healed, the site of the wound often having no bearing on the diseased part that improved. Over several decades, points were mapped out on the body that had an influence on certain internal organs and parts of the body if they were stimulated by pressure, needle (originally made from bamboo) or burning. These points were called *acupuncture points, acupoints, xue* or *tsubo*.

Acupoints on the body that possessed a similar internal organ or system affinity were 'joined together' in a series of invisible energy lines called *meridians* or *channels*. Each of the meridians was named after the internal organ or system that it appeared to influence. The meridians housed the vital force or chi (ki or prana) and by affecting the acupoint the chi was sedated or stimulated. Until just a few years ago it was widely thought that the meridian system could be likened to a canal waterway system, and the acupoints to lock gates. When the acupoint is stimulated the lock gate is opened and the water flows through, energy once more flowing freely through the system.

The eleven meridians that are named after the internal organs they influence are; Large Intestine (LI), Small Intestine (SI), Stomach (ST), Gall Bladder (GB), Bladder (BL), Lung (LU), Heart (HT), Spleen (SP), Liver (LR), Kidney (KI) and Pericardium (PC). Added to these was the Triple Energizer (TE) channel. These twelve all exist as bilateral meridians. There are a further eight 'extraordinary' meridians, six of which are composites of the original twelve, plus two unilateral channels named Governor (Gov) and Conception (Con).

Traditional forms of acupuncture and acupressure are not confined to China. Ayurvedic medicine has given us the amazing concept of the major and minor chakras that are considered to be whorls of energy that stem from a single acupoint on the physical body and permeate the layers of the subtle auric bodies. There are also Marma points – another traditional Ayurvedic concept which states that there are 107 vital acupoints in the body that link the energy channels of the nerves, muscles and joints. These points are mostly used with pressure and incorporated into massage techniques but may be used in acupuncture as they seem to exist as a combination of meridian, non meridian, trigger and reflex points.

Yin and Yang

Although this 'concise' book will not deal with acupuncture analysis and diagnosis or deeper aspects of philosophy, it is important that these two terms are understood as changes in the chi energy affect Yin and Yang each time an acupoint is influenced. These two words (properly pronounced 'inn' and 'arng') are the two poles of chi and are opposite and yet complementary to each other. Yin and Yang philosophy forms the backbone of traditional Chinese, Japanese, Indian and tribal medicines (although they are sometimes known by different names). The ideas behind Yin and Yang developed from observing the physical world. It was observed that nature appears to group into pairs of dependent opposites. Thus, the concept of 'night' has no meaning without the concept of 'day'. As you will know, there is no such thing as absolute Yang or absolute Yin and an increment of one always appears in the other. The organs and meridians are either predominantly Yin or Yang (called Zang and Fu) – the Yin organs being mostly solid in nature, and mostly essential to life, whereas the Yang organs are hollow and often peristaltic in nature. The Yin meridians are generally positioned along the antero-medial aspects of the limbs and torso and the Yang meridians on the postero-lateral. The Yin meridians therefore 'ape' the organs in that they appear to be 'protected'. Further divisions will be mentioned later in the chapter.

Yin	Yang
Winter	Summer
Cold	Heat
Female	Male
Dark	Light
Chronic	Acute
Flaccid	Spastic
Stiffness	Mobility
Oedema	Inflammation
Hypotension	Hypertension
Vital organs	Hollow organs

Table 1.1 Yin and Yang equivalents (shortened version).

Acupuncture Nomenclature

In 2003 the World Health Authority decided to standardize acupuncture nomenclature so that each practitioner used the same names and initials. Until then it had been a hotchpotch of different titles and initials. The Pericardium meridian had been known as Heart Constrictor and even Circulation-Sex by kinesiologists. The Triple Energizer had also been known as the San Jiao, Triple Warmer or Three Heater. The initials used have also been through a number of changes before they were standardized. They now consist of all upper case initials.

Modern Concepts

The reason why the practice of acupuncture has proliferated in the West over the past couple of decades is that a great deal of its physiological rationale has been scientifically proven beyond doubt. It is certainly the reason why it is practiced in publicly funded medical organisations as well as those that are privately run. Medical acupuncture is not practiced on the foundation of vital force or any 'archaic' diagnostic procedures such as tongue and pulse diagnosis, but rather by using formulaic procedures for given conditions or pain syndromes. Traditionalists would argue that this noble art (note – not science) has been denigrated and watered down by removing that part of the philosophy that enabled the person to be treated holistically as opposed to merely easing the symptoms. It is an argument that will run and run. Rather than obstruction in the flow of circulation and chi described in the traditional texts, disease is understood to be caused by micro-organisms, metabolic failure, changes in DNA structure or signalling, or a breakdown in the immune system.

Modern studies have indicated that acupuncture stimulates some of these signalling systems, which may increase that rate of the healing response. Research has indicated the primary signalling system affected by acupuncture is the central nervous system, which not only transmits signals along the nerves but also a variety of bio chemicals that influence other cells of the body. Acupuncture analgesia seems to be mediated by the release of enkephalin and beta-endorphins. Although modern science has proven how pain relief works *ad nauseum*, it has failed to show how non-pain syndromes are helped. These would include improving the wellbeing of a patient, emotional imbalance, non-painful respiratory, skin, cardiac and other internal organ imbalance.

Acupoints and Reflex Points

There has been much debate over whether or not there is any correlation between acupoints and reflex points. It has been shown that meridian acupoints, non meridian acupoints and the major reflex points (some of which are classical trigger points) seem to be points on the body that show a lower electrical resistance compared to the surrounding tissues. My own research has shown that there is no actual difference between acupoints and reflex points except that acupoints are used more widely in acupuncture than reflex points. All of these points are, after all, reflected points of internal organs or other parts of the body and exhibit tenderness when there is an energy imbalance within the body part. This Concise book will concentrate on the most used meridian acupoints but will also include some useful non-meridian acupoints and reflex points.

Deqi

Each time an acupoint is needled, the practitioner should evoke the sensation of deqi within the patient's tissues. Deqi literally means 'acquiring the qi' (or chi). The patient may feel a myriad of sensations when a needle is correctly inserted into the acupoint. These could include an ache, a spreading sensation into the local tissues of travelling down the meridian channel, numbness, tingling, pulling, heaviness or warmth. Experienced patients will always let the practitioner know if the needle is 'spot on' and, quite frankly, it is a waste of time performing acupuncture unless deqi has been felt. The practitioner will also sense deqi. The acupoint will often 'grab' the needle and seem to suck it in, it amazingly hangs on to the needle until the treatment has been effective, after approximately twenty minutes. The practitioner may also sense an alteration in the patient's breathing rate, pulse rate, or body temperature. It may also bring about abdominal rumbling, sighing, sweating, itching or crying. Therefore correct needle insertion must influence the patient's autonomic nervous system. An area of redness around the needle insertion will often appear after a few seconds. In traditional acupuncture philosophy this is said to represent '*fong*' or *perverse energy* and would indicate correct acupuncture treatment. Some patients have stronger reactions than others and some acupoints react more forcefully than others. The strongest fong reaction points appear to be on the torso and abdomen. Fong is just a histamine reaction within the patient's tissues, which varies widely from person to person.

What Can We Do With an Acupoint?

In attempting to affect the flow of chi, you may use the following methods:

- Needle in sedation or stimulation mode
- Needle stimulated with an electro-acupuncture instrument
- Plum Blossom needle stimulation
- Press needle or stud as used in auriculotherapy
- Prismatic needle or scarifier for blood letting
- Moxabustion either directly on the point or above it using a moxa stick
- Electronic machine stimulation such as TENS
- Laser stimulation
- Magnets
- Cupping
- Finger pressure in sedation or stimulating mode (acupressure, shiatsu or tuina)

Acupoints may even be injected with substances (especially homoeopathic tinctures) that possess the same vibrational frequency as the point. This is called 'homoeo-puncture' and is a technique that is popular in France and Belgium. There are also several different portable electronic instruments that both detect the existence of acupoints as well as stimulating them. To add a little esotericism to the plot here, it is also possible to stimulate the 'auric' acupoint either by needle or finger stimulation. If acupoints are considered to be vortices of energy, then each acupoint must possess an etheric position as well. The most popular ways to affect acupoints though are by needle, moxabustion and acupressure and it is these three that will be discussed.

Needle

Needles are usually made from stainless steel but occasionally are made from specialized metals such as gold, zinc and copper. They may be inserted by means of a metal or plastic guide tube if the handle of the needle will accommodate this. By far the most common needling practice in the West is to use pre-sterilized blister packs and each one is disposed of after use. As recently as the late 1980s it was impossible to do this and every needle needed to be sterilized by autoclave or glass bead sterilizer after use. The most commonly used needles are between half an inch and three inches in length. The much longer fine needles that are up to eight inches long are used to thread along a superficial meridian along the scalp (very specialized).

Needling Techniques

As practitioners will acknowledge, it is not just a question of inserting a needle at the correct angle to the body into an acupoint and 'leaving it there'. Where chi is deficient, the needle needs to be stimulated by a range of different methods such as lifting, thrusting, rotation, flicking or stroking the handle. This is called *reinforcing* or *stimulation* and is designed to create a surge of chi flow where little existed before. The reducing or sedating technique is to insert the needle and leave it in situ for up to twenty minutes in order to reduce an excess of chi. There is also a neutral (or even) technique when there is neither insufficiency nor excess and the acupoint is needled to affect a distal region.

Needling Angles

The angle at which the needle is inserted is dependent upon the anatomical site of the acupoint, the desired result and the patient's underlying condition. There are three main angles of insertion; perpendicular, oblique and transverse. Perpendicular insertion is at 90 degrees to the skin and is the most commonly used. It is especially suitable for fleshy areas. Oblique or slanted insertion (30 to 60 degrees) is suitable where the flesh is thin or where an internal organ or vessel lies deep to the location. Transverse insertion (5 to 20 degrees) is suitable for thin areas with very little flesh and for subcutaneous needling. Many of the facial and neck points are needled in this fashion or where two points are needled at the same time.

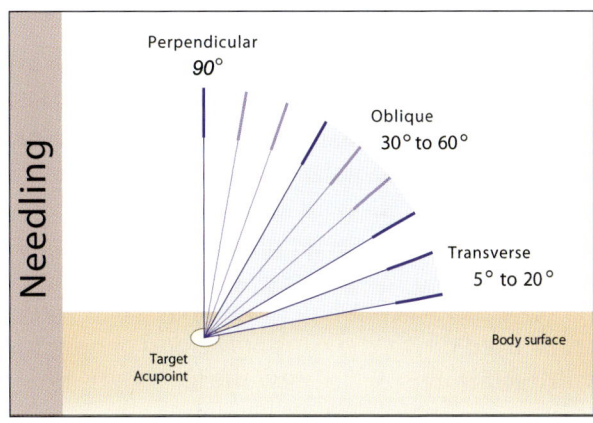

Figure 1.1: Needling angles.

Needling Depth

The depths that are recommended in this book are for the 'average' adult size. The depth of insertion should be modified for children (shallower), overweight and obese patients (longer needle required) and very slim adults where the needling is more superficial. The golden rule in all needling is to affect the acupoint and obtain the sensation of deqi (sometimes called *te qui*).

Needling Contraindications

Needles should not be applied to; scar tissue, open wounds, swellings such as lipomas, cysts, skin growths, boils or infected areas. Adjacent points along the same meridian should be chosen instead. Certain acupoints are also 'forbidden' in pregnancy and patients with certain psychotic tendencies. Needling should not be considered in patients with bleeding and clotting disorders or who are taking anti-coagulant drugs. Unless the point is a recognized standard acupoint, the skin should not be punctured. It also goes without saying (but I shall) that needling is also contraindicated in patients who do not want invasive acupuncture – their wishes must be respected at all times. One can administer acupressure, magnets, cupping, TENS and many more types of non-invasive acupuncture to achieve the same results. Be very careful of needling around the lungs and pleura deeper than a centimetre. The nipple (ST 17) and umbilicus (Con 8) should be considered as 'no go' acupoints to needle although there are many more that are potentially dangerous and hazardous. These will all be indicated in the text.

Moxabustion

Moxabustion (often referred to as moxibustion) is as old if not older than needling. It is a process of burning a dried herb, usually mugwort (*Artemisia vulgaris*) on the acupoint. Mugwort is used as it burns slowly and evenly. It is performed when there is a deficiency of chi in the acupoint, meridian or corresponding internal organ. Thermal energy is easily taken up by the body. Certain acupoints are forbidden to moxa and these are highlighted in the text. Moxa may be used directly or indirectly to affect an acupoint.

Direct Moxabustion
This may be performed in several ways:

- By making a cone from loose moxa punk. The small rolled up ball is placed on the acupoint and lit by means of a taper. The patient is instructed to say 'ouch' or some other acceptable incantation when he or she feels a sharp flash of heat and the practitioner removes quickly.
- Packed moxa inside a paper tube about half an inch thick and tall is placed on the acupoint and lit using a match or taper. This method intrudes thermal energy on a much more even and slower rate that the moxa ball. The ash is then removed following up to five 'moxas'.
- Loose moxa punk or a packed moxa pack as previously described may be placed on the end of a special copper-handled long needle that has previously been inserted into an acupoint. The moxa is lit and heat is transferred down the copper (a good conductor) handle thus giving heat to the acupoint. Chronic arthritic joints or deep muscular lesions may be helped enormously by this method.
- On acupoints that are forbidden to needle or moxa, moxabustion may still be applied by using a medium between the moxa and the patient's skin. Salt is often placed in Con 8 (umbilicus) and the moxa is burned on the layer of salt. Slices of garlic and ginger may be used as a mugwort substitute in any acupoint.

Indirect Moxabustion
Thermal energy may be applied indirectly to an acupoint by the following:

- A moxa roll is a long cigar-shaped paper tube filled with compacted mugwort. The end is lit and allowed to burn for a few seconds and is introduced to the vicinity of the acupoint approximately one to two centimetres above the skin. The patient is asked to report when he/she feels the warmth. A similar technique may be applied with an ordinary taper.
- A moxa box appears in various designs but works on the common principle of allowing heat from the moxa to be distributed over a large area. This is ideal to treat a large area of the lower spine.

Moxabustion Cautions
The following precautions must be taken:

- Precautions must be taken to avoid burning, so care must be taken in not stimulating the acupoint too much.
- Areas of numbness and febrile diseases are contraindicated.
- Do not use moxabustion to the lower spine or abdomen in pregnant women.
- Do not give moxa on areas of oedema and varicosities.
- A burn may be treated by using a proprietary branded 'burn ointment' after the part has been doused in cold water. Hydrocortisone cream or homoeopathic *calendula* ointment may also be tried.

Acupressure

The use of pressure with the fingers on an acupoint is older than the use of needles or moxabustion. Various methods of manual techniques include acupressure (several approaches), reflexology (several types), shiatsu (Japanese), tuina (Traditional Chinese), anma (Traditional Japanese) and daoyin (strictly a mind/body exercise). There are scores of variations of these, some of which combine acupoints into the treatment regimen and others that do not.

Methods of finger acupressure (using the word as a generic term) are:

- Light touch on a point
- Deep touch on a point
- Gentle massage on a point
- Stimulating massage on a point
- Light massage on an area or meridian
- Stimulating massage on an area or meridian

These methods are used to stimulate or sedate the acupoint and the surrounding tissues and influence the controlling meridian, thus affecting the local area or the reflected area.

Acupressure Contraindications

Pressure and massage treatment should not be performed during the first three months of pregnancy or anywhere on the abdomen during the whole of pregnancy. Pressure should not be applied to any area of open wounds, swellings, cysts and lipomas or any area of varicosities. The acupoints of Gov 28 (mouth), ST 17 (nipple) and Con 1 (perineum) are obvious no go areas. Please also be aware that you do not have to be 'pin-point' accurate when applying pressure and that there is an 'area of influence' surrounding the point. Some therapists imagine that acupressure is a 'watered down' cheap imitation of needle acupuncture – nothing is further from the truth. The great advantage of acupressure (performed correctly) is that you can feel what is occurring within the patient's tissues as the treatment is progressing.

Traditional Relationships of Acupoints

The relationship of acupoints is the cornerstone of traditional acupuncture and separates the philosophies of Chinese, Japanese and Ayurvedic traditional acupuncture systems from those of modern Western acupuncture that concentrate on formulaic and symptomatic approaches.

There are several traditional acupuncture relationships and approaches that may be employed, and below is a flavour of what exists, it is not though a total breakdown as that would fall outside the remit of this book.

Traditional Chinese medicine approaches include:

- Great points
- Source points
- Accumulation points
- Connecting points
- Gathering points

- Five Transporting points
- Tonification, Sedation and Horary points
- Back Transporting points
- Front Collecting points
- Eight Opening points

Traditional Ayurvedic medicine philosophy (combined with my own research) includes:

- Physical aspects of the seven major chakras (anterior and posterior)
- Physical aspects of the twenty-one minor chakras
- Marma points

Traditional Chinese and Japanese philosophy usually associated with reflected areas:

- Vertical zones incorporating specific acupoints
- Parallel points

Modern Western acupuncture and pressure/massage also use the scores of active and latent Trigger points

Great Points

The term 'Great' point is a relatively modern interpretation of possibly the twelve most commonly used acupoints in acupuncture. This represents one acupoint per meridian even though some meridians would contain two or more commonly used points. They are considered to be the 'polychrest' of acupoints in that each of these points may be used in at least three different ways. These must be learned in order to be able to perform even the most basic forms of successful acupuncture. They are:

Yang points   **LI 4; ST 36; SI 3; BL 66; TE 5** and **GB 41**
Yin points   **LU 7; SP 6; HT 7; KI 3; PC 6** and **LR 3**

Source Points

The Source or Yuan points for each of the twelve meridians are located around the ankles and wrists. They are said to have a direct link with the associated organ or system represented by the meridian and, as such, are those points used to stimulate the energy in the organ. They are:

Yang points   **LI 4; ST 42; SI 4; BL 64; TE 4** and **GB 40**
Yin points   **LU 9; SP 3; HT 7; KI 3; PC 7** and **LR 3**

Accumulation Points

The Accumulation or Cleft-Xi points generally treat an excess of chi (yang) in the organ or meridian, particularly when there is pain. They are:

Yang points	**LI 7; ST 34; SI 6; BL 63; TE 7** and **GB 36**
Yin points	**LU 6; SP 8; HT 6; KI 5; PC 4** and **LR 6**

Connecting Points

The Connecting or Luo points are used to balance or harmonise chi between the paired yin-yang meridians, usually from a yin channel to its yang counterpart. They are:

Yang points	**LI 6; ST 40; SI 7; BL 58; TE 5** and **GB 37**
Yin points	**LU 7; SP 4; HT 5; KI 4; PC 6** and **LR 5**

Gathering Points

There are eight Gathering (sometimes called Influential or Meeting) points. They appear to have a direct influence on various systems of the body and should be used in conditions where the specific system is deficient. They are:

Chi	**Con 17**	Bone	**BL 11**
Blood	**BL 17**	Tendons	**GB 34**
Vessels	**LU 9**	Yin organs	**LR 13**
Marrow	**GB 39**	Yang organs	**Con 12**

Five Transporting Points

The five Transporting (sometimes called Command) points are five points on each meridian between the fingers and elbows and between the toes and knees. They are linked to the Law of Five Elements or Transformations. Each of the five points represents a different depth of chi flow where the meridian may be likened to a river flowing with water. From the distal to the proximal, i.e. finger or toe to the elbow or knee the points are named Tsing (Well), Ying (Spring), Shu (Stream), Jing (River) and He (Sea). Figure 1.2 represents this.

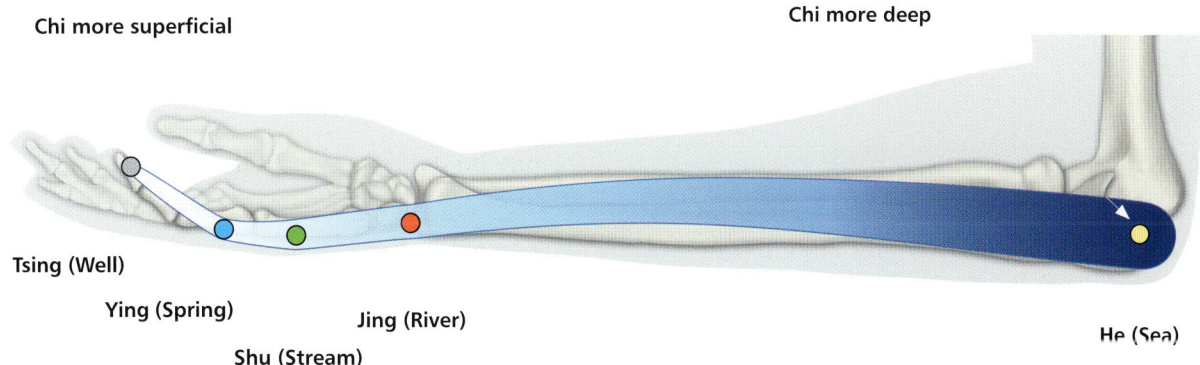

Figure 1.2: Schematic representation of the Five Transporting points.

The *Tsing* points are located at the distal end of the meridian and are sometimes called the *nail* point. Here, the chi is at its most superficial and is often where the energy of the associated yin/yang meridians alters its polarity. On the yin meridians they are points on the Wood element and on the yang meridians they are on the Metal element.

The *Ying* points are located at the base of the fingers and toes and have a deeper energy flow to the Tsing *points*. On the yin meridians they are points on the Fire element and on the yang meridians they are on the Water element.

The *Shu* points are located at the wrists or ankles and represent a deeper flow of energy than the other two. On the yin meridians they are also the Source points and the Earth element, and on the yang meridians they are on the Wood element.

The *Jing* points are located on the forearm and lower leg. The flow of chi is much deeper and stronger in these points. On the yin meridians they are on the Metal element and the yang meridians are on the Fire element.

The *He* points are located at the elbows and knees and represent the most harmonising points of the five. On the yin meridians they are allocated to the Water element and on the yang meridians they are part of the Earth element.

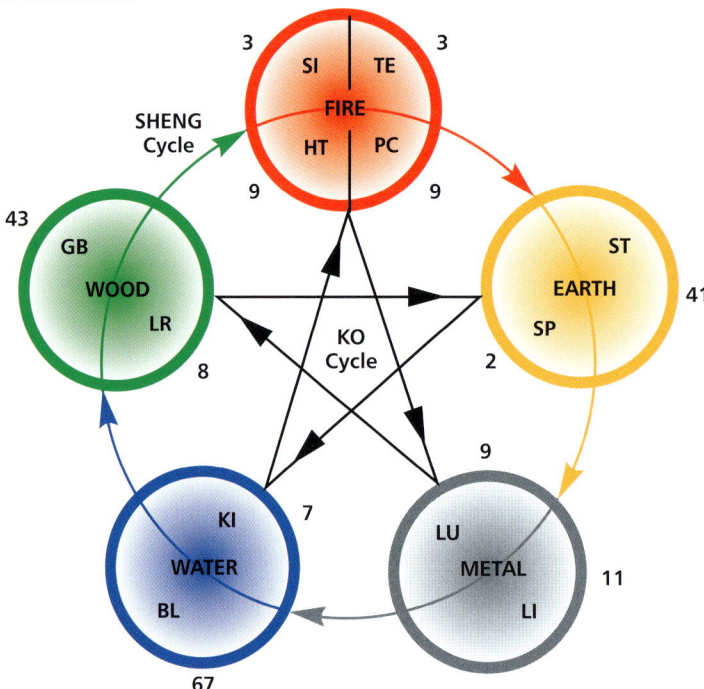

Figure 1.3: The internal organs and seasons in relation to the Five Elements in the Creation, Controlling and Rebelling cycles.

Tonification, Sedation and Horary Points

These sets of points are linked to the traditional concept of the Law of Five Elements or Transformations (Phases). This comprehensive and far reaching part of traditional philosophy remains one of the cornerstones of traditional acupuncture and is well known to all who practice this noble art. As there are so many erudite tomes on this Law, it is merely illustrated here and the acupoints shown. Figure 1.3 shows an illustration of the Law with the internal organs colour-coded showing the *Tonification* points. These are points that are used (on either the Sheng cycle yang or Sheng cycle yin) to transfer chi energy from one organ to another i.e. from the 'mother' to the 'son'. They are often used at the end of a treatment session to create a balance of energy within the patient. They are:

Yang Sheng cycle   **ST 41; LI 11; BL 67; GB 43; SI 3** or **TE 3**
Yin Sheng cycle   **SP 2; LU 11; KI 7; LR 8; HT 7** or **PC 9**

Where there is an excess of chi energy within the organ/meridian, the *Sedation* points are used to disperse chi from the 'son'. They are:

Yang acupoints   **ST 45; LI 2; BL 65; GB 38; SI 18** and **TE 10**
Yin acupoints   **SP 5; LU 5; KI 1; LR 2; HT 7** and **PC 7**

The *Horary* points are those points that reinforce chi in an organ/meridian by using the same Element point as the organ, e.g. the Fire point to stimulate the Small Intestine or the Metal point to reinforce the Lung. In clinical practice this is most beneficial if it coincides with that time of the day when there is most chi in a particular organ compared with the rest of the 24 hours (Chinese Clock). They are:

Yang points   **LI 1; ST 36; SI 5; BL 66; TE 6** and **GB 41**
Yin points   **LU 8; SP 3; HT 8; KI 10; PC 8** and **LR 1**

Back Transporting Points

The Back Transporting (also known as Back-Shu or Associated Effect) points are those points on the 'inner' Bladder meridian on the posterior aspect of the trunk that seem to have a direct energy link to the internal organs, probably by an autonomic nervous system link. They are ideal points used in pressure and massage techniques but extensively used with needle. They are excellent points to use in chronic energy imbalances. Figure 1.4 illustrates these points.

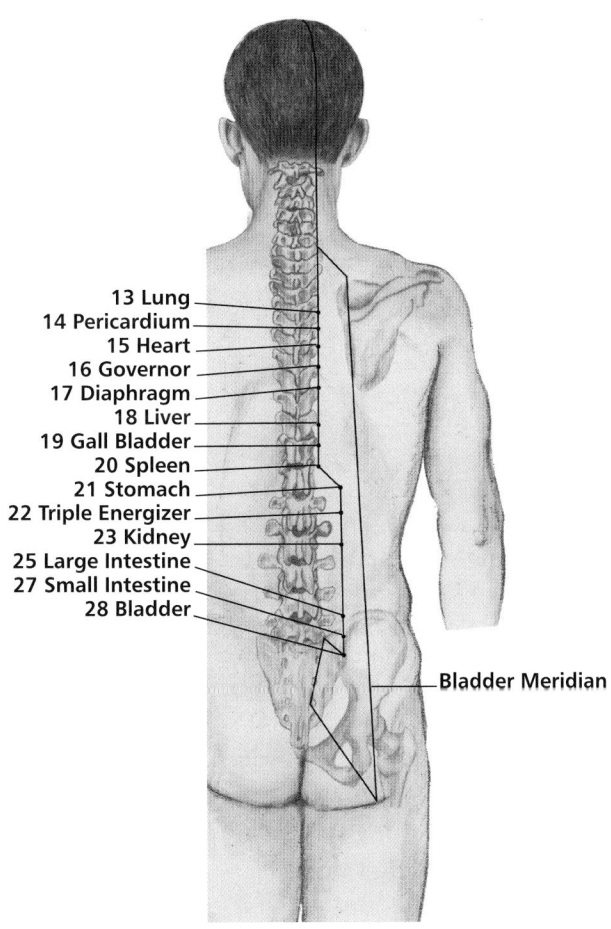

13 Lung
14 Pericardium
15 Heart
16 Governor
17 Diaphragm
18 Liver
19 Gall Bladder
20 Spleen
21 Stomach
22 Triple Energizer
23 Kidney
25 Large Intestine
27 Small Intestine
28 Bladder

Bladder Meridian

Figure 1.4: Back transporting points.

Front Collecting Points

The Front Collecting (also known as Mu or Alarm) points are located on the chest and abdomen. They are sensitive points when the corresponding organ is in a state of stress and are often used in First Aid situations and acute conditions. Figure 1.5 illustrates these points.

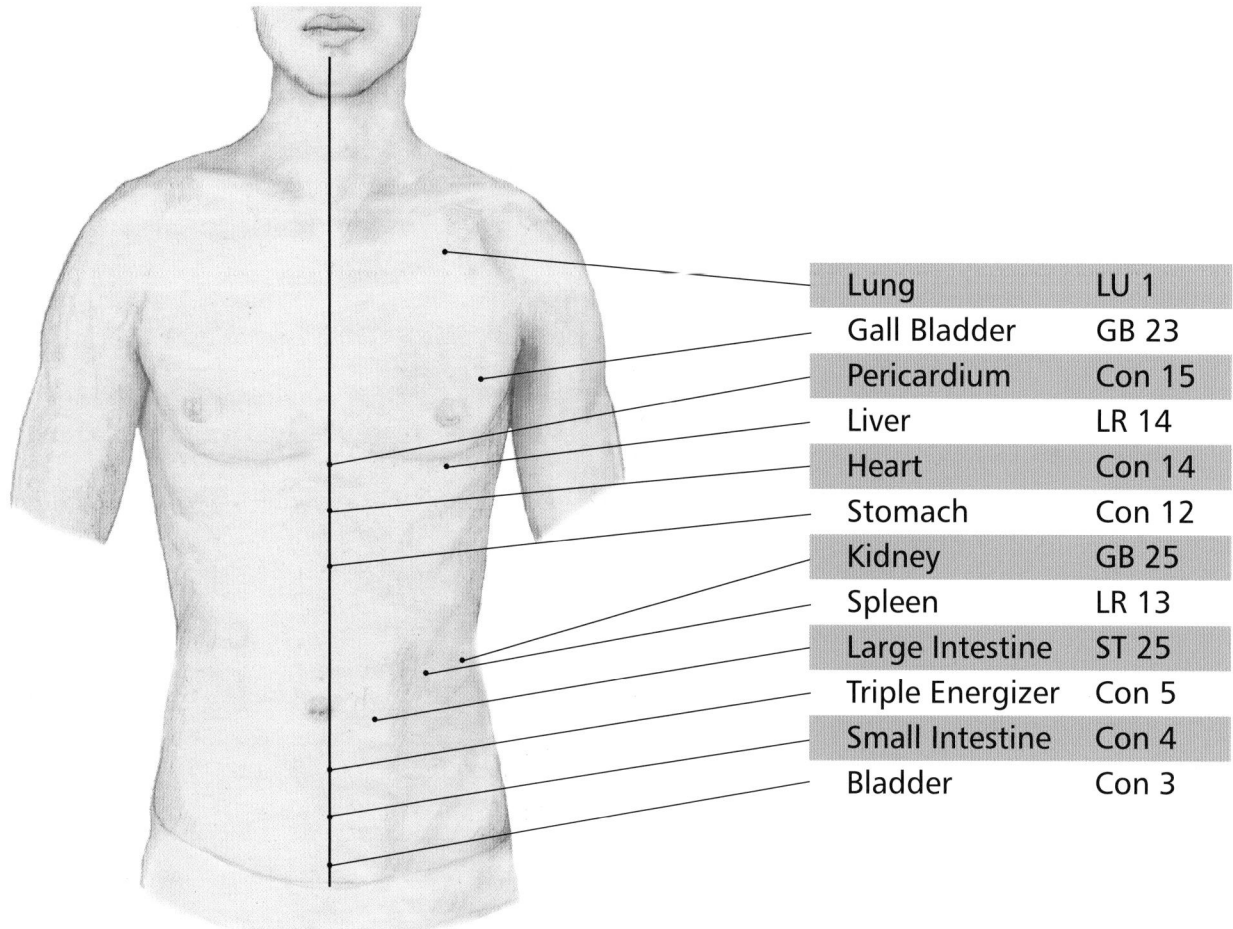

Lung	LU 1
Gall Bladder	GB 23
Pericardium	Con 15
Liver	LR 14
Heart	Con 14
Stomach	Con 12
Kidney	GB 25
Spleen	LR 13
Large Intestine	ST 25
Triple Energizer	Con 5
Small Intestine	Con 4
Bladder	Con 3

Figure 1.5: Front Collecting or Alarm points.

Eight Opening Points

The Eight Opening (also known as Key) points are those points that seem to 'open up' the eight extraordinary meridians. These meridians are not directly linked to internal organs and only two of them Conception and Governor have acupoints dedicated just to them. The other six use acupoints of other meridians. The key points on these channels may be used with needle, pressure and magnets as they seem to work powerfully in hormonal and chemical imbalance. The eight points are usually treated as four couples and remain a powerful tool for practitioners worldwide. They are:

- Governor (Du Mai) **SI 3** coupled point **BL 62**
- Conception (Ren Mai) **LU 7** coupled point **KI 6**
- Vital Vessel (Chong Mai) **SP 4** coupled point **PC 6**
- Girdle Vessel (Dai Mai) **GB 41** coupled with **TE 5**
- Yang Motility (Yangchiao Mai) **BL 62** coupled with **SI 3**
- Yin Motility (Yinchiao Mai) **KI 6** coupled with **LU 7**
- Yang Regulator (Yangwei Mai) **TE 5** coupled with **GB 41**
- Yin Regulator (Yinwei Mai) **PC 6** coupled with **SP 4**

Physical Aspects of the Seven Major Chakras

The word *chakra* means 'wheel' in Sanskrit. These are considered to be *force centres* or whorls of energy permeating from an acupoint on the physical body through the layers of the subtle bodies in an ever-increasing fan-shaped formation. They are rotating vortices of subtle matter and are considered to be focal points for the reception and transmission of energies. With the exception of the Crown chakra, each of the major chakras has both spinal and ventral aspects with corresponding acupoints. Strictly speaking the Base chakra is situated at Con 1 or Gov 1 but these two points are not readily accessible or acceptable to being treated for obvious anatomical reasons. Con 2 and Gov 2 may therefore be used as each point is still within the area of influence that is required. The acupoints are as follows:

Chakra	Spinal Level	Spinal Acupoint	Ventral Acupoint
Crown	–	Gov 20	Gov 20
Brow	Occipito-Atlas	Gov 16	Extra 1 (Yintang)
Throat	C7–T1	Gov 14	Con 22
Heart	T6–T7	Gov 10	Con 17
Solar Plexus	T12–L1	Gov 6	Con 14
Sacral	L4–L5	Gov 3	Con 6
Base	Sacro-Coccyx	Gov 2	Con 2

Physical Aspects of the Twenty-one Minor Chakras

The minor chakras or centres are considered to be reflected points of the major chakras. They are, though, powerful energy points in their own right even though there is not the depth and range that are exhibited by the majors. Twenty of them (ten bilateral points) are used to treat pain syndromes with needle, pressure and magnets. The exception is the Spleen chakra which is sometimes considered to be the eighth major chakra and it is used mostly with the Solar Plexus and Sacral chakras. They are:

Positions	Minor Chakra	Acupoint
1	Spleen chakra	SP 16 (left)
2 and 3	Foot chakra	KI 1
4 and 5	Hand chakra	PC 8
6 and 7	Knee chakra	BL 40
8 and 9	Elbow chakra	PC 3
10 and 11	Groin chakra	ST 30
12 and 13	Clavicular chakra	KI 27
14 and 15	Shoulder chakra	LI 15
16 and 17	Navel chakra	KI 16
18 and 19	Ear chakra	TE 17
20 and 21	Intercostal chakra	SP 21

Each of the major and minor chakras is associated with one or two meridians and has a Key point, which may be used to 'open up' the chakra energy flow. Further information about this fascinating energy system can be found in my two books '*Healing with the Chakra Energy System – Acupressure, Bodywork and Reflexology for Total Health*' and '*Acupuncture and the Chakra Energy System – Treating the Cause of Disease*'. Each of these books is published by North Atlantic Books. Figure 1.6 illustrates the position of the major and minor chakra acupoints.

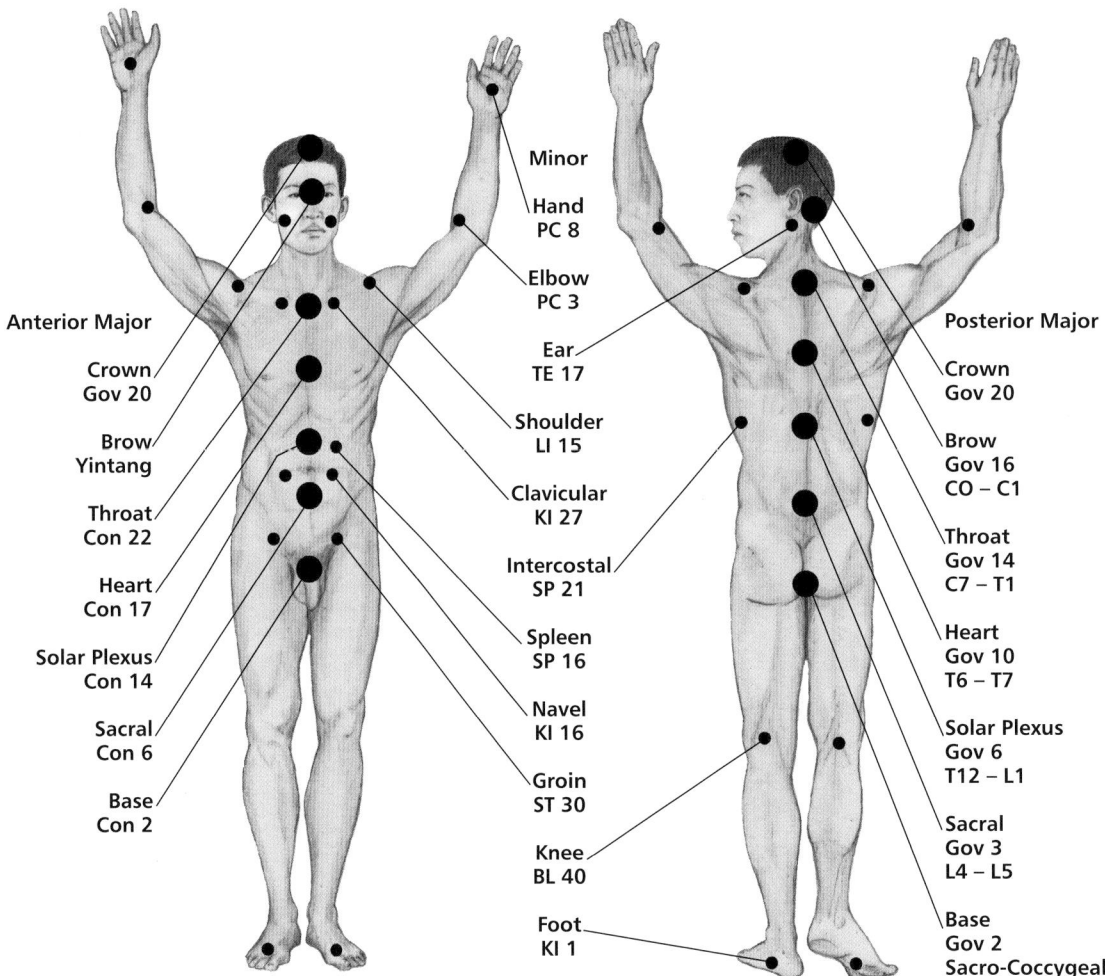

Figure 1.6: Position of the major and minor chakra acupoints.

Marma Points

Marma points appear to be the 'new kid on the block' although their philosophy is aligned to traditional Ayurvedic therapy. They consist of one hundred and seven points that link energy channels, nerves, muscles and joints and are used to treat mainly musculo-skeletal conditions. The main technique is with finger pressure and Ayurvedic massage but it is possible to use them with acupuncture. They appear to be composite acupoints – some meridian, some non meridian and some trigger points.

Vertical Zones: Reflected Acupoints

Although Zone therapy is as old as reflexology and acupuncture, the modern practice of zone therapy began with an American ENT specialist, Dr. William Fitzgerald. He noticed that patients who had performed their own kind of 'painful point therapy' on their feet fared better than those who had not. He discovered that the body may be divided into ten equal vertical sections (five on each side of the body) that cut through the underlying internal organs as well as the skin. Figure 1.6 shows these invisible energy pathways. In simple terms, when a part of the body becomes painful, check in which vertical zone the pain appears and use an acupoint distal to the pain site on the same vertical zone. Examples are; little finger discomfort (zone 5) which may be treated with little toe, outer aspect of knee, outer aspect of trunk or outer aspect of face acupoints. Try it – it works!

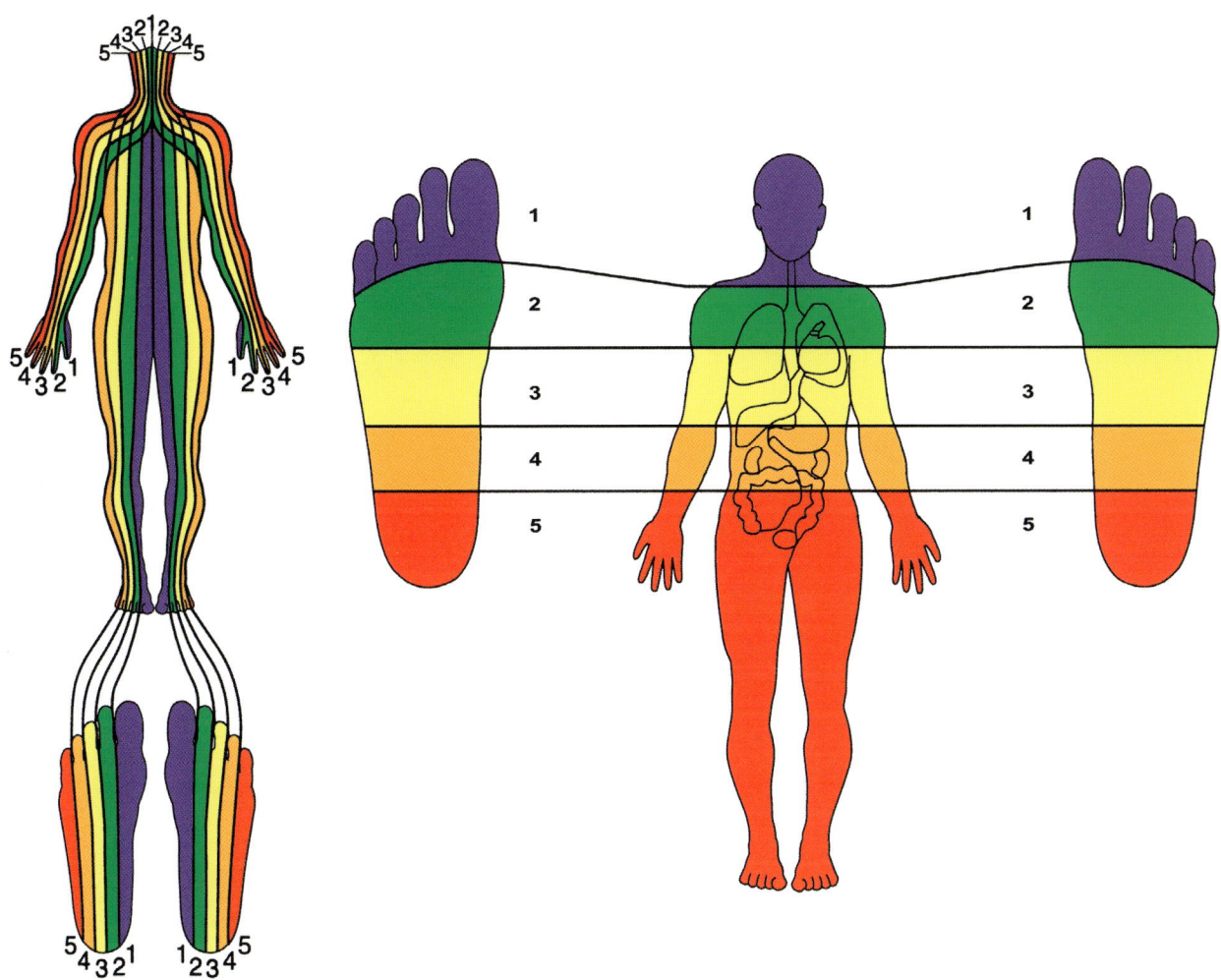

Figure 1.7: a) Body and feet zones, b) level of reflexes on the feet.

Parallel Acupoints

Another aspect of reflexology philosophy that may also be used with needle acupuncture is parallel points. This is based on the very simple concept of parallel joints and works in either of two ways:

- Pain in one joint (or part of the body) may be treated by affecting (by pressure, needle or magnet) the exact same point on the opposite side of the body, e.g. a left shoulder pain may be treated by placing a needle in the opposite LI 15 for example. This is particularly effective when the body part is inaccessible either due to a skin lesion or ulcer or in cases of amputation.
- Pain in a joint may be treated by using an acupoint in the parallel joint. These are: Shoulder – Hip; Elbow – Knee; Wrist – Ankle; Hand – Foot; Occiput – Sacrum, etc. Wherever a pain exists, a reflected area or point will always show tenderness and it is the tender point that requires treatment. As an example pain on the lateral aspect of the knee may be treated by a tender acupoint on the lateral aspect of the elbow e.g. LI 11. Figure 1.8 shows the parallel areas.

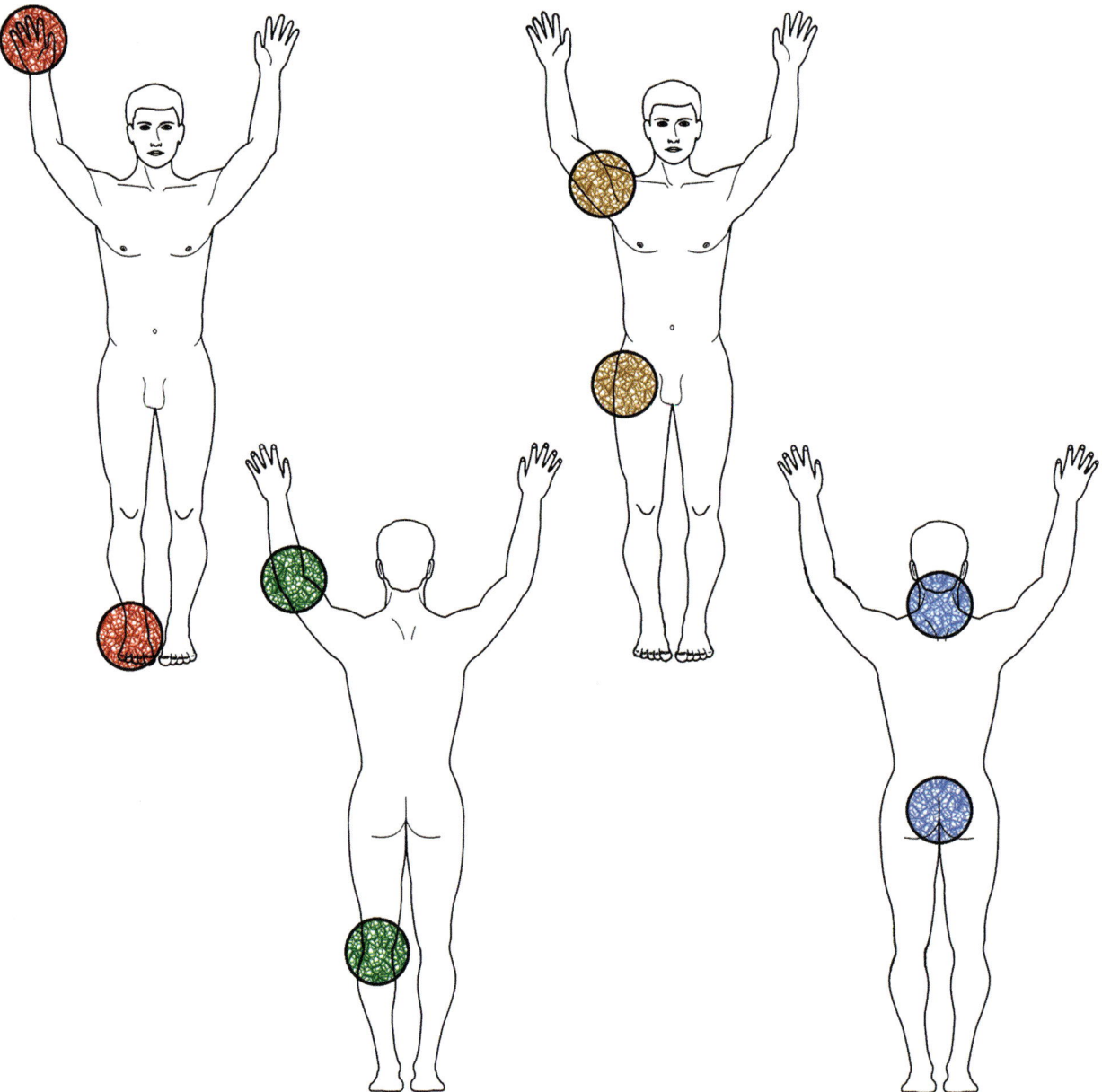

Figure 1.8: Parallel acupoints.

Trigger Points

The so-called trigger points are described as hyperirritable spots in skeletal muscles that are associated with palpable nodules in taut bands of muscle fibres. They appear to be small contraction knots within the muscle. There are two types; active and latent, both of which are acutely painful to the touch. *Active trigger points* are those which have, historically, been mapped out on the body as being linked to certain pain syndromes. An example of this would be Erb's point which is to be found in the upper quadrant of the trapezius muscle close to the second thoracic vertebra – this is linked to pain and inflammation in C5–C6. *Latent trigger points* are those that exist as sore spots that only show exquisite tenderness when heavily palpated. These points are not necessarily associated with classical pain syndromes. Needle acupuncture should be used for very short 'bursts' and needles are not in situ for very long.

Cun Measurement

In the times when Traditional Chinese medicine was in its infancy, patients were all shapes and sizes – fat and thin, short and tall. Where was the yardstick to produce accurate measurements, since it could not be based upon standard units or imperial measure? The patient's own body was therefore used in a method that still exists today. The cun (or pouce or AMI) is a very accurate way of measuring where acupoints exist on the body. One cun is the length of the middle phalanx of the patient's index finger or the width of their thumb. Some simple examples are:

* Two fingers width represent 1.5 cun.
* Four fingers width represent 3 cun.
* Distance from the greater trochanter on the hip to the upper border of the fibula represents 19 cun. Figure 1.9 shows the cun or pouce measurements.

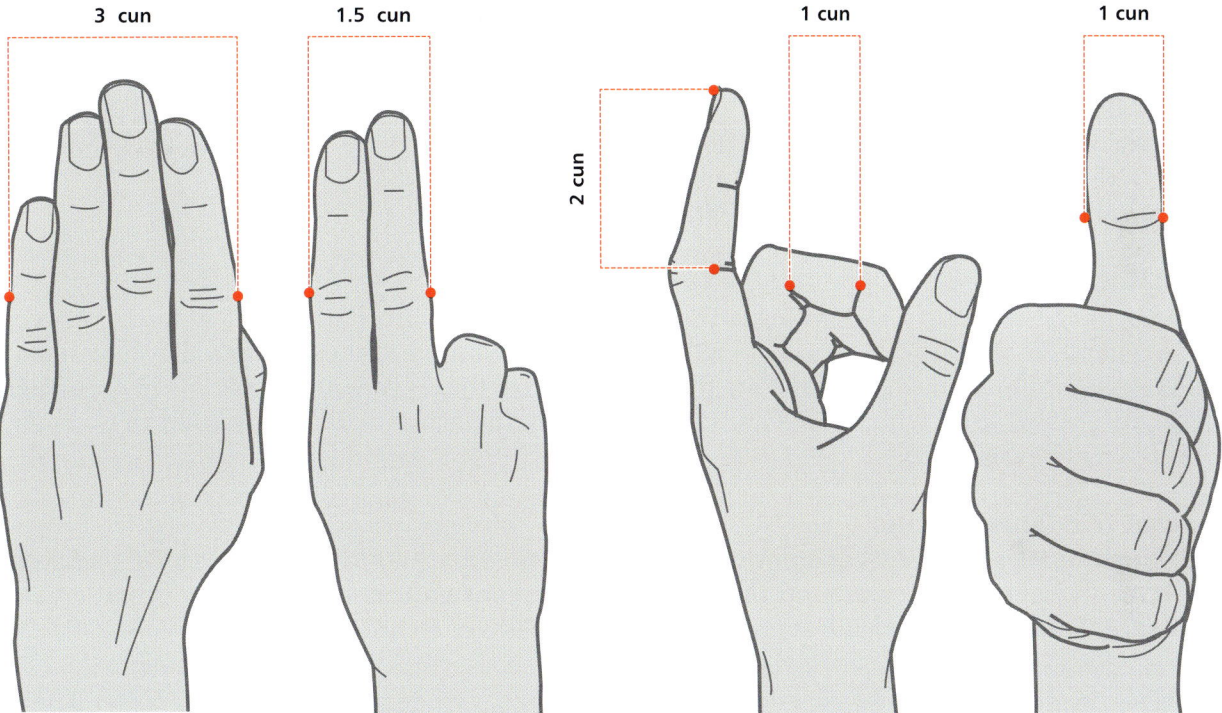

Figure 1.9: The cun or pouce measurements.

Principles of Point Selection

This book is aimed at all acupuncturists; the traditional, the Western trained or medical acupuncturist, the acupuncture student as well as the physical therapy and bodywork practitioner. It is therefore impossible to give a complete list of the principles of point selections; this would cover a whole book in its own right! Acupoints are selected using various parameters, which include:

- Local acupoints
- Distal acupoints
- Acupoints chosen for various disease syndromes – both according to traditional and modern (formulaic) methods
- Trigger points
- Major and minor chakra points

A description of each of the chosen acupoints will include the following:

- Location
- Needle with contraindications
- Moxa and pressure with contraindications
- Actions and indications (Traditional and Western)
- Special properties (only certain acupoints)

Star Ratings

Unique to this book is a star rating attributed to each acupoint. Each point is rated between 2 (★★) and 5 (★★★★★). The ★★★★★ rating is awarded to those points that have many different indications and actions and are the most useful in the body. Some acupoints may be rated differently when used with needle and pressure. Only the acupoints that are used in everyday practice will be described.

About the Illustrations

The illustrations aim to be as anatomically accurate as possible and to show the relevant adjacent structure. A light blue area around the 'dot' of an acupoint indicates a narrow or broad area of influence that may be used with acupressure and/or massage techniques.

The Fourteen Meridians

There are several depths or layers to each of the meridians. The most superficial 'layer' is the tendino-muscular meridian (TM) that carries the Wei energy. The acupoints for these meridians are usually the Command Points found between the finger and elbow and between the toe and the knee and are exactly the same as those of the main channels. The main (or surface) meridians contain Yong energy and, as such are slightly deeper than the TM meridians. The Lo meridian is the channel that connects each of the yin/yang couples. There is also an inner or deeper channel that uses traditional philosophy to show how the meridian is associated with its own internal organ as well as sometimes that of its coupled meridian and other organs. This introduction is not meant to confuse the reader but rather to enlighten them to the many 'layers' of energy existing within the body. The knowledge of the deeper meridians or channels should serve to enlighten the reader as to many of the indications of a given acupoint.

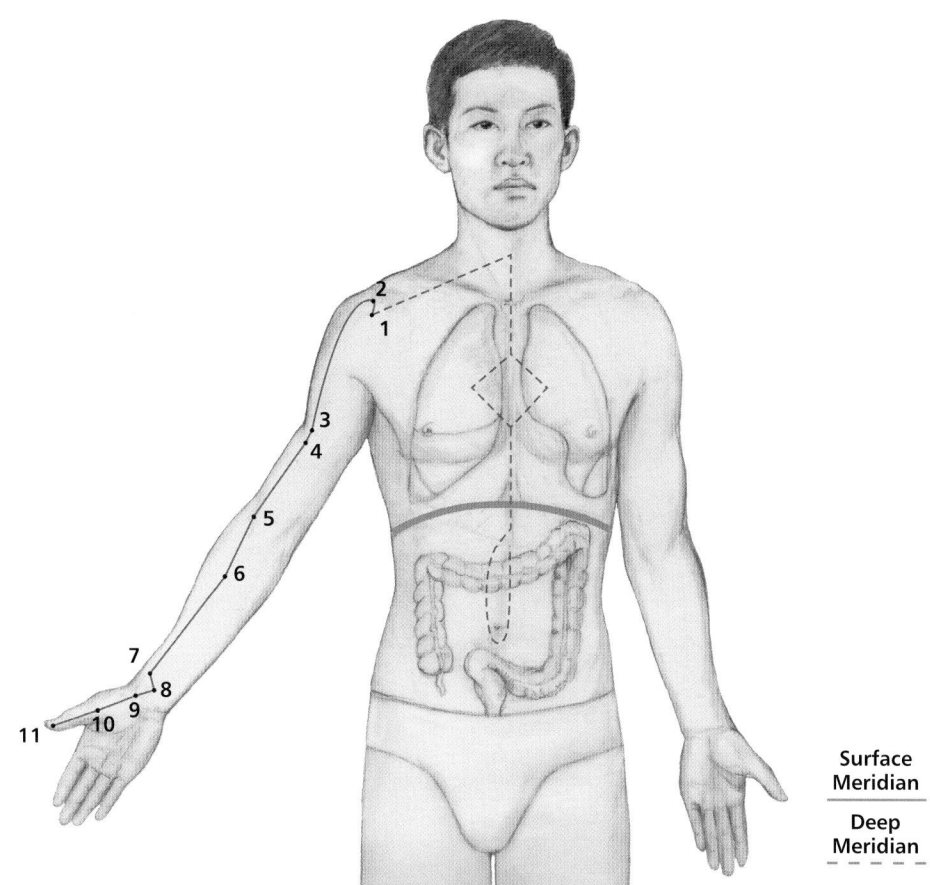

The Lung channel is the Yin aspect of the Metal element. There are eleven (11) acupoints on the main (surface) meridian. The deeper part of the Lung channel originates in the Zhongjiao or the middle of the abdomen. It runs downwards to connect with the large intestine (its Yang couple), passes through the diaphragm and penetrates the lungs, trachea and pharynx and leaves the chest cavity beneath the clavicle at acupoint LU 1. The surface meridian runs along the antero-lateral aspect of the upper arm and forearm, passing over the thenar eminence to end at the lateral edge of the thumb.

Only five of the eleven acupoints on this channel warrant description, as these are the most commonly used: LU 1, LU 5, LU7, LU9 and LU 11. The other acupoints on the meridian are not as commonly used as those described.

LU 1 *Zhong Fu* (Central Palace)

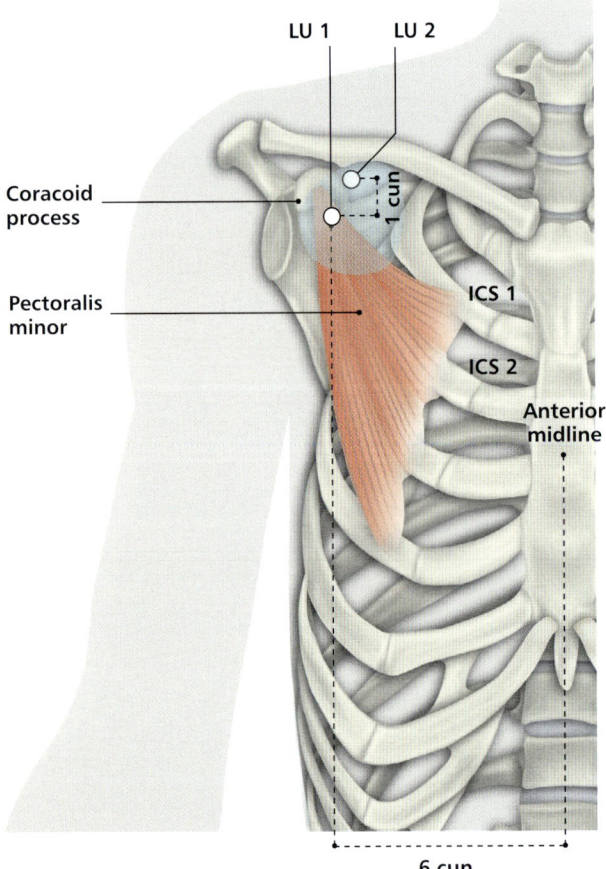

Location

Situated at the level of the 1st intercostal space, 6 cun lateral to the midline and 1 cun inferior to the inferior edge of the clavicle. This is a very important point but can be difficult for beginners to locate. The best way is to firstly locate LU 2 (beneath the clavicle) and move the locating finger 1 cun inferiorly to locate LU 1. The patient may help you by lying supine with the arm at approximately 45 degrees in abduction.

Needle

Superficial needling only is used with this point – approximately half a cun using an oblique and lateral insertion.

> There is a danger of lung puncture and possible pneumothorax if deeper medial needling is used. Also, even if the direction is correct, there is a danger of puncturing the cephalic vein or one of the brachial plexus tributaries if the needling is too deep.

Moxa and pressure

Light stimulation with moxa may be useful in order to raise the chi levels. Pressure techniques should adopt a light touch so as not to affect the underlying structures.

Indications

LU 1 is a very important and extensively used point for many types of breathing disorders, especially coughing and dyspnoea. It is used to treat tightness of the chest, cough, fullness of the chest and hiccough. It is also used as a self-help point when persistent niggling coughing prevents lying down. It is also a very good 'local' point for anterior shoulder pain and fullness, stiff and sore pectoral muscles and frozen shoulder. There is also a lesser action for some skin and abdominal conditions (mainly skin allergies and rashes and irritable bowel syndrome).

Special properties

LU 1 is the Alarm point of the lungs and as such is used as a diagnostic and analytical point as well as for treatment. The point is always acutely tender when the Lung meridian or the lungs themselves require treatment. A deep channel of the Spleen passes through LU1 as it continues on to supply the throat and mouth.

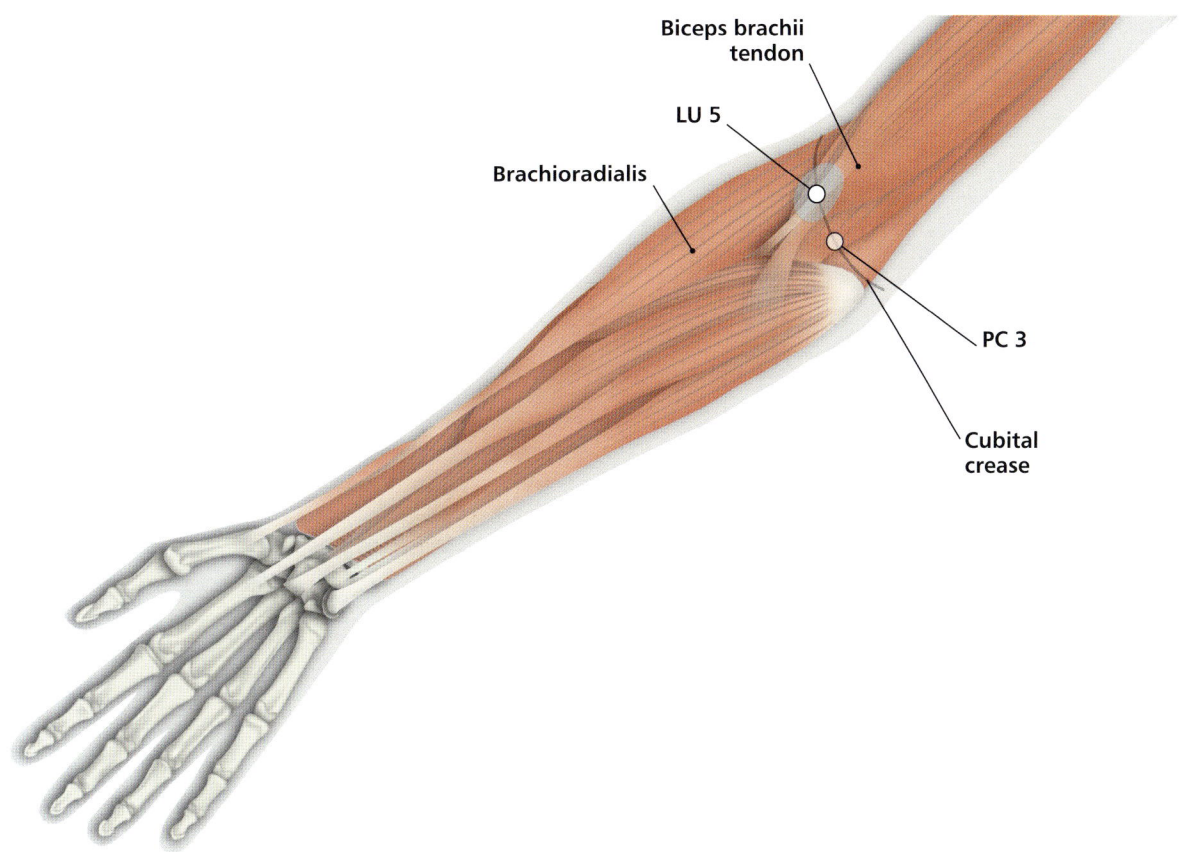

Biceps brachii tendon

LU 5

Brachioradialis

PC 3

Cubital crease

Location
Situated on the cubital crease of the elbow joint, in the depression on the radial side of biceps brachii muscle.

Needle
Up to 1 cun with perpendicular insertion.

> Deeper insertion may puncture the cephalic vein or even the lateral cutaneous nerve.

Moxa and pressure
Light to medium stimulation only with moxa. Stimulating acupressure may be applied to affect the inferior aspects of the biceps brachii muscle.

Indications
LU 5 is a significant acupoint in the treatment of the following:

- Sore throat, cough, bronchitis, fullness of the lungs, frequent sneezing.
- Chest and sinus infections, mild fevers.
- As a local point it relaxes the tendons and ligaments around the antero-lateral aspect of the elbow and may be used in conjunction with LI 11 in tennis elbow.

Special properties
- LU 5 is the 'water' point of the Lung meridian and, as such may help in the treatment of kidney pain, frequent urination, urinary retention and oedema.
- It is also the 'sedation' point and helps in the treatment of dry mouth, vomiting, painful and swollen abdomen and haematemesis.

LU 7 *Lieque* (Broken Sequence or Narrow Gap)

列缺 ★★★★★

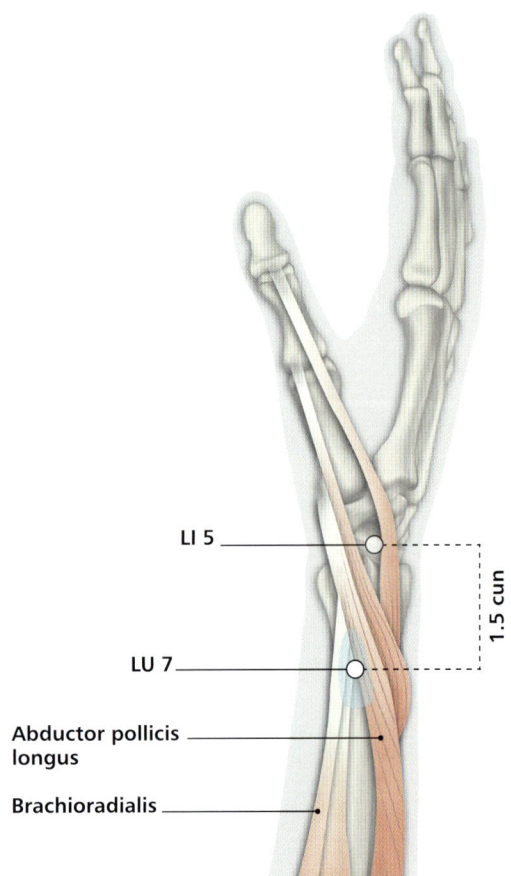

LI 5

1.5 cun

LU 7

Abductor pollicis longus

Brachioradialis

Location

Situated 1.5 cun above the wrist crease in the depression below the radial styloid, in the cleft between the tendons of the brachioradialis and abductor pollicis longus muscles.

Needle

Up to 1 cun with transverse needling proximally. Note: It often helps to pinch the skin and subcutaneous tissue to insert the needle.

Deeper or perpendicular needling may puncture the radial artery or vein.

Moxa and pressure

LU 7 can take quite a bit of stimulation with direct or indirect moxa. Acupressure may be performed using stimulation to the point to aid breathing or by gentle touch in conjunction with KI 6 to help utilize the eight extra meridians (see Special properties).

Indications

LU 7 is one of the great acupoints with several functions. Some of its indications are:

- Lack of energy – tonification with needle or moxa helps here.
- Coughing with phlegm (loose or tight). LU 7 is sometimes called the 'oxygen' point of the Lung meridian and it is the most beneficial point to aid correct breathing – especially in emergencies such as acute asthma. It is helpful in promoting sweating, in sore throats and dry mouth, sinusitis and rhinitis.
- An excellent acupoint (in combination with others) in the treatment of the symptoms of hemiplegia with deviation of the mouth and eyes.
- May be used as a local point in anterior wrist pain – especially tenosynovitis of the pollicis tendons.
- It is an excellent point (in combination with others) for emotional conditions – especially in dealing with grief, sadness and worry.

Special properties

- It is the Connecting Luo point with the Large Intestine meridian via LI 4 and, as such, may be used in pain syndromes and large bowel conditions.
- It is the Key (Opening) point of the Conception (Ren Mai) channel and nourishes yin and fluids throughout the body. It helps with night sweats, insomnia, sensitive skin, scant urination and weakened sexual functions. It helps with oedema and urinary incontinence. Since it is the Key point of the Conception, it is often used in conjunction with KI 6 (Yinchiao Mai) with biomagnets. (See Introduction on the topic of the eight extraordinary meridians.)
- It is also the Command point of the head and neck and should be considered in all cases of musculo-skeletal conditions of that area. Symptoms treated are headaches, neck stiffness, facial pain, toothache and facial paralysis.
- As previously mentioned it has a strong emotional influence and particularly helpful in the resolution of grief (together with Con 22), excessive weeping and depression. It has recently been introduced as a powerful point in the treatment of addictions.

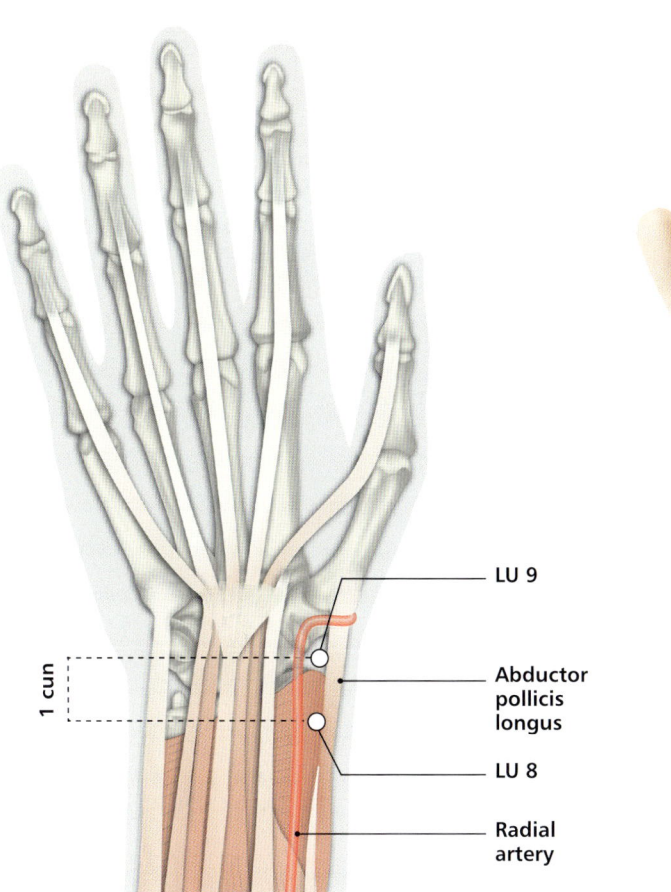

- LU 9
- Abductor pollicis longus
- LU 8
- Radial artery

1 cun

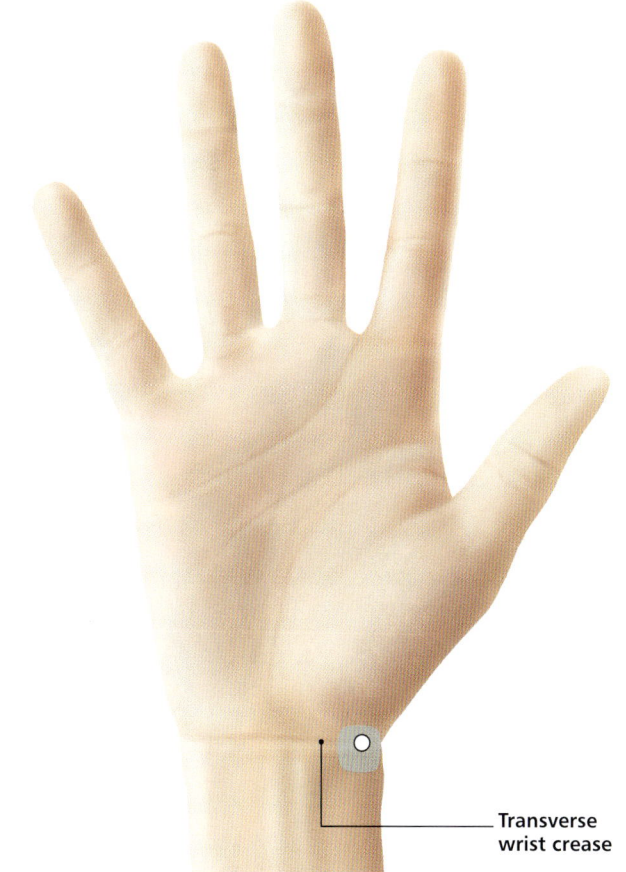

- Transverse wrist crease

Location
Situated on the radial end of the inferior wrist crease on the lateral side of the radial artery.

Needle
Superficial needling only up to 0.5 cun using a perpendicular approach.

> Be very careful not to puncture the radial artery by needling too medially.

Moxa and pressure
This point is excellent as a self-help acupoint with professional singers to strengthen the vocal chords.

> Moxabustion contraindicated. Avoid strong acupressure due to the adjacent artery.

Indications
The indications for LU 9 are very similar to the previous Lung meridian points in that it tonifies the lung and general chest chi, thus benefiting respiration, alleviating coughing and strengthening the voice. The extra action for this point is that it is used in very chronic conditions to boost lung energy. This is particularly effective with patients recovering from chest infections or a long bout of bronchitis.

LU 11 *Shao Shang* (Lesser Metal) 少商 ⭐⭐ Needle ⭐⭐⭐ Pressure

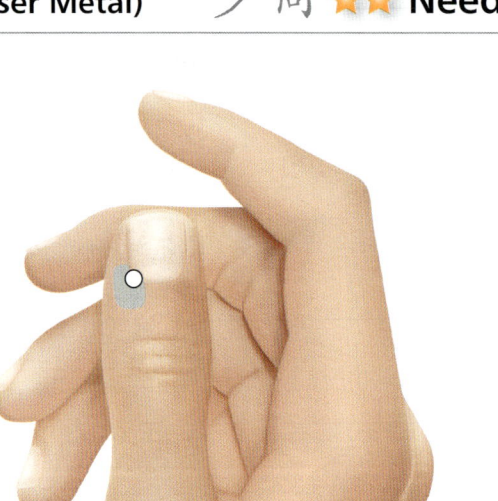

Location
Situated on the radial (lateral) side of the thumb 0.1 cun superior to the corner of the nail.

Needle
0.1 to 0.2 cun with perpendicular insertion.

Moxa and pressure
Small moxa punk cones are recommended on most 'nail' or Tsing points (be careful that they do not roll off before lighting!). Acupressure is strongly indicated with this point either by the therapist or in self-help. It is one of the better points for easing a sore throat. Please be careful not to exert too much pressure though as the tissues will be made very sore and could bleed.

Indications
As previously stated LU 11 is useful in the treatment of sore throats, swollen and painful tonsils, laryngitis and pharyngitis.

Special properties
LU 11 helps to pacify the heart and useful in self-help therapy for grief. It is also useful as an adjunctive point in the treatment of hemiplegia.

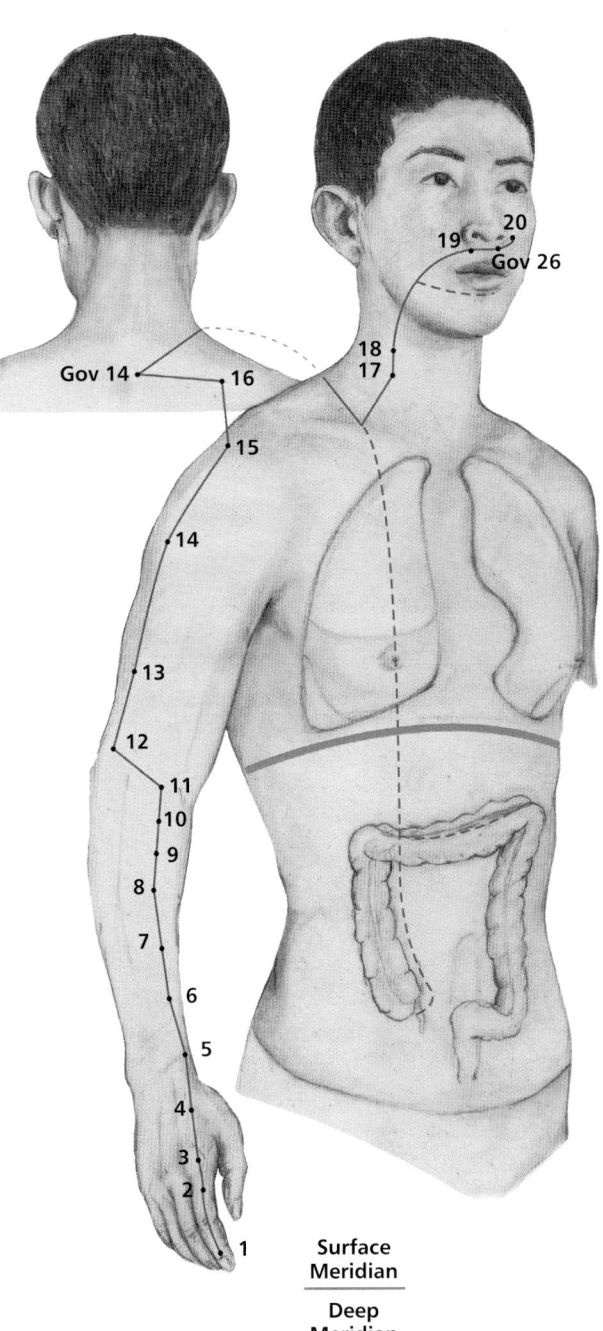

Surface
Meridian

Deep
Meridian
- - - - -

The Large Intestine channel is the Yang aspect of the Metal element. There are twenty (20) points on the surface pathway of the channel. The meridian commences at the radial side of the tip of the index finger, passes through the anatomical snuffbox and over the superior part of the lateral aspect of the forearm to the lateral side of the elbow. It continues up the antero-lateral side of the arm to the outside of the shoulder. The channel then girdles to just below the 7th cervical vertebra at acupoint Gov 14 and returns to the anterior aspect of the chest and enters the ribs via a deep channel connecting to the lungs. The deep channel then passes through the diaphragm to enter the large intestine. The surface pathway continues from the supraclavicular fossa past the lower neck to the corners of the mouth and onto the opposite naso-labial groove. Another deep channel also supplies the lower mouth and gums as well as uniting with the Stomach channel. It has always been hotly debated as to whether or not the superficial channel crosses the midline under the nose or remains on the same side at LI 20. Personally I do not think it matters – the really important thing to remember is that it unites with Gov 14 and also the lower mouth. You may also wonder if the bilateral channels of the large intestine meet at Gov 14 and return to the same side or cross over – who knows! It is a pity that modern meridian charts do not show the deeper channels.

The following 8 acupoints will be described: LI1, LI4, LI5, LI10, LI11, LI15, LI16 and LI 20.

LI 1 *Shang Yang* (Metal Yang) 商陽 ★★ Needle ★★★★ Pressure

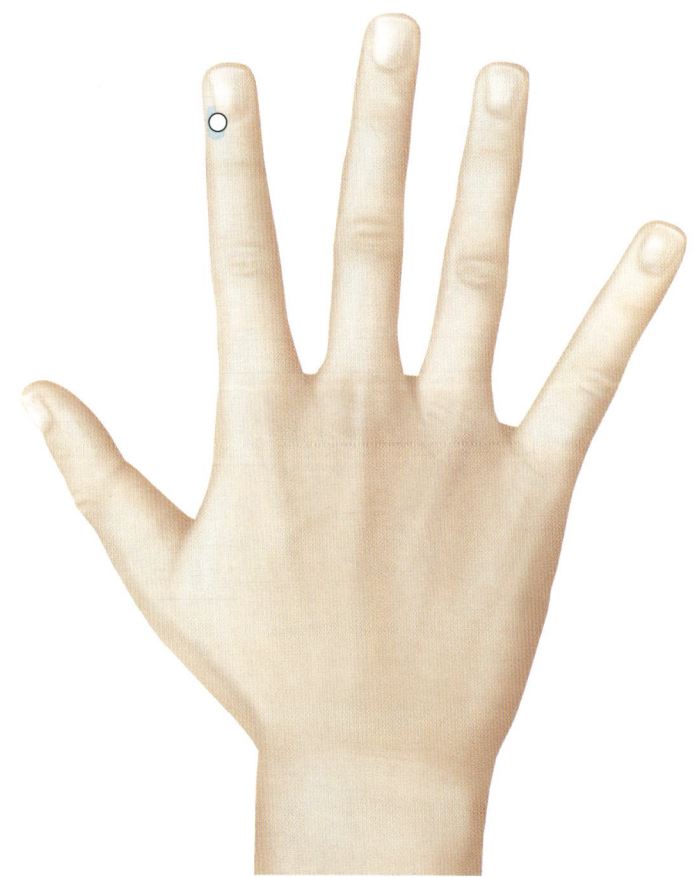

Location
Situated 0.1 cun from the radial border of the index finger nail.

Needle
Very superficially (0.1 cun) using perpendicular insertion.

Moxa and pressure
Moxa should only used as an energy restorative treatment following syncope or faint feeling. Acupressure is very important with this point – see 'indications'.

Indications
This point is used in the treatment of acute sore throats. Its use with acupressure is much more impressive and is used in two distinct ways. It may be used as self-help in toothache (especially of the lower mouth), treated using the opposite thumb nail or similar – works wonders if stimulation is continued (remember that over stimulation produces distal sedation). The second use in acupressure (and to a lesser extent with needle) is in the first aid treatment of shock, syncope and fainting.

Special properties
As LI 1 is the Tsing point (and Metal point), there is an affinity with the treatment of emotions (especially grief and instability).

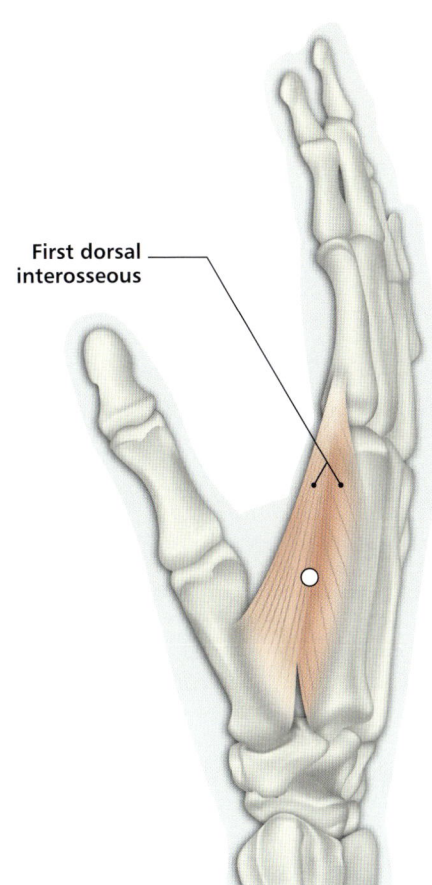

First dorsal interosseous

Location

Situated on the dorsum of the hand to the side of the midpoint of the second metacarpal bone, in the first interosseous muscle. As this is such a well-used point, there are many variations of securing its location. The best one that I have found is for the patient to bring their thumb and forefinger together to produce the mound of the first interosseous muscle. Place your forefinger perpendicularly on this mound and ask them to take the thumb away from their forefinger. Your finger will fall into the point.

Needle

This point is usually affected up to 1 cun in depth using a perpendicular approach. An oblique insertion may be attempted at 1.5 cun depth directing the needle towards LI 3.

This point is very powerful and is often used to induce menstruation and labour, so is contraindicated to needle in menstruation and pregnancy. Never use strong stimulation in patients who have a weak vital force. The point can also induce 'needle shock' in some patients.

Moxa and pressure

Moxa is very effective on LI 4 to improve the patient's general vital force – though no more than 10 moxas in any one treatment session. Pressure is effective when used as a self-help point in pain relief (see below).

Indications

This acupoint is possibly the most used in the whole body due to its indications in the treatment of many syndromes. A few of its many indications are:

- This point is colloquially called 'the great eliminator' and, as such, is used to 'eliminate' pain and discomfort. It is the great pain relief point and is used in conjunction with other points in acupuncture anaesthesia (more later).
- It is used for painful syndromes of the face, head, throat, upper chest, shoulder and arm.
- It is used in the treatment of upper respiratory tract infections, chills and fever, sneezing, sinusitis and throat conditions.
- As well as easing pain around the face and head it is used for syndromes around that area such as facial paralysis, stiffness of the jaw, mouth abscesses, toothache and migraine.
- It is, naturally, thought of when treating conditions associated with the excretory organs of the bowel and skin.

Special properties

- LI 4 is the Source point of the organ and has a direct affinity with the large bowel.
- When coupled with LR 3 it gives a powerful four needle (known as the Four Gates) treatment in pain syndromes as well as offering relaxation of the mind and body. [LR 3, which is situated between the great toe and second toe is often called the LI 4 on the foot and mimics its positioning.]
- When combined with other points, is used in acupuncture anaesthesia. It is combined with LI 11 in facial pain, LR 3 in emotional and general pain, SP 6 in gynaecological pain and so on. Its versatility makes it such a useful point.
- This point is contraindicated in pregnancy, yet it is used in the very late stages of pregnancy to ease labour and aid the birth process.
- It is a major point in the treatment of hemiplegia and most neurological conditions.

LI 5 *Yang Xi* (Yang Stream)

陽谿 ★★★

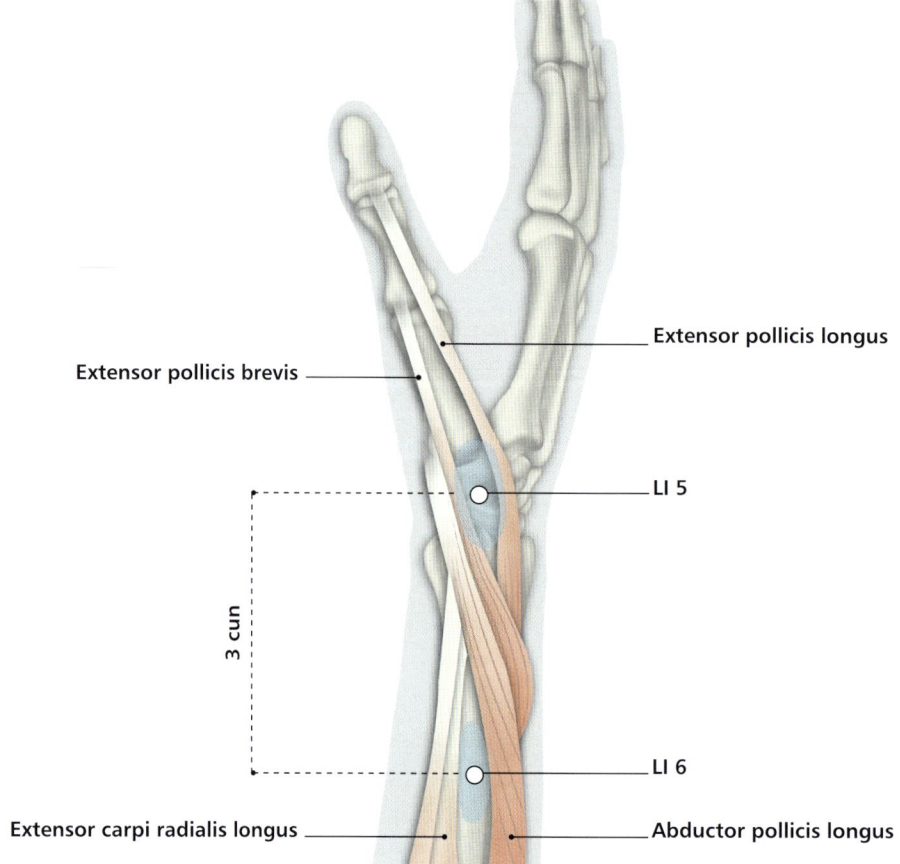

Extensor pollicis longus

Extensor pollicis brevis

LI 5

3 cun

LI 6

Extensor carpi radialis longus

Abductor pollicis longus

Location
Situated on the radial side of the dorsal wrist crease, in the centre of the anatomical snuffbox formed by the tendons of the extensor pollicis longus and brevis muscles.

Needle
Up to 1 cun depth angled towards the wrist joint.

Do not needle any deeper as there is a danger of piercing the cephalic vein.

Moxa and pressure
Light or medium moxa stimulation only due to underlying veins and nerves. When used with acupressure, it is a very effective point used locally for tenosynovitis. This is a favourite point with some therapists to exert pressure with transverse frictions – it seems to work well but can be a little harsh for the patient.

Indications
This is a very important point, used locally, in wrist pain and tenosynovitis. It is an excellent acupoint used in conjunction with LI 4 in local pain and swelling following scaphoid or radial fracture consolidation.

Special properties
LI 5 is the Fire point of the Large Intestine meridian and, as such, may be used in aiding discomfort around the heart or in treating painful shoulder girdle syndromes with burning pain.

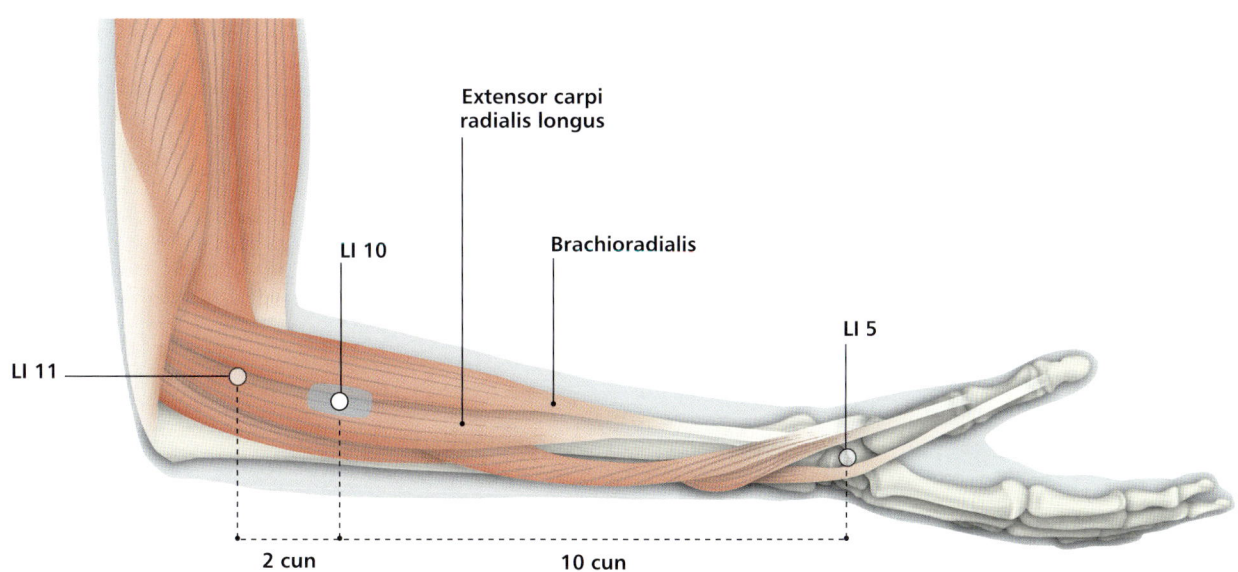

Extensor carpi radialis longus

Brachioradialis

LI 10

LI 11

LI 5

2 cun   10 cun

Location

Situated in a depression 2 cun distal to LI 11 on a line aimed towards LI 5 and 10 cun proximal to the wrist crease.

Needle

As this acupoint lies in the extensor carpi radialis longus muscle, depth may be up to 1.5 cun using a perpendicular insertion.

> Deeper needling may puncture the posterior interosseous nerve.

Moxa and pressure

Mild stimulation with moxa only. Practitioner led or self-help acupressure should be firm, so as to affect the point.

Indications and special properties

This acupoint is not one that the old texts suggested had much of an indication compared to its close ally – LI 11. There are three significant properties:

- LI 10 is the arm equivalent of ST 36 on the leg, and has similar actions in increasing blood flow and warmth to the extremities. It is therefore an excellent point in the treatment of cold hands (an excellent point to teach the patient to self-help with acupressure) Pressure must be sustained for up to five minutes.
- It is a very good point to treat pain, stiffness and motor impairment when combined with muscular atrophy or spasm and is excellent in hemiplegia treatment.
- As mentioned before, when combined in treatment with ST 36, it produces energy and harmony to the extremities.

LI 11 *Qu Chi* (Pool at the Crook or Pond at the Bend)

曲池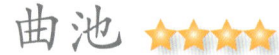

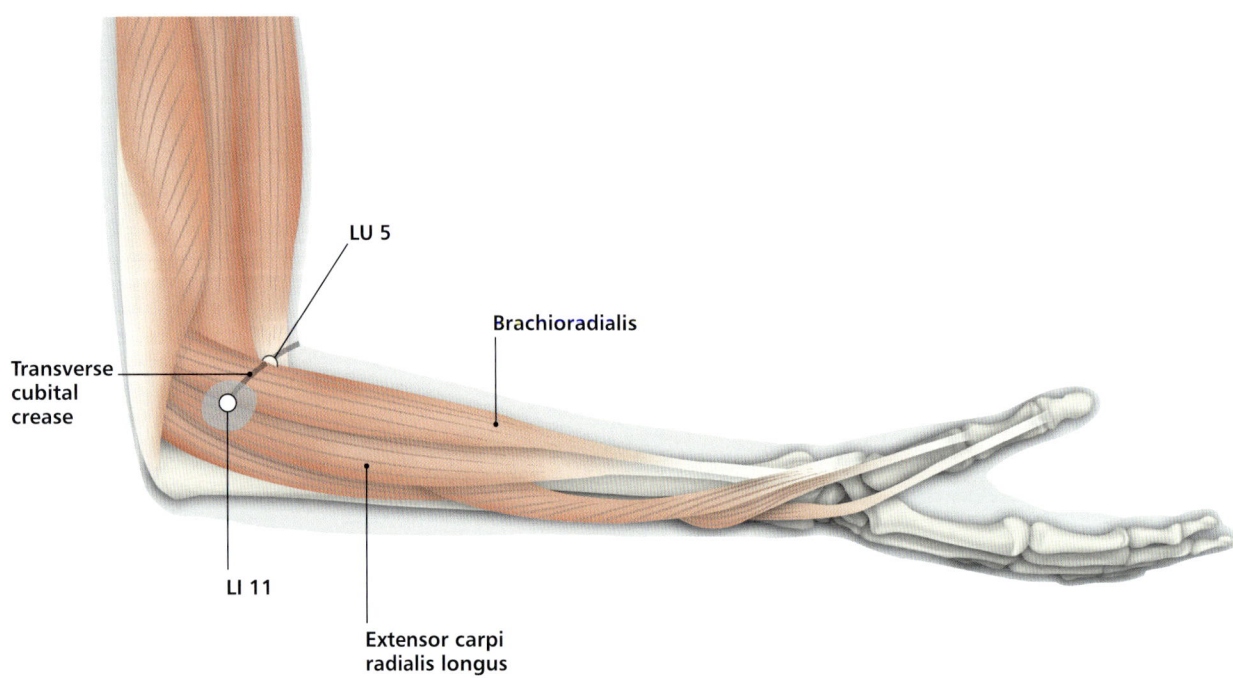

Location
Situated at the lateral edge of the transverse cubital crease when the elbow is flexed. It is imperative that the patient flexes the elbow in order to locate it.

Needle
It is fairly deep so needling need be up to 1.5 cun with a perpendicular approach.

Moxa and pressure
It answers well to a lot of stimulating direct and indirect moxa for general (as well as lung/large intestine) energy improvement. Moxa must be carried out with a slightly flexed elbow so the moxa balls do not fall off. Acupressure works on a local or general way. Localised conditions such as tennis elbow may be treated in combination with other points.

Indications
- It is used in conjunction with other points in elbow and forearm conditions including tennis elbow, elbow arthritis, pain and stiffness of the elbow and shoulder and muscle cramps caused by neurological conditions.
- It is one of our best points in the treatment of skin conditions such as eczema and acne.
- It is indicated in fever, headache, red or inflamed eyes, nasal obstruction, sore throat, earache, toothache and fullness of the chest. This point is often called the poor man's LI 4 as it is used in many of the syndromes where LI 4 is employed. The two points work well together.
- In emotional conditions it is helpful in depression, restlessness and irritability.

Special properties
- LI 11 is the 'Earth' point of the Large Intestine meridian and, as such, deals with several stomach conditions and sensitivity along the midriff of the body. It is very helpful to teach this point to patients to use it as part of a self-help strategy in diaphragmatic tension and spasm – this works much better with acupressure than with needle.
- This point is also the Key point of the Naval chakra (based at KI 16) which confirms its use in stomach related conditions.

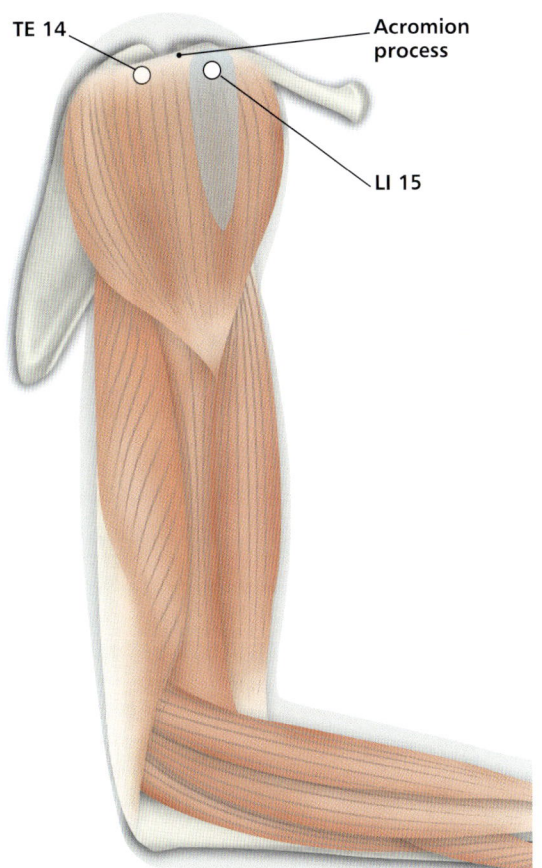

Location

This point is found at the lateral aspect of the shoulder at the level of the acromio-clavicular joint in the large hollow when the arm is abducted.

Needle

The best (of many) ways to needle this point is with the patient's arm at their side, up to 1 cun with a perpendicular approach. The needle should enter the space between the subacromial bursa and the acromion process.

Moxa and pressure

This point answers well to either direct or indirect moxa and will accept a lot of stimulation. It is ideally used with a moxa stick as many acupoints in the area may be treated in the same session. This technique is ideal in the treatment of stiff shoulders. This point is not very accessible to stimulating acupressure but may be used to great advantage with sedating pressure – see below.

Indications

The main classical indication for this acupoint is in localised conditions. It is useful for most shoulder conditions including pain and stiffness, frozen shoulder if the cause is injurious, supraspinatus and biceps tendonitis, and periarthritis of the shoulder joint.

Special properties

LI 15 is the physical acupoint of the Shoulder chakra. This is a minor chakra that is associated with both the Throat chakra (major) and the Naval chakra (minor). This triad of points – LI 15, Con 22 and KI 16 is very useful in all cases of lack of expression and excretion (see more comments when Con 22 is discussed). The point answers very well to very gentle acupressure. Both LI 15 points may be treated at the same time with the therapist sitting proximal to the patient's head with them in supine lying. You may place either the finger pads on the points or even the whole of the hands as long as the focus and intention is on LI 15. It is ideal for general relaxation and ending a treatment session.

LI 16 *Ju Gu* (Great Bone)

巨骨 ★★★

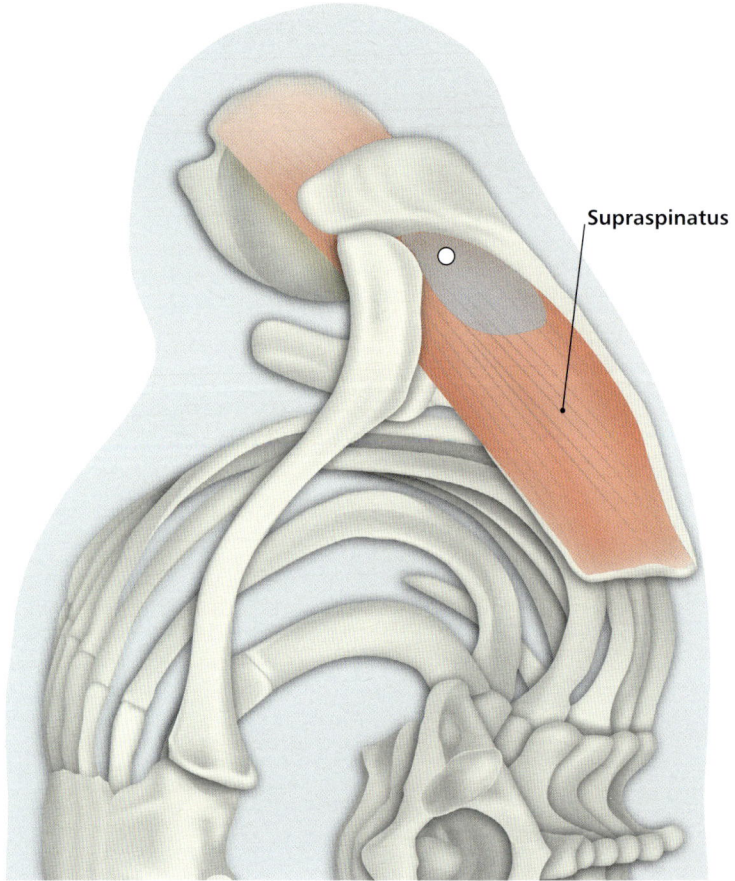

Supraspinatus

Location
Situated in the depression between the lateral end of the clavicle and the spine of scapula, medial to the acromion process.

Needle
This acupoint is relatively easy to locate and is mostly exquisitely tender. Needle up to 1.5 cun in a perpendicular direction.

> Be careful not to needle too deeply as the lung tissue above the clavicle may be pierced.

Moxa and pressure
Moxa is usually performed (as stated with the previous point) indirectly with a moxa stick. Sustained gentle acupressure is useful for localised shoulder inflammation.

Indications
This is a powerful point in treating pain and impaired mobility of the shoulder and arm. It is also indicated in conditions of the thyroid gland (goitre and hypothyroidism) and also relaxes and opens the chest and is effective in clearing phlegm and stasis.

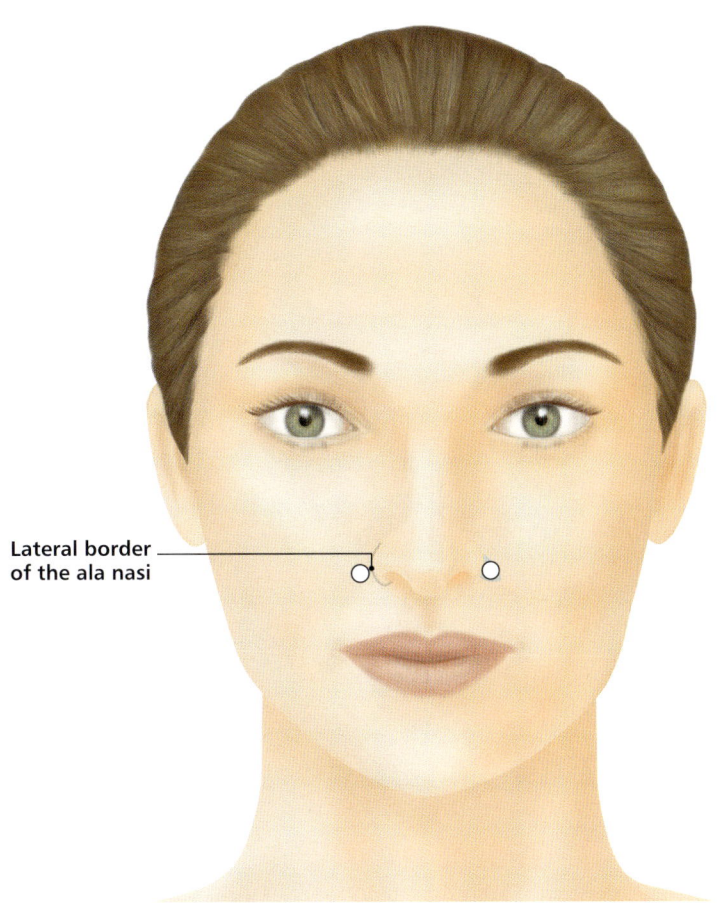

Lateral border
of the ala nasi

Location
The end point of the Large Intestine meridian is situated in the nasolabial sulcus, level with lateral border of the ala nasi.

Needle
Needle up to 0.5 cun with perpendicular insertion or up to 1.5 cun with transverse insertion directed downwards along nasolabial sulcus.

Moxa and pressure
Self-treatment can be particularly effective on this point using light stimulation in clearing the nasal passages and aiding breathing.

Moxa is forbidden on this acupoint.

Indications
This is a major point in opening up the nasal sinuses and aiding breathing. It may also be used in nasal obstruction, nosebleed, loss of smell, rhinitis and sinusitis. It has secondary effects on some facial paralysis, mouth abscesses and toothache.

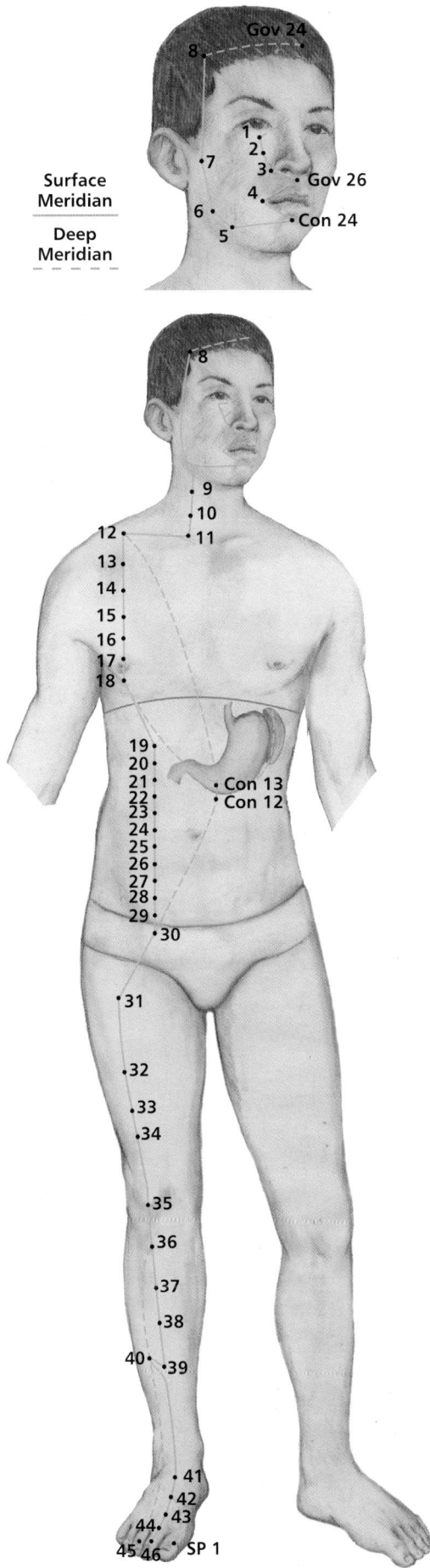

The Stomach channel represents the Yang aspect of the Earth element. There are forty-five (45) points on its surface pathway. The Stomach meridian is a long and complicated one that travels from the head to the foot. It is unique in that it is the only yang channel to lie on the anterior aspect of the chest and abdomen.

ST 1 is situated on the lower edge of the eye socket. Some traditional charts give ST 8 as the first point of the meridian, which I feel makes more sense! The two strands of the channel form one channel to descend to the side of the neck to the upper clavicular fossa and laterally across the upper aspect of the clavicle. There are internal pathways through to Gov 20, Gov 26 and Con 24. An inner pathway descends from ST 12 through the diaphragm, supplies the stomach and becomes superficial at Con 13/12 before proceeding internally towards the groin at ST 30. The surface pathway descends from ST 12 down to just below the nipple where it travels medially and then straight down to the side of the rectus abdominus muscle to ST 30. The surface pathway runs down the antero-lateral aspect of the thigh to the side of the patella and then via the anterior aspect of the lower leg and foot dorsum terminating at the lateral aspect of the second toenail. Deeper pathways emerge from ST 36 and ST 40. We shall discuss only those points that are the most popular and effective.

ST 2 *Si Bai* (Four Whites)

四白 ★★ Needle ★★★ Pressure

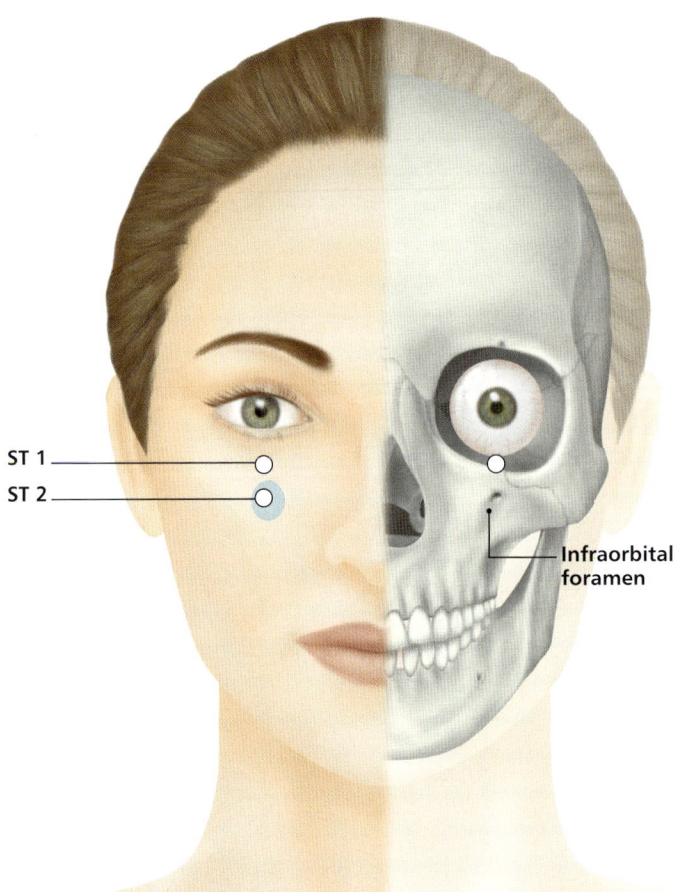

ST 1
ST 2

Infraorbital foramen

Location
Situated approximately 0.3 cun directly below ST 1 in the infraorbital foramen depression.

Needle
Very superficial needling – up to 0.2 cun with perpendicular insertion.

> Do not insert any deeper as there is a possibility of affecting the eyeball.

Moxa and pressure
Although moxa is not contraindicated, it is not usually performed due the adjacency to the eye. For pressure techniques, see under 'special properties'.

Indications
This point is important in the treatment of many eye disorders. These include easing heavy eyes, 'grittiness', painful syndromes, excessive lacrimation and general inflammation. A secondary use of this point with needle is in cosmetic acupuncture treating under eye puffiness, swelling and dark circles.

Special properties
According to applied kinesiology philosophy this point and ST 1 (Cheng Qi) may be used with gentle acupressure techniques to weaken excess tonicity in muscles that are associated with stomach energy. These muscles, historically, are the pectoralis major (clavicular portion), biceps brachii, neck muscles and brachioradialis. This is extremely important with some neurological conditions and especially with self-treatment. Some martial arts suggest that by just touching this point (or even staring at it with intent) will weaken the opponent sufficiently so as to disarm them and weaken their whole system. Using this technique obviously requires experience and is not to be attempted without experience.

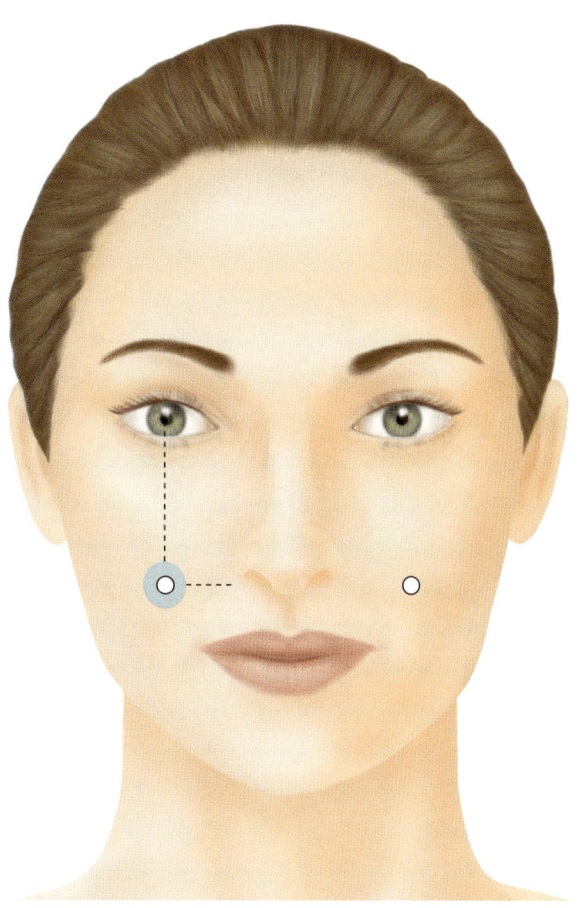

Location
Situated below the zygomatic arch directly below ST 2 in line with the ala nasi.

Needle
Needling is fairly superficial (0.2 to 0.5 cun) perpendicular.

Moxa and pressure
As with most facial points moxa is not usually employed directly on to the skin but is useful indirectly using a moxa roll – be careful that smoke does not go into the patient's eye! Self-help pressure is most useful (with other local points) in all cases of nasal and sinus obstruction.

Indications
This point is indicated in nasal obstruction and inflammation, sinusitis and cheek pain, epistaxis, allergic rhinitis, toothache and trigeminal neuralgia. This point is usually treated along with LI 20 and has very similar properties.

ST 6 *Jia Che* (Jaw Bone)

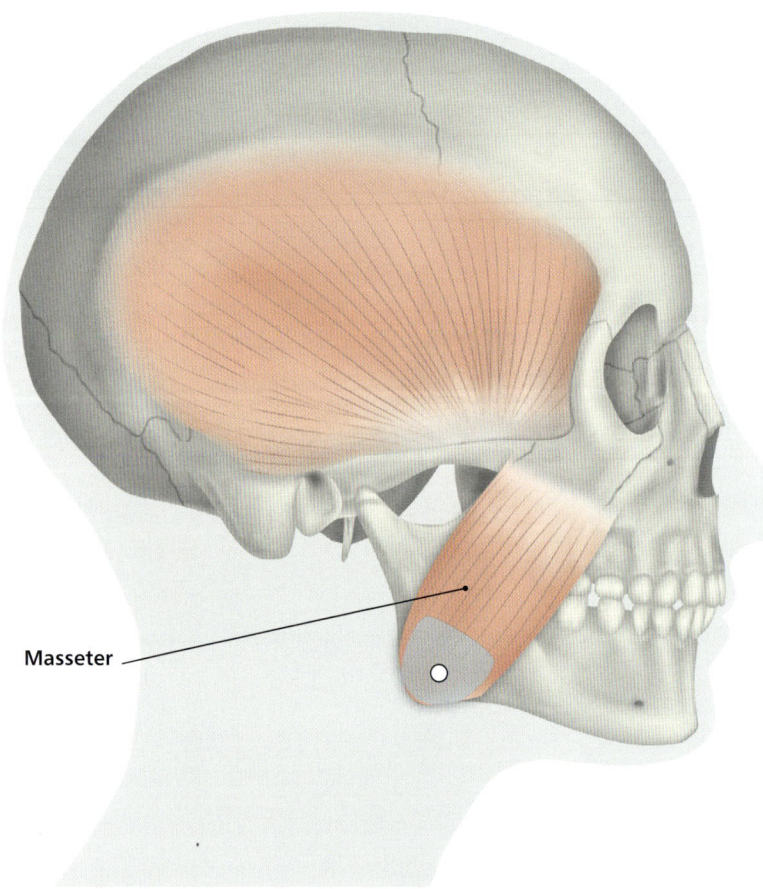

Masseter

Location
Situated in the depression at the prominence of the masseter muscle, approximately one finger-width superior to the angle of the mandible. Ask the patient to clench the teeth in order to find the point.

Needle
This point may be inserted using 0.5 cun depth with perpendicular direction or up to 2 cun using a transverse insertion towards ST 4.

> Be careful not to puncture the buccal branch of the facial nerve.

Moxa and pressure
Lightly applied moxa may be used in cases of masseter muscle spasm. Pressure is extremely effective in cases of masseter spasm, weakness and jaw pain due to tension. The point is pressed gently with pressure using no stimulation whatsoever. As heat is produced locally and the muscle starts to relax, the point is pressed slightly deeper until relaxation of the area occurs – this is a first-rate procedure either by the therapist or as self-help.

Indications
The main indication is in its local use in the treatment of jaw and TMJ disorders in that it relaxes the supporting muscles and tendons and clears inflammation. Tension here may be caused by teeth grinding, clenching, tension headaches, migraine, trigeminal neuralgia, mouth deviation and facial paralysis.

Special properties
ST 6 is an excellent 'calming' point and is used in easing stress and relaxing the head and neck. It may also be used to treat excessive salivation – particularly so in hemiplegia cases.

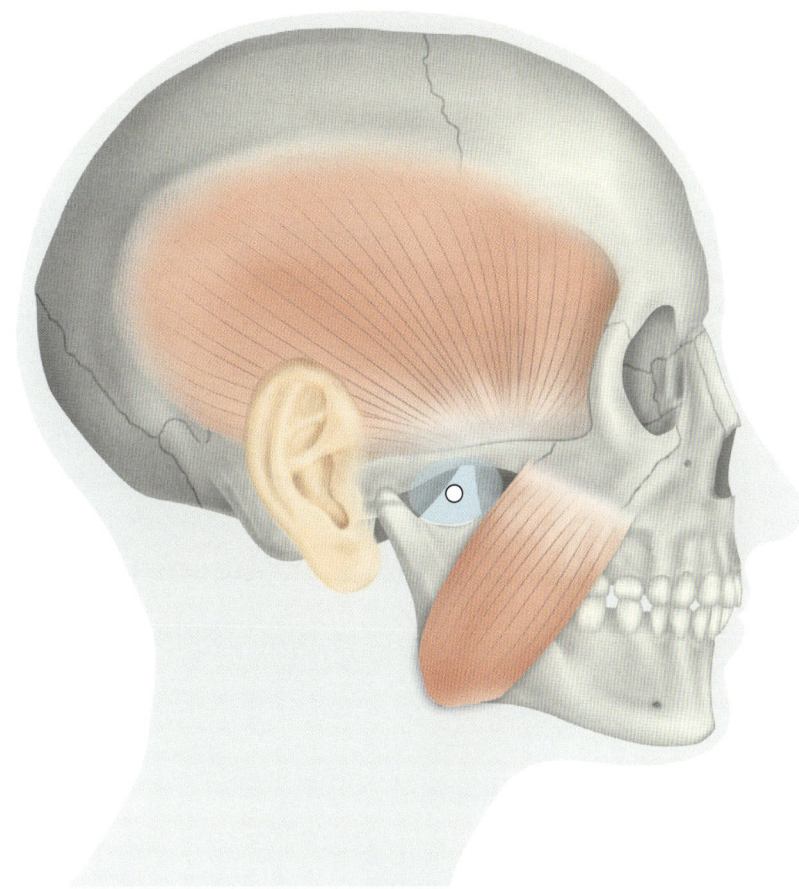

Location

Situated in the depression between the zygomatic arch and the condyloid process of the mandible. This point may only be found when the mouth is closed but 'disappears' in an open mouth.

Needle

This point should be needled up to 1 cun with a perpendicular action.

Do not needle any deeper as there is a danger of puncturing the facial nerve, artery or vein.

Moxa and pressure

Pressure is very effective, used with similar effect to ST 6.

Direct moxa is forbidden.

Indications

This point is used mostly in localized conditions of the TMJ including spasm, pain and swelling. It is also effective in trigeminal neuralgia, facial neuralgia, facial paralysis, toothache and tinnitus. Because of the tension that is usually held in the TMJ, this point (coupled with other local TMJ points) is excellent in the general treatment of stress related conditions. This point is also connected with the Gall Bladder meridian and may be used as such.

ST 8 *Tou Wei* (Head's Binding)

頭維 ★★★

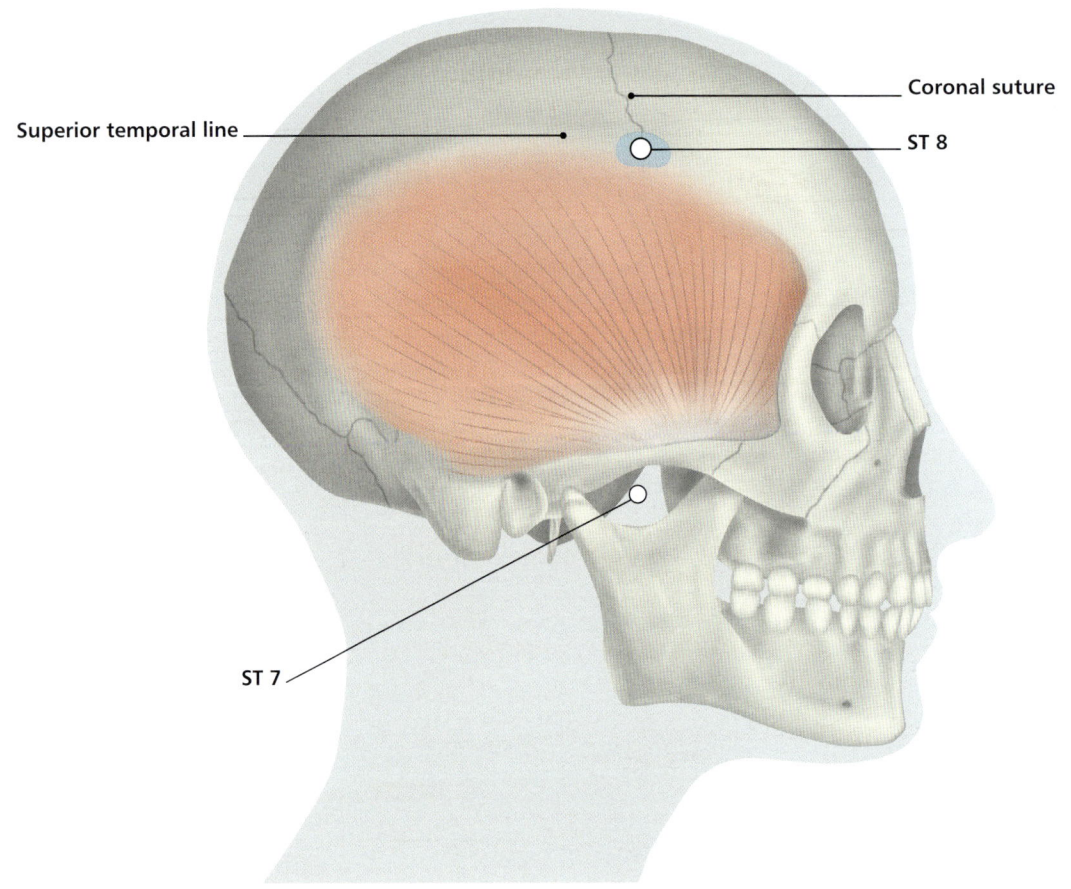

Coronal suture

Superior temporal line

ST 8

ST 7

Location
Situated in the depression at the corner of the forehead, at the superior margin of the temporalis muscle, 0.5 cun within the anterior hairline, 4.5 cun lateral to the anterior midline at Gov 24.

Needle
Needling is either perpendicular 0.1 to 0.2 cun (pinch the forehead skin first) or up to 1 cun using a transverse insertion posteriorly.

Moxa and pressure
Pressure techniques can be very effective in the treatment of headaches and stress. Please note that this point is tender to the touch and only gentle touch should be employed.

> Moxa is forbidden.

Indications
This very useful acupoint may be used in headaches and the 'brain fog' type of heavy headaches. It is also used in vertigo, poor concentration, facial pain and paralysis, excessive lacrimation and eye twitching.

Special properties
- In common with many other stomach meridian points, ST 8 is excellent in the treatment of depression and other emotional disorders either with pressure or needle. It is particularly effective as a point used in indian head massage.
- This acupoint used to be named as ST 1 as it was thought to have a direct link to the upper extremities of the stomach. It is extremely effective in the treatment of hemi cranial headaches that are brought on by consuming foods and liquids that disagree or by having drinks that are too cold.

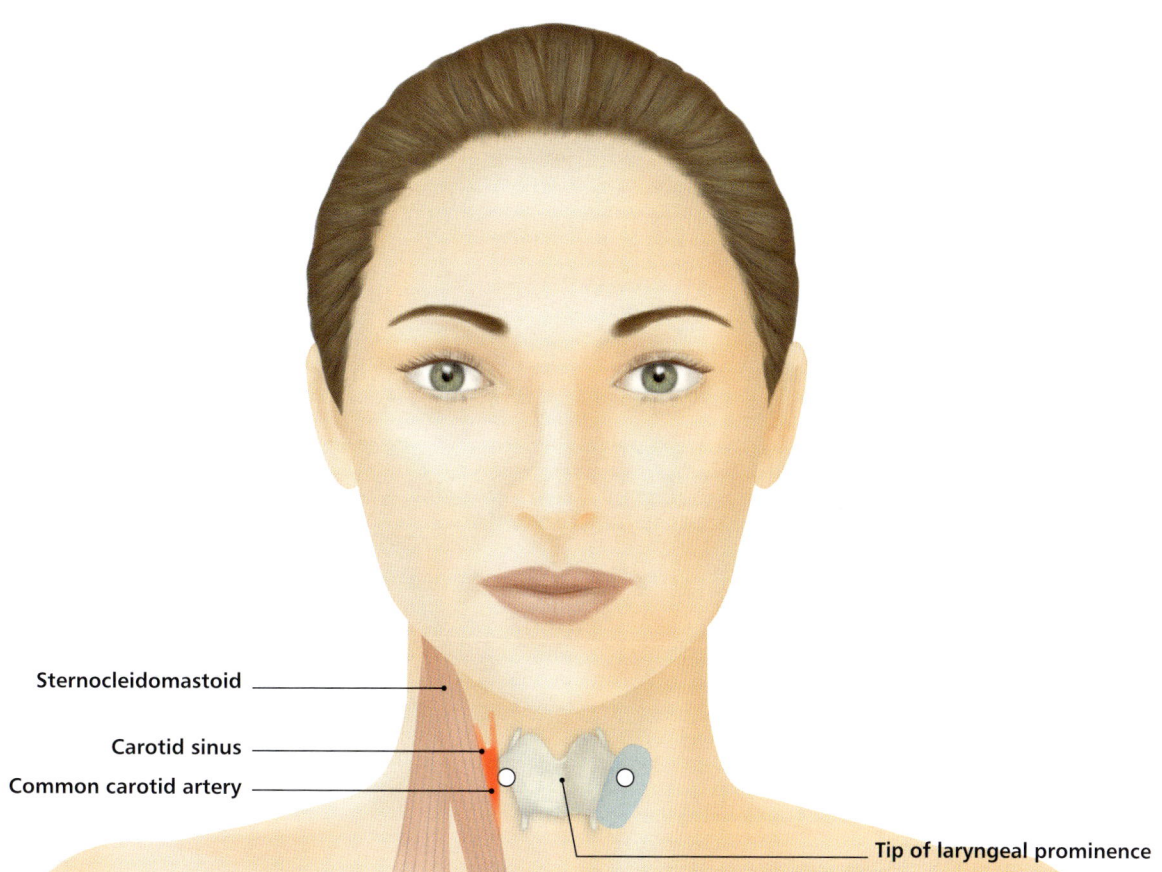

Sternocleidomastoid

Carotid sinus

Common carotid artery

Tip of laryngeal prominence

Location

Situated on the anterior aspect of the sternocleidomastoid muscle, 1.5 cun lateral to the Adam's apple. Great care should be taken in locating this point as it can be extremely dangerous if the point is not located properly either by needle or pressure.

Needle

Some old texts clearly state that needle is forbidden due to the adjacency of the carotid artery and carotid sinus. Up to 1 cun perpendicular insertion may be performed by experienced acupuncturists only.

Moxa and pressure

For pressure techniques, see below.

Moxa is forbidden.

Indications

This is an important acupoint in dry mouth, sore throat, headache, palpitations and tachycardia (see special properties), fright, panic attack, tight chest, difficult swallowing and oesophageal obstruction.

Special properties

The main special property of this point is that it is a first aid point in palpitation, tachycardia, panic attacks and generalized sympathetic nerve hyperactivity. Stimulation of the point affects the vagus nerve that has the effect of helping to restore a sinus rhythm following tachycardia. Ironically, when used in a non first aid manner, if it is treated with gentle touch (by therapist or patient) it can create relaxation of the whole body by decreasing hypertension and lowering the heart rate by increasing the vagus (parasympathetic) nerve action.

Only perform these techniques if you are competent and experienced.

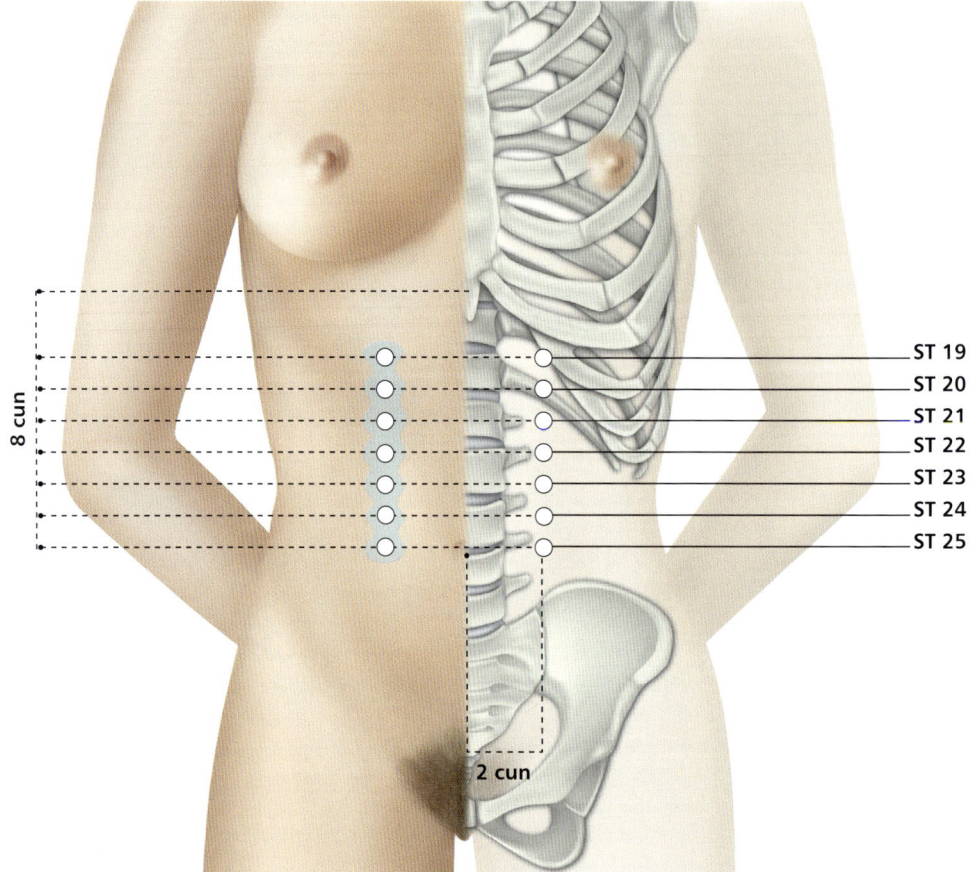

ST 19
ST 20
ST 21
ST 22
ST 23
ST 24
ST 25

8 cun

2 cun

Location
Situated 2 cun lateral to Con 12 which is 4 cun above the umbilicus.

Needle
1 to 1.5 cun using perpendicular insertion. Do not needle any deeper where the patient is very thin or frail in case of internal organ damage.

Moxa and pressure
This point answers well to stimulating moxa and pressure in patients where there is low stomach chi. Do not tonify where nausea is present.

Indications
This point regulates chi balance in the stomach and small bowel and is therefore used in both acute and chronic gastritis. Symptomatology includes gastritis, hardness of the abdomen, bloating with gas, heartburn, pain of hiatus hernia, loose stool and stomach rumbling.

Special properties
Although it is not designated as being the Alarm point of the stomach (that honour falls to Con 12), experience has shown that this acupoint is a much better stomach chi indicator. It is therefore very tender to the touch in all cases of acute gastritis.

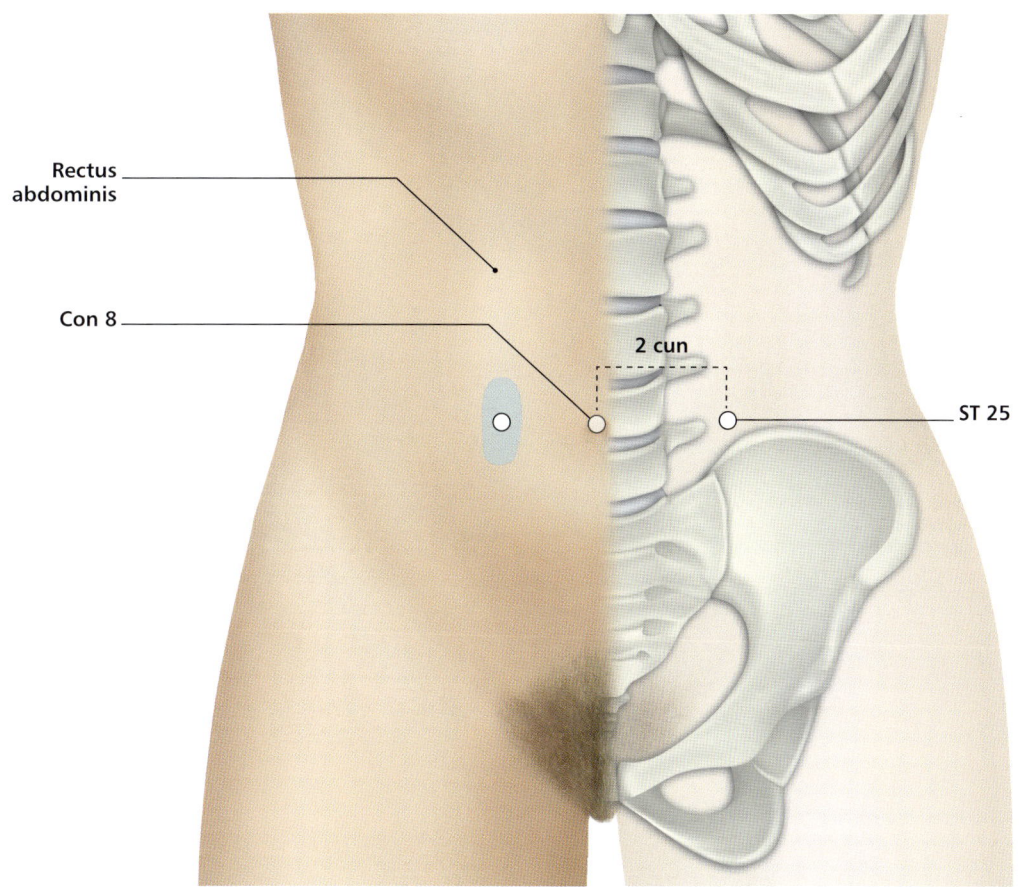

Location

Situated 2 pouce lateral to the umbilicus (Con 8) in the rectus abdominis muscle.

Needle

Up to 1.5 cun depth using a perpendicular approach. Do not needle any deeper in thin and frail patients.

Moxa and pressure

This point answers very well to moxa and pressure techniques. Gentle finger tip pressure may be self-applied in cases of gastritis.

Indications

This acupoint is, by far, the best 'local' stomach point to use in all cases of acute or chronic abdominal related conditions. Symptoms include abdominal distension, swelling and pain, gastroenteritis, diarrhoea, foul smelling stools, mucous or blood in the stool, constipation, nausea, vomiting, irregular menstruation and dysmenorrhoea.

Special properties

This point is significant in two other ways:

- It is the Alarm point of the Large Intestine and, as such, is the best indicator there is to indicate acute large bowel conditions.
- It is the physical aspect of the Naval chakra, which is a minor chakra associated with the Shoulder chakra (LI 15) and the Throat chakra (Con 22). This very important triad of points may be used together in all aspects of excretion, elimination and expression syndromes.

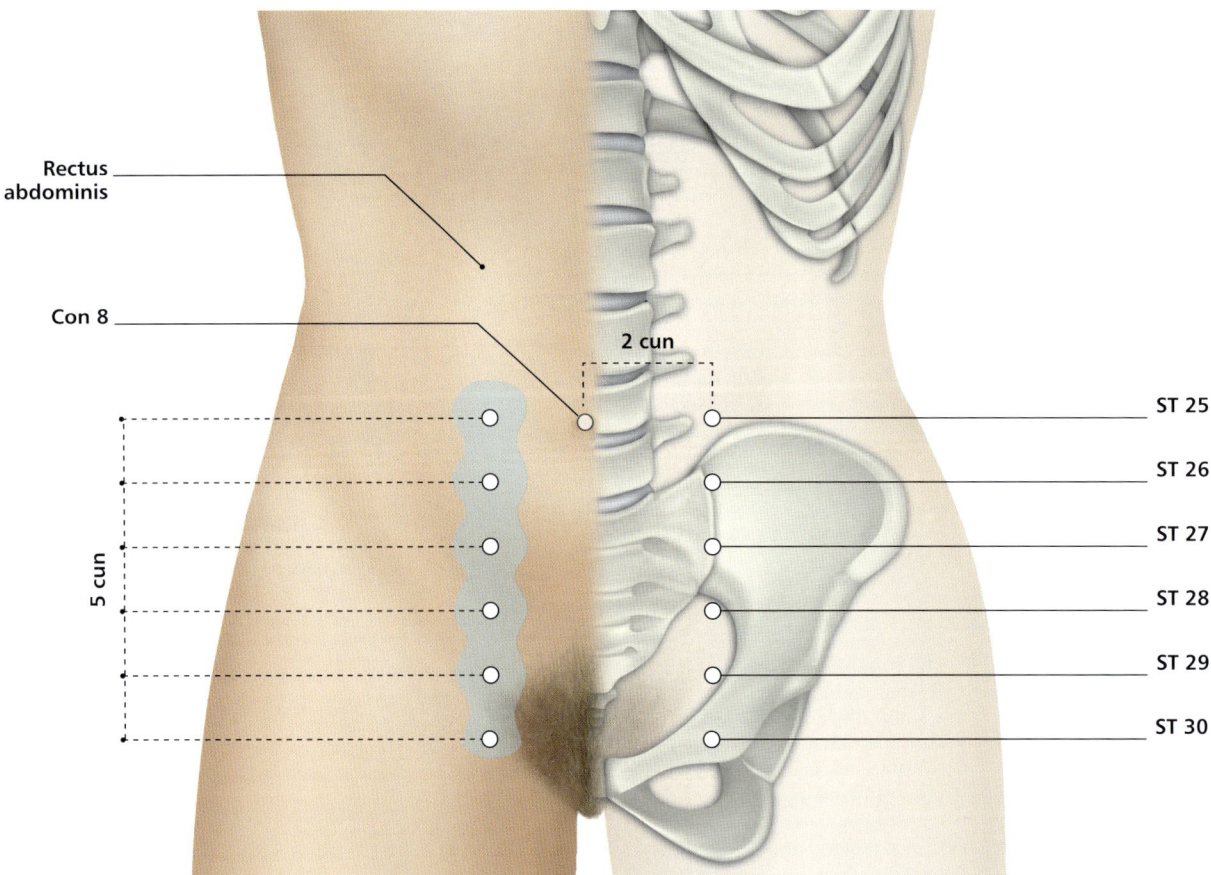

Rectus
abdominis

Con 8

2 cun

5 cun

ST 25

ST 26

ST 27

ST 28

ST 29

ST 30

Location

Situated in the groin region, 2 cun lateral to the midline and 5 cun inferior to ST 25.

Needle

0.5 to 1.0 cun using a perpendicular insertion.

> Do not needle any deeper as it could affect the femoral vein or artery.

Moxa and pressure

Only use very light moxa due to the adjacency of many important vessels beneath.

> Do not use any stimulating acupressure.

Light touch acupressure is acceptable and is an excellent local point in the treatment of groin strain.

Indications

This acupoint is extremely effective in general and local syndromes. It is indicated in infertility, irregular menstruation, uterine prolapse, pain in the external genital area, upper groin strain, frequent urination, inguinal hernia and testicular retraction.

Special properties

This very important acupoint has two other properties:

- It is said to be the emerging point of the Chong Mai meridian (Vital channel), which is one of the eight extraordinary meridians. This channel commences within the pelvic girdle, emerges at ST 30 and travels up the Kidney meridian towards KI 27 and upwards to the mouth. For this reason it is used in genito-urinary and some sex organ syndromes.
- The point is also the physical aspect of the minor chakra known as the Groin chakra. This chakra point is associated with the Clavicular chakra (KI 27) and the Brow chakra (Yin Tang). This triad of points is used with all the symptoms of ST 30 plus lack of mental focus, irritability and stress.

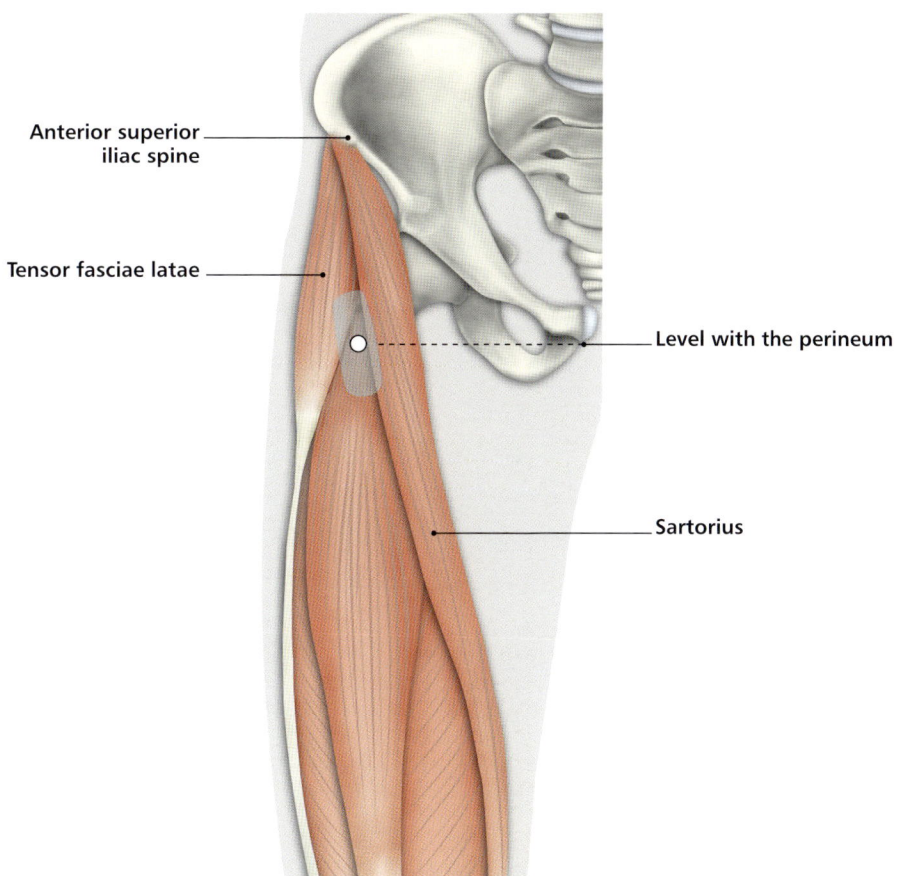

Anterior superior iliac spine

Tensor fasciae latae

Level with the perineum

Sartorius

Location

Situated at the level of the inferior gluteal fold, between the sartorius and tensor fascia latae muscles, approximately level with the perineum and directly below the anterior superior iliac spine.

Needle

With the patient either in side lying or with the knee slightly flexed in supine lying it is up to 2.5 cun depth with perpendicular insertion. This is one of the deepest acupoints in the body.

Moxa and pressure

Mild moxa stimulation only except when used on the end of a copper (fire) needle. Acupressure techniques are given below.

Indications

This is a useful point for localized conditions of the hip such as hip pain, osteoarthritic changes, thigh muscle spasms, coldness in the knee, and hip stiffness. It is also one of those points that seem to increase chi and circulation downwards. It is therefore excellent for cold knees and feet. It has limited generalized indications.

Special properties

This represents a brilliant point in acupressure for easing anterior hip pain and joint stiffness. The technique is to apply gentle pressure initially and allow your finger pads to go deeper as the patient's tissues become more 'pliable'. The point sometimes needs to be held for up to five minutes.

ST 36 *Zu San Li* (Leg Three Miles)

足三里 ★★★★★

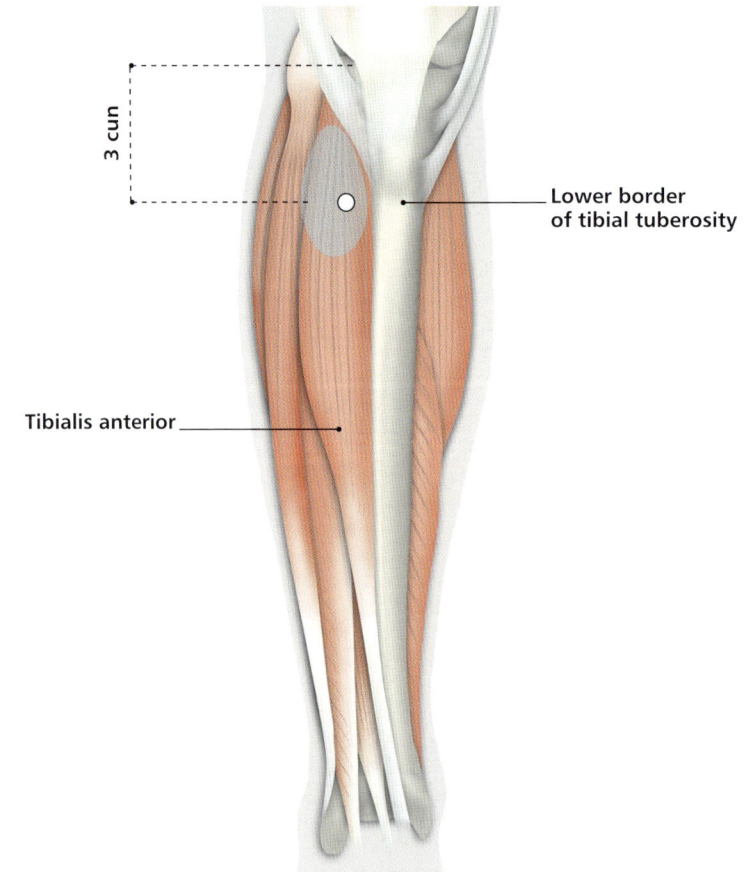

3 cun

Lower border
of tibial tuberosity

Tibialis anterior

Location

Situated within the fibres of the tibialis anterior muscle, approximately one finger-width lateral to the tibial crest level with the lower border of the tibial tuberosity (quadriceps insertion).

Needle

Needle between 1 and 1.5 cun depth with a perpendicular insertion. Please note that when this acupoint is needled correctly there is quite a marked de qi sensation down the tibialis anterior towards the ankle. A patient who is not used to acupuncture at this point will inform you that you have 'hit a nerve'.

Moxa and pressure

This point answers well to strong moxa, both directly and by moxa stick. This point represents one of the most effective to use with acupressure in the treatment of stomach conditions and for general energy depletion; it is an excellent point for use with self-help.

Indications

Digestive: Afflictions of the mouth, bitter taste, frequent vomiting, gastralgia and gastroenteritis, chronic constipation and diarrhoea, colic and diaphragm spasms.

General: Anxiety, hypertension, dyspnoea, urethritis, incontinence and difficulty in urination, inflammation of the skin, nervous system afflictions, headaches, vertigo, pain in general, weakness of the legs and oedema.

Special properties

As well as being used in isolation or combination with many other points in very many syndromes, this point is one of our greatest points for the treatment of tiredness, lethargy and general lack of fibre. It is therefore treated with some aggression with either moxa or tonifying needle. The exception to this is in acute gastritis when sedation techniques should be employed. It is an excellent 'pre-event' acupoint in athletes in order to boost energy to the legs and the system in general. It truly is one of our most dynamic and widely used points in the body.

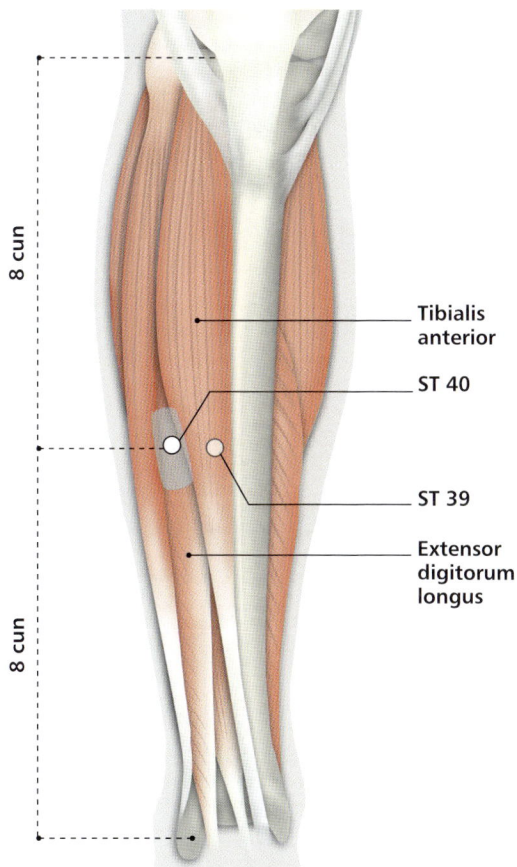

Tibialis anterior

ST 40

ST 39

Extensor digitorum longus

8 cun

8 cun

Location

Situated on the anterolateral aspect of the leg, 8 cun proximal to the lateral malleolus, 1.5 cun lateral to the tibial crest. The point is situated in the fibres of the extensor digitorum longus.

Needle

Up to 1.5 cun with a perpendicular insertion. Do not needle too enthusiastically in frail and weak patients.

Moxa and pressure

Use moderate moxa only. For pressure techniques, see below.

Indications

This point is one of the most important points we have in resolving phlegm and is particularly important in treating throat conditions. These include productive cough, tightness in the chest, asthmatic wheezing and bronchitis. General symptoms include mental restlessness and anxiety, lethargy, palpitations, shoulder pain, headache and leg pains.

Special properties

This point is the Key point of the Shoulder chakra (LI 15) and is therefore used to treat shoulder pain, arthritis, or frozen shoulder. When using acupressure, it may be useful to combine this point with ST 38 (one finger-width medially) and consider them both to be one acupoint. It is the most effective distal point in shoulder conditions because the area in the mid position of the fibula is considered to be the shoulder reflex on the leg.

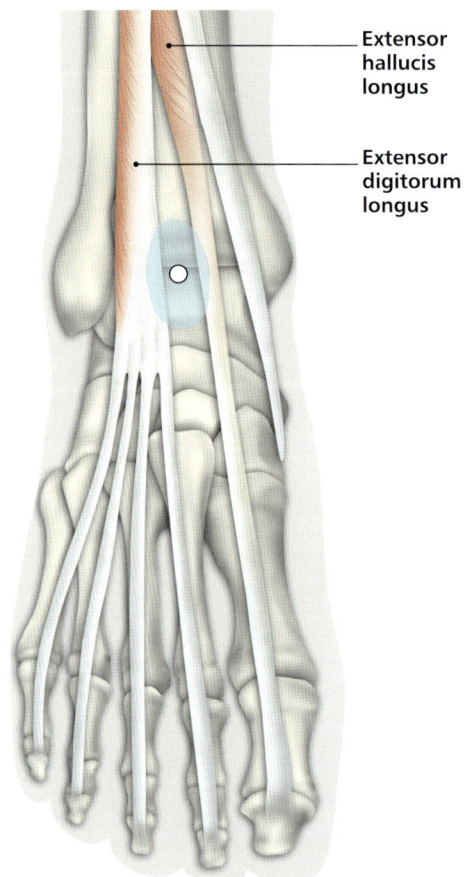

Extensor
hallucis
longus

Extensor
digitorum
longus

Location
Situated on the front of the ankle joint midway between the medial and lateral malleolus.

Needle
Needle up to 1.5 cun using perpendicular insertion.

Do not needle any deeper as there will be a danger of puncturing the anterior tibial artery.

Moxa and pressure
Use light moxa only on this point (no more than 6 cones). Acupressure is particularly effective in treating localized ankle joint conditions. This point is the reflex point of the centre of the wrist joint and may be used to treat wrist conditions.

Indications
As this point is directly over the ankle joint, it is therefore effective in treating ankle pain, arthritic changes and interosseous ligament strain. The general symptomatology includes dispersing stomach heat, clearing heaviness from the eyes, thirst, constipation, vertigo, restlessness and insomnia.

Special properties
This point is the Fire and Tonification point on the Stomach channel. It is therefore used to dispel heat, redness and inflammation from any region over which the Stomach channel passes. It is also used to 'transfer' energy around the Sheng cycle to the Large Intestine meridian.

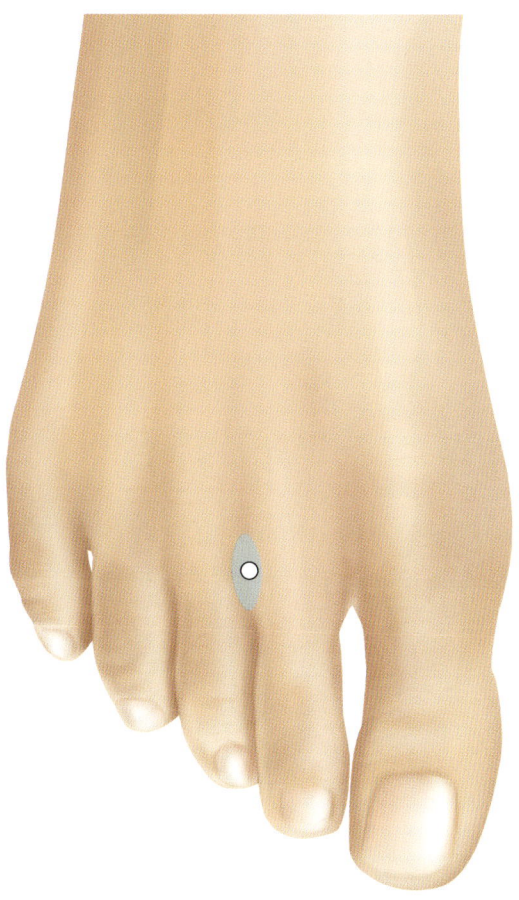

Location
Situated between the second and third toes, proximal to the margin of the web (at the end of the crease).

Needle
Needle only to 0.5 cun using perpendicular insertion between the second and third metatarso-phalangeal joint.

Moxa and pressure
Use medium strength moxa only. This point answers well to pressure techniques, especially stimulation in the treatment of facial and mouth symptoms.

Indications
These are wide ranging, and include epigastric pain, abdominal distension, enteritis, gastritis, heartburn, halitosis, bleeding gums and other mouth symptoms, pain along the course of the stomach meridian especially of the face and neck, deviation of the mouth and localized metatarsal pain.

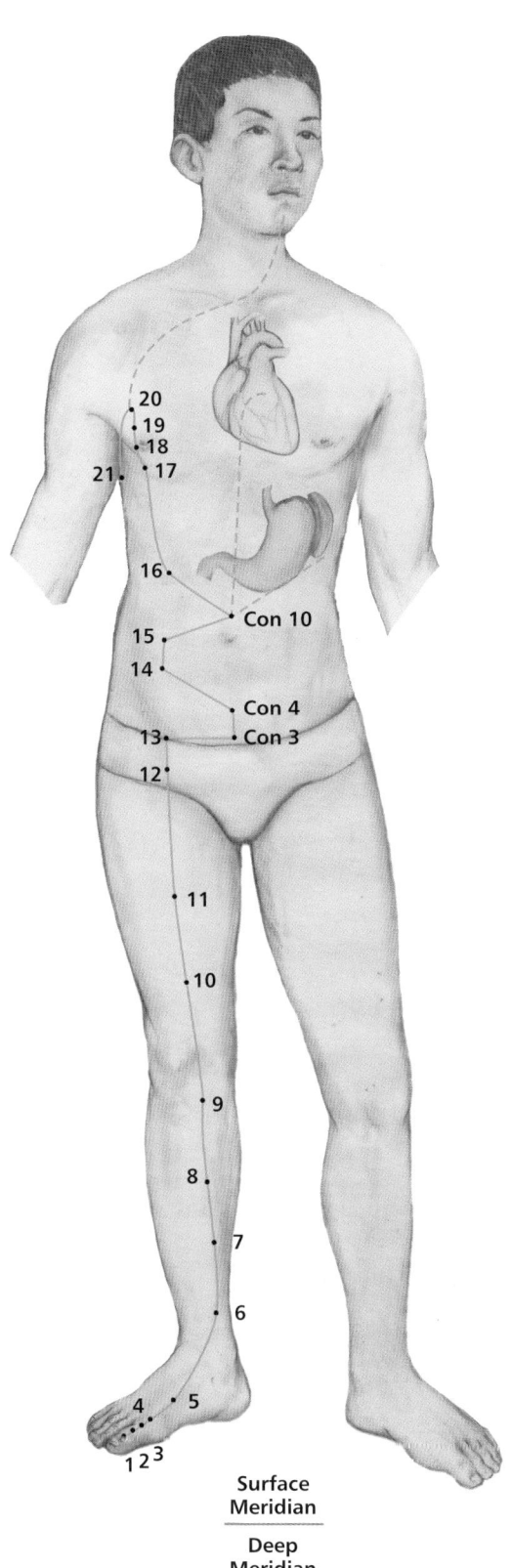

Surface
Meridian
_____

Deep
Meridian
- - - - -

The Spleen meridian represents the Yin aspect of the Earth element. There are twenty-one (21) points on its surface pathway that travels from the big toe to the side of the chest. The meridian commences at the nail point on the medial aspect of the great toe and ascends the instep and up the medial aspect of the lower leg and knee where it runs antero-medially up the leg to above the groin. The channel then dives deep and travels medially through Con 3 and Con 4 acupoints before travelling laterally again towards SP 14. The channel then ascends and again deviates medially towards Con 10. From Con 10 the deeper channel goes on to supply the stomach, spleen and heart. The surface pathway at Con 10 moves laterally towards SP 16 where it ascends on the antero lateral aspect of the chest to SP 20 before ending at SP 21 in the 6th intercostal space in the mid axillary line. At SP 20 a deep channel travels towards the throat and ends in the lower aspect of the tongue.

We shall discuss the following Spleen acupoints: SP 1, SP 3, SP 4, SP 6, SP 9, SP 10, SP 16 and SP 21.

SP 1 *Yin Bai* (Hidden White)

隱白 ★★

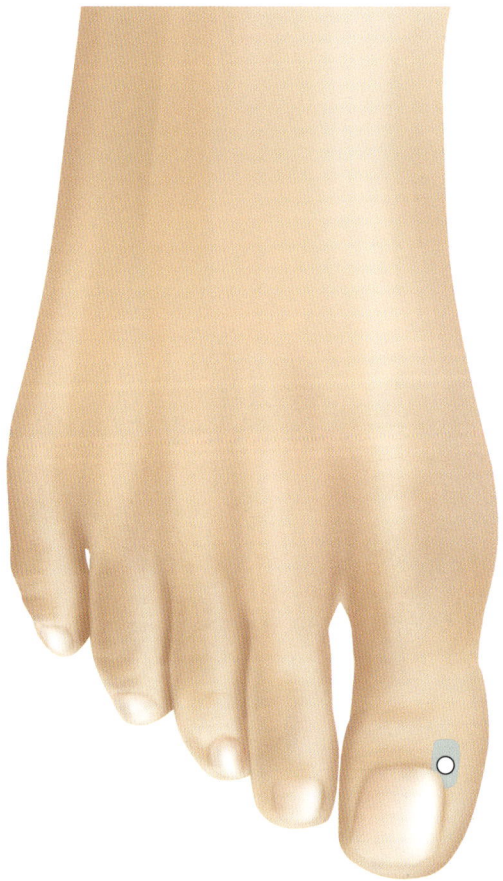

Location
The Tsing (nail) point of this meridian is situated on the medial aspect of the great toe.

Needle
Extremely superficial needling required; 0.1 cun with perpendicular angle.

Moxa and pressure
For pressure details, see 'special properties'.

> Moxa is forbidden.

Indications
As with most Tsing points, SP 1 is an excellent point in helping to calm the mind and for dizziness, vertigo, fainting and insomnia.

Special properties
This point is usually used as a first aid point to arrest bleeding and haemorrhage anywhere in the body. Stimulating pressure only has to be applied until the bleeding is halted. Some texts insist that stimulating moxa may also be used for this purpose, although in a true emergency situation, moxa is either not always to hand and takes considerably longer to apply than stimulating massage!

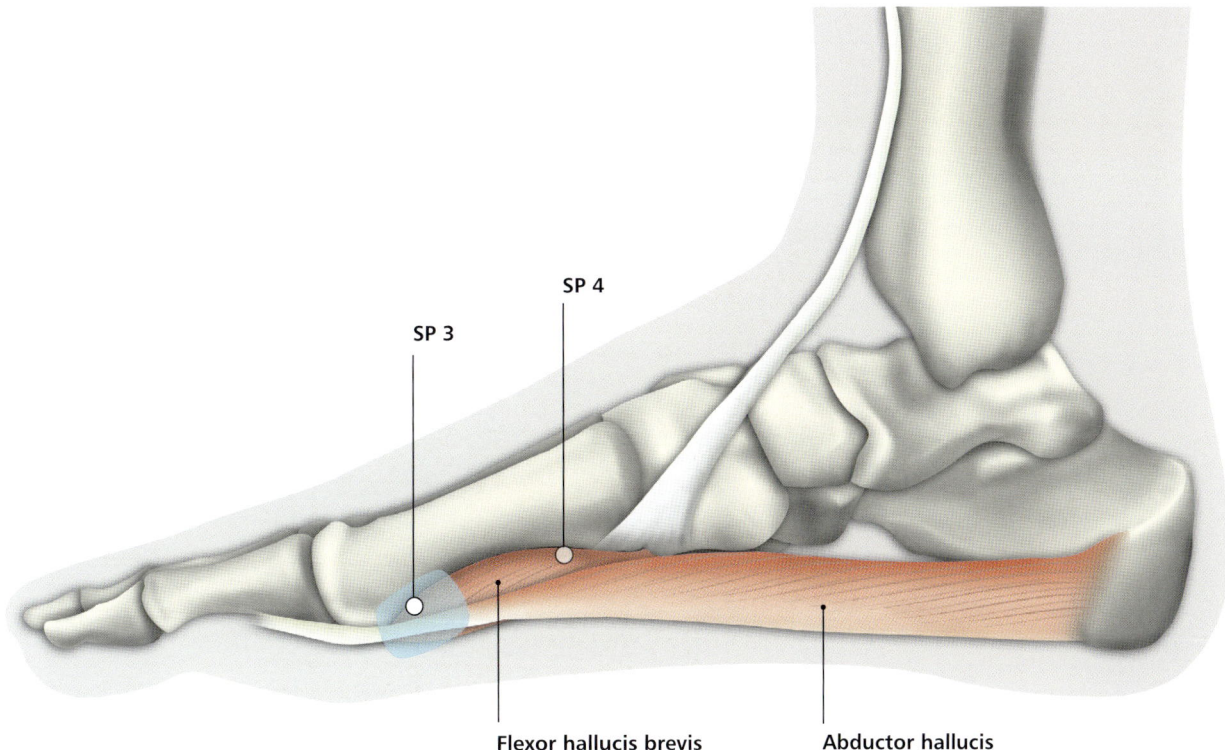

SP 4

SP 3

Flexor hallucis brevis

Abductor hallucis

Location

Situated below the zygomatic arch directly Situated in the depression proximal and medial to the first metatarso-phalangeal joint on the medial surface.

Needle

Accessed using a perpendicular insertion up to 1 cun in depth.

Moxa and pressure

This point will take quite a lot of moxa stimulation. The patient will need to change position to avoid the moxa falling off. Acupressure here aids in the treatment of abductor hallucis and flexor hallucis brevis tendonitis. The point also represents the upper thoracic spine in reflexology.

Indications

This is an important acupoint with the following indications:

- Tiredness, weakness of the limbs and general lethargy.
- Poor appetite, obesity, altered eating habits, abdominal distension, stomach ache and heartburn, candidiasis, diarrhoea and constipation.
- Vaginal discharge, vaginitis, frequent urination, dysuria and cystitis.
- Cough with profuse sputum.

Special properties

This point is the Earth (Horary) as well as being the Source (Yuan) point. It therefore has a direct link with the spleen. It also has an affinity in thought processes, and is used in improving mental functions and concentration and poor memory, sleepiness, heaviness and muzziness.

SP 4 *Gong Sun* (Grandfather-Grandson)

公孫 ★★★★

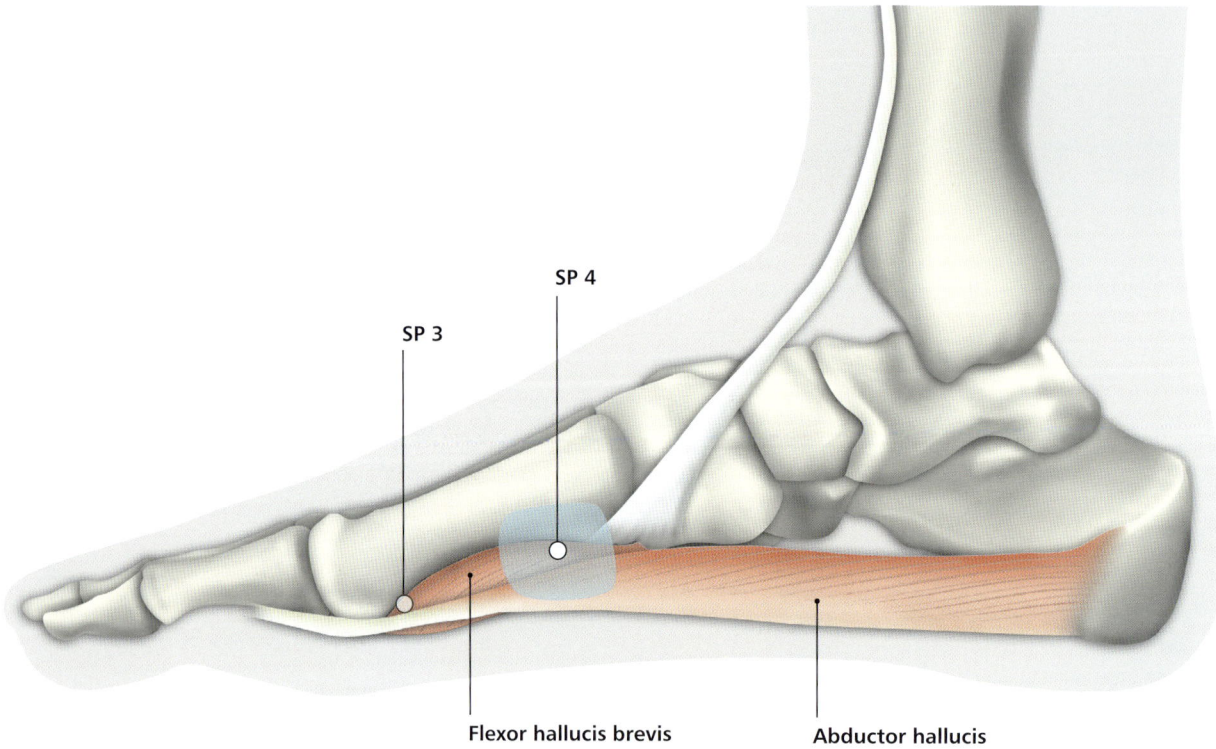

SP 4

SP 3

Flexor hallucis brevis

Abductor hallucis

Location
Situated distal and inferior to the base of the first metatarsal bone at the junction of the skin of the plantar and dorsal surface.

Needle
This point is situated within the flexor hallucis brevis muscle and is therefore deeper than SP 3. Needling is up to 1.5 cun using a perpendicular insertion.

> Beware that the needle does not pierce the tendons of the abductor hallucis.

Moxa and pressure
Moxa either by direct or indirect methods can be very effective. Acupressure has similar uses as SP 3.

Indications
This acupoint is a very influential one and has many facets:
- It boosts spleen and stomach energy, helping to dispel dampness and swelling.
- It is extremely important in gynaecological conditions as it regulates menstruation and strengthens the uterus. Symptomatology includes irregular menstruation, premenstrual tension, endometriosis, excessive menstrual bleeding and some cases of infertility.
- It strengthens the digestive system and helps with gastritis, bloating, irritable bowel syndrome, constipation, gastroenteritis, heartburn, indigestion and morning sickness in pregnancy.
- This point also eases tight chests, regulates the heart and calms the mind and is used in many types of emotional conditions.

Special properties
SP 4 is the Key point of the Chong Mai meridian (Vital channel) and is nearly always linked with PC 6, which is the key point of the Yin Wei Mai (Yin regulating channel). The two points may be used in unison with needle, pressure and magnets. Biomagnets are particularly effective – the negative magnet placed on SP 4 and the positive one on PC 6. This duo of points is excellent in treating many gynaecological conditions, oedema, nausea and in generally balancing chi in blood conditions.

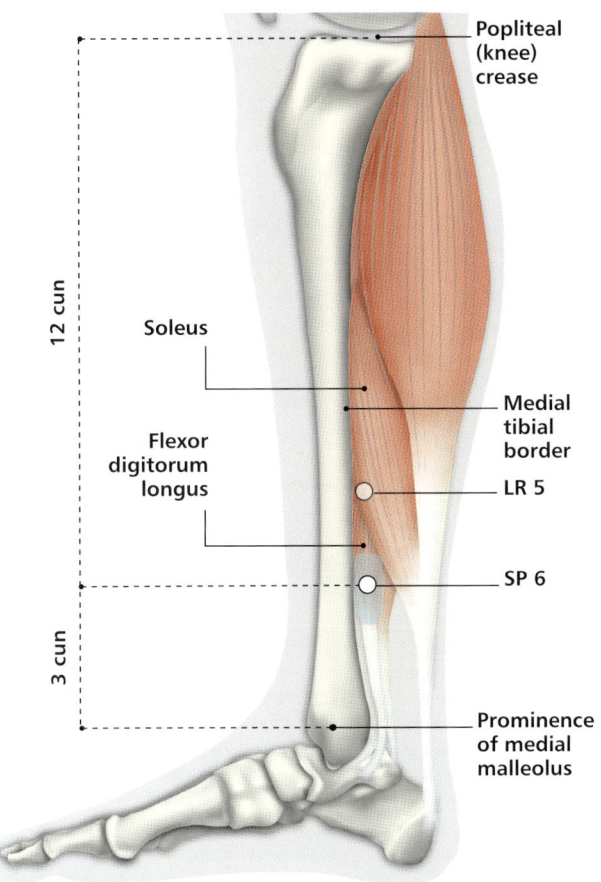

Location
Situated 3 cun proximal to the prominence of the medial malleolus, dorsal to the medial crest of the tibia.

Needle
Use a perpendicular approach and 1.5 to 2 cun depth.

> Deeper insertion may pierce the great saphenous vein or the posterior tibial artery. Also do NOT needle during the first eight months of pregnancy (see 'special properties') and in heavy menstrual bleeding.

Moxa and pressure
Due to underlying blood vessels, use medium stimulation only. This point is nearly always tender to the touch, especially during menstruation and early pregnancy. It may be used as a very good self-help point in many pain and gynaecological conditions.

Indications
- It is used in general cases of regulating chi and blood. It is therefore used in chronic tiredness, exhaustion, blurred vision, tinnitus, oedema and ascites.
- It is probably best used in gynaecological conditions as it regulates uterus and menstrual chi. It is therefore indicated in dysmenorrhoea, delayed menstruation, infertility, vaginal discharge, genital itching, urethritis and incontinence. It may also induce labour (see 'special properties').
- It is helpful in digestive conditions – see SP 3 for the same symptoms.
- SP 6 cools and nourishes Yin and calms the mind. It is therefore useful in dizziness, tinnitus, vertigo, headache, night sweats, palpitations, insomnia and depression (especially if it caused by hormonal imbalance).

Special properties
- SP 6 is one of the great points on the body. It is said to be at the intersection of the three Yin vessels of the leg: spleen, kidney and liver, and as such, helps any condition associated with these three organs. It is colloquially called the 'Great Yin'.
- In combination with other acupoints it is one of the most used anaesthetic acupoints and is used in pain relief especially in gynaecological conditions.
- It is also used in the last few days of pregnancy to aid labour (only experienced acupuncturists should use this).

SP 9 *Yin Ling Quan* (Fountain of the Yin Hillock)

陰陵泉 ★★★

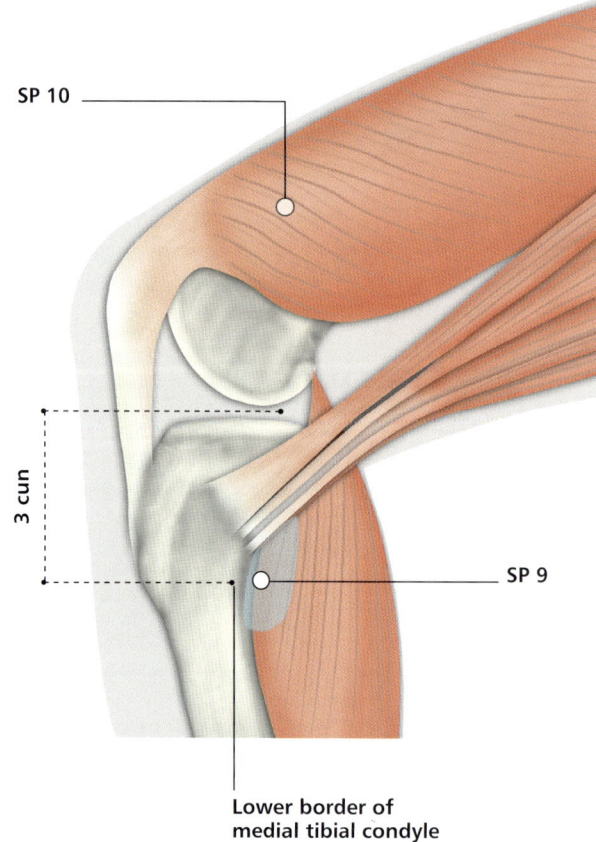

SP 10

3 cun

SP 9

Lower border of
medial tibial condyle

Location
Situated in the depression, distal and dorsal to the tibial medial condyle.

Needle
Perpendicular insertion of 1 cun is required.

Deeper needling could affect the deep saphenous nerve or vein.

Moxa and pressure
Use medium strength moxa due to the underlying vessels. Pressure techniques can be effective and used for medial knee conditions as well as pain along the medial aspect of the leg. Particularly good is to do an energy balance between SP 9 and SP 6 along the medial aspect of the tibia. This helps in leg pain, uterine cramps and aids relaxation.

Indications
To a certain extent SP 9 is a watered down version of SP 6 (in a similar way that LI 11 is subservient to LI 4). In some ways this is true in that anything that SP 6 is used for SP 9 makes an excellent companion and is used for all the symptoms that SP 6 is used for.

Special properties
SP 9 is the Water point of the Spleen meridian and affects the body's water balance. It is therefore indicated in urethritis, cystitis, loose stools, sweating, oedema and menstrual flooding.

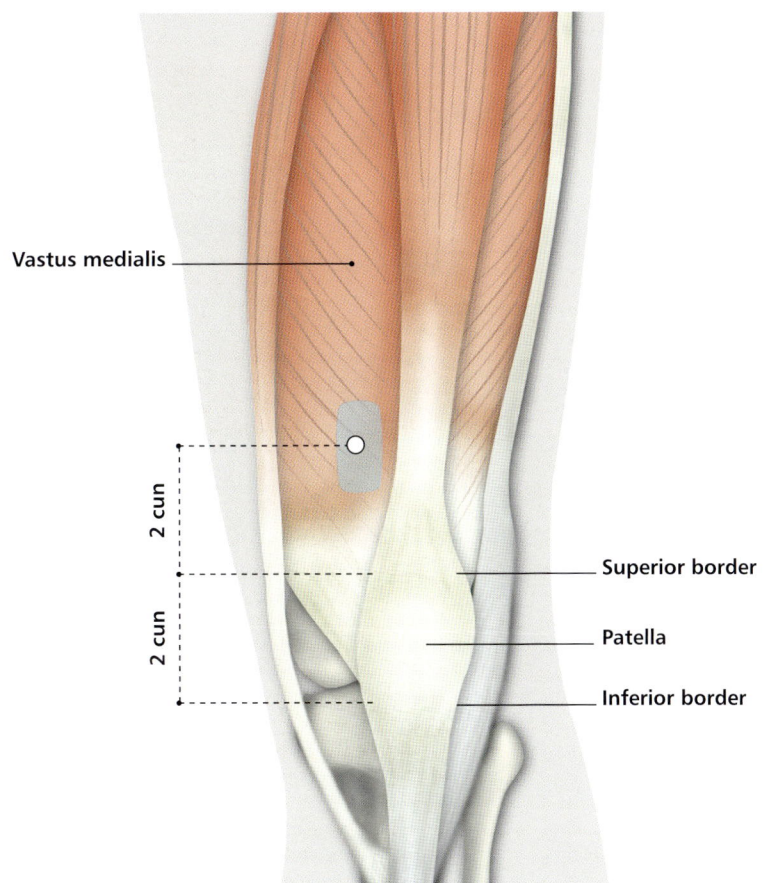

Vastus medialis

2 cun

2 cun

Superior border

Patella

Inferior border

Location

Situated in the depression on the protuberance of the vastus medialis muscle, 2 cun proximal to the medial superior border of the patella. It is directly above SP 9 and should be found with the patient's knee in a flexed position.

Needle

As this point is within the belly of the vastus medialis, deep needling of 2 cun is required with perpendicular insertion.

Moxa and pressure

Use medium moxa stimulation only. Due to its easy location this point is often used as a self-help point in gynaecological conditions. The point is deep so some pressure is required.

Indications

This point may, obviously be used as a local point in proximal knee conditions. It is used extensively though in cases of excess bleeding, especially uterine. It is also used in cases of oedema and anywhere in the body that has 'fluid' imbalance.

Special properties

Due to its effect on cleansing blood, this point is excellent in the treatment of some skin conditions where cleansing and purifying is required. It helps with itchy skin, ulceration, eczema, urticaria and some allergies.

SP 16 *Fu Ai* (Groaning of the Abdomen)

腹哀 ★★★

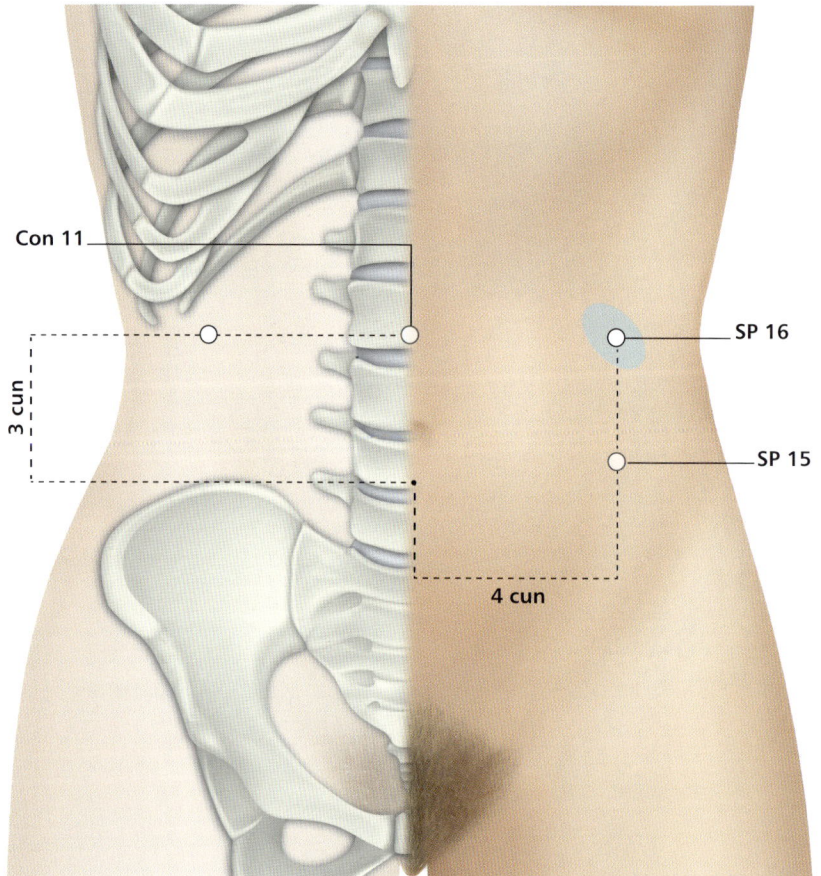

Location

Situated in the large depression directly below the costal arch, lateral to the rectus abdominis muscle, 4 cun lateral to the midline and 3 cun superior to the level of the umbilicus.

Needle

This point may be needled up to 1.5 cun deep with a perpendicular insertion.

> Do not needle any deeper as there is a possibility of affecting the peritoneum and piercing the spleen (left) or the liver (right).

Moxa and pressure

Heavy moxa may be used with this point. Acupressure is very effective in self-help. Do not use heavy pressure when the stomach is distended (see 'special properties').

Indications

This point is used to treat digestive disorders including abdominal distension, abdominal rumbling, diarrhoea and constipation. This point traditionally harmonises the spleen and large intestine.

Special properties

SP 16 on the left is said to be the physical positioning of the Spleen chakra. This chakra is reckoned to be the most important of the minor chakras and is often used in conjunction with the Sacral and Solar Plexus chakras in many conditions. To 'activate' this point, the Key point is Gov 8.

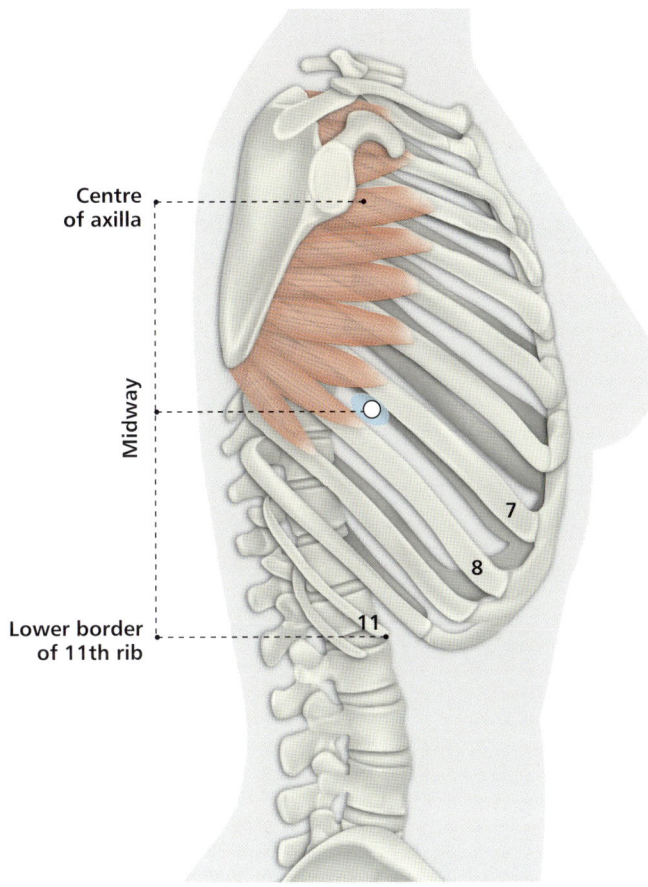

Location

Situated on the lateral aspect of the trunk, approximately 3 cun inferior to the axilla in the 6th intercostal space.

Needle

> Only needle up to 0.5 cun to avoid puncturing the lung.

Moxa and pressure

Moxa can be very effective in the treatment of pain and circulation disorders. Acupressure techniques are extremely effective both practitioner based and as self-help in helping stress conditions and providing body relaxation.

Indications

This point helps in cases where the chest is tight, intercostal neuralgia, rib pain, coughing, generalised joint pains and weakness of the limbs.

Special properties

- SP 21 is the Luo point of the Spleen meridian and is connected to the Heart meridian, thus helping in anxiety and stress conditions.
- It is also the Intercostal chakra. This is a minor chakra that is associated with the Ear chakra (minor) and the Heart chakra (major) to give a triad that helps in stress conditions amongst others. Its Key point is GB 37.

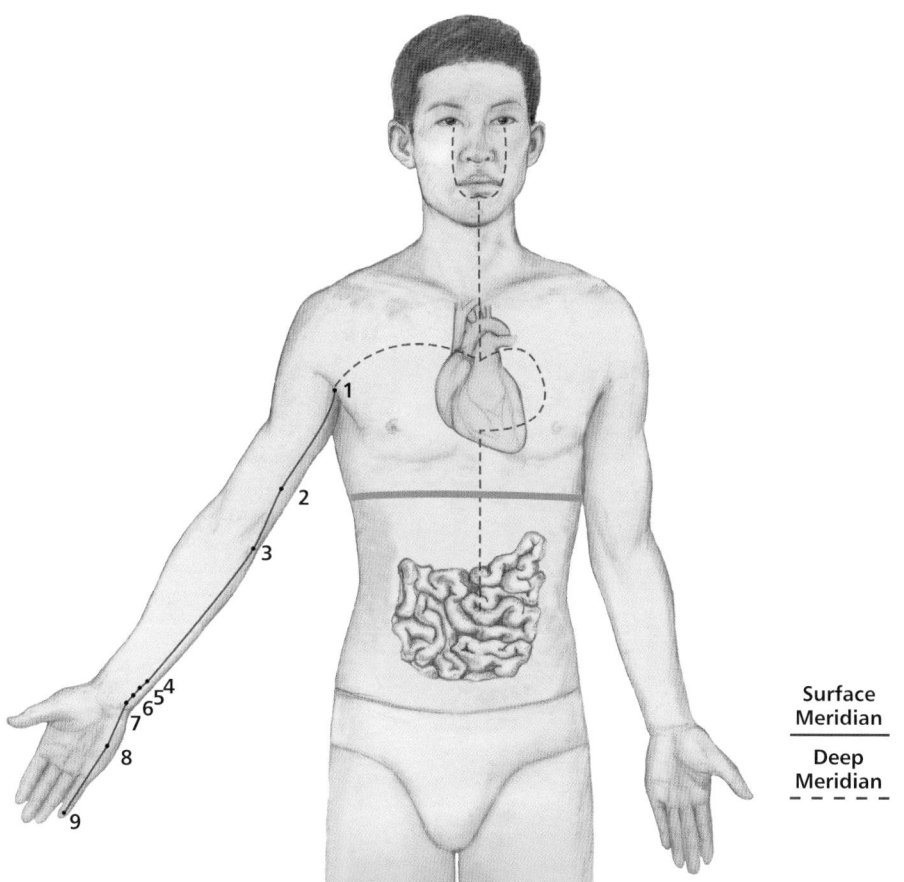

The Heart meridian represents one of the two Yin aspects (together with the Pericardium meridian) of the Fire element. The surface meridian is the shortest of the fourteen and has only nine (9) points. The deeper channel commences in the heart and small intestine and supplies the diaphragm and oesophagus ascending to the mouth and eyes. A connecting deep pathway runs from the midline in the chest to the axilla where it emerges as the first surface point. The surface meridian runs to the medial aspect of the arm to the inside of the elbow joint and to the antero-lateral aspect of the lower arm. At the wrist joint it runs radially past the pisiform bone through the palm and ends on the lateral nail point of the little finger. We shall discuss the following acupoints: HT 1, HT 3, HT 5, HT 6, HT 7 and HT 9.

HT 1 *Ji Quan* (Summit Spring) 極泉 ★★ Needle ★★★ Pressure

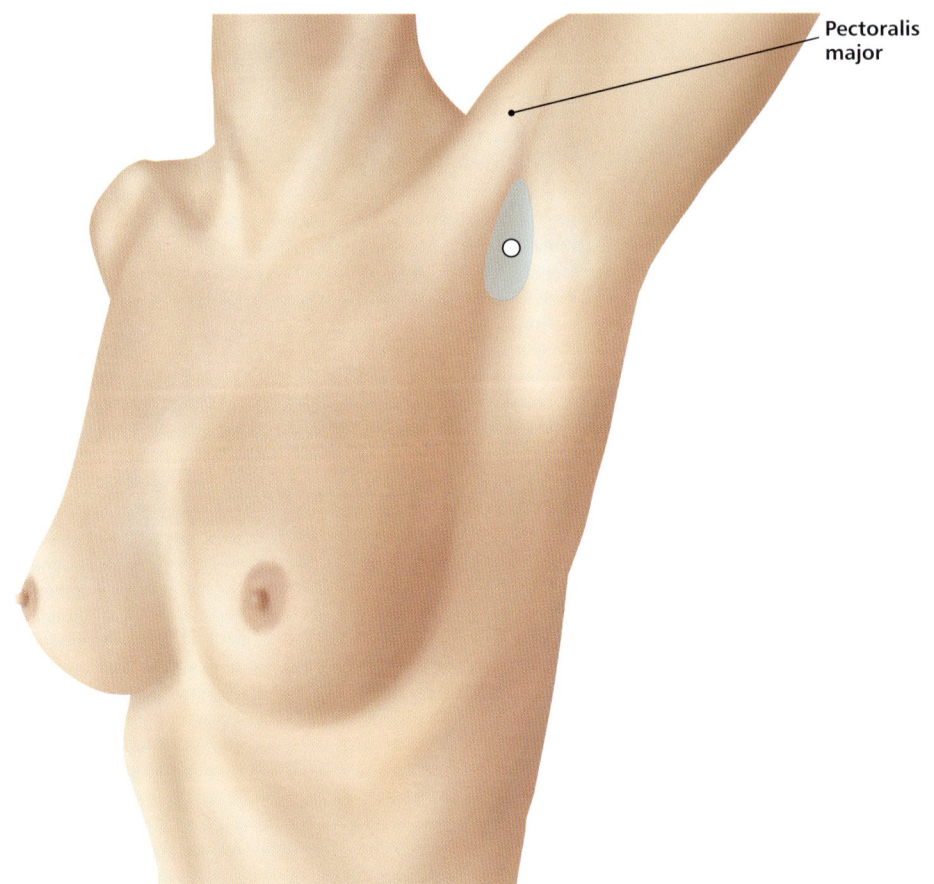

Pectoralis major

Location
Situated in the centre of the axilla medial to the axillary artery. Ask the patient to raise their arm in order to locate and treat.

Needle
The older texts indicate no problems with needling this point, yet some modern ones say that it is forbidden to needle. As there are many axillary vessels underneath it is wisest for inexperienced practitioners not to needle but to concentrate on pressure techniques. Needle only 0.5 cun perpendicularly.

Moxa and pressure
Use mild stimulation only when using a moxa stick. Do not use any stimulating massage on this acutely sore point. It answers very well though to sedation acupressure.

Direct moxa is forbidden.

Indications
This is a very useful (if slightly inaccessible) acupoint. It is indicated in axillary and shoulder pain, intercostal neuralgia, excessive sweating, lymphatic obstruction and mastitis. It is also indicated in some conditions of the heart and chest such as fullness, arrhythmia and palpitations.

Special properties
HT 1 is the Key point of the Heart chakra and is used to 'open up' the energies of the chakra that rules circulatory and emotional conditions.

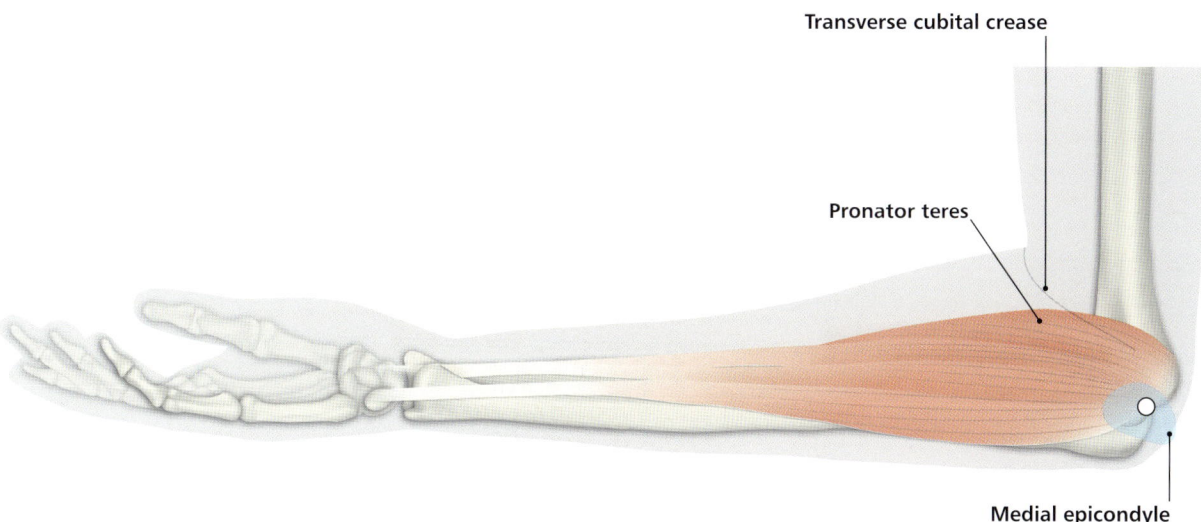

Transverse cubital crease

Pronator teres

Medial epicondyle

Location

Situated midway between the medial end of the cubital crease and the medial epicondyle of the humerus. Locate and treat with the elbow in flexion.

Needle

0.5 to 1 cun depth using a perpendicular approach.

> Danger of puncturing basilica vein or branches of the ulnar nerve if penetration is too deep.

Moxa and pressure

> Direct moxa is forbidden.

Use mild stimulation only using a moxa stick. Acupressure can be very effective as a local point in the treatment of golfer's elbow.

Indications

These fall into the categories of local and general. As a local point it is used for pain and stiffness on the medial aspect of the elbow, golfer's elbow, weakness and trembling of the forearm. As a general point it is effective in the treatment of insomnia, depression, mental agitation, epilepsy, chest pains, toothache, headache and fever.

HT 5 *Tong Li* (Door to the Interior) 通里 ★★★

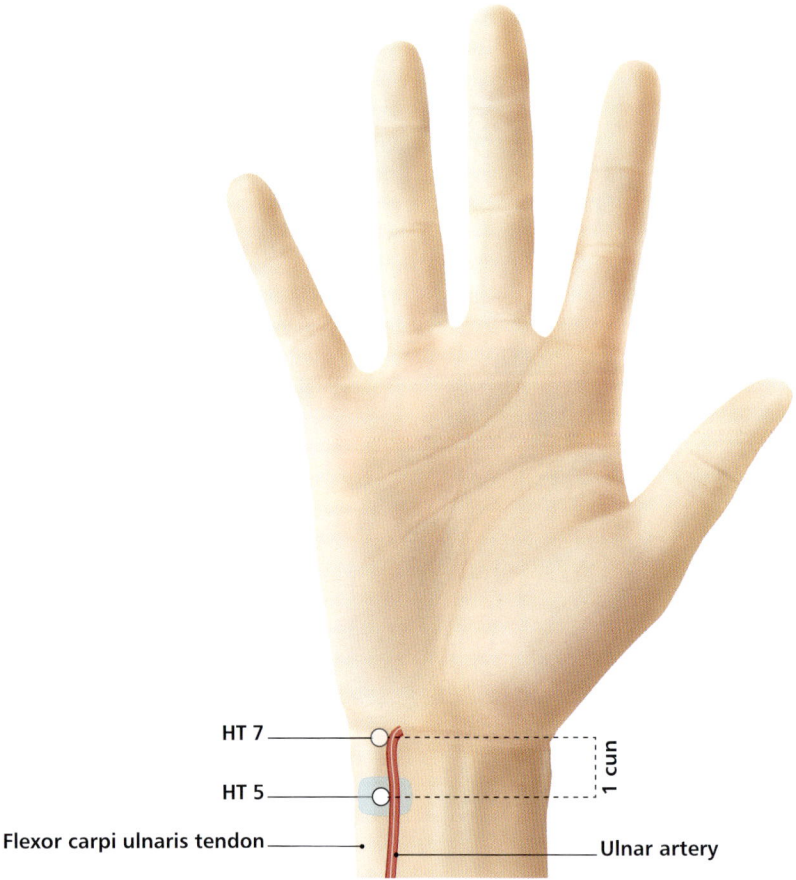

HT 7

HT 5

1 cun

Flexor carpi ulnaris tendon

Ulnar artery

Location
Situated 1 cun proximal to the distal wrist crease on the radial side of the flexor carpi ulnaris tendon.

Needle
Use very shallow needling if perpendicular – 0.3 to 0.5 cun. One of the most popular techniques is to use an oblique 'thread' incorporating three out of the four heart meridian points around the medial aspect of the wrist.

Moxa and pressure
Acupressure is used but, again, usually in combination with the other heart points.

Moxa is forbidden.

Indications
HT 5 is an important and widely used point to tonify Heart chi and to calm the mind. Symptoms include palpitations, chest pains on exertion, mental tiredness, dizziness, epilepsy, grief, fright, shock and hysteria. HT 5 is also the Luo point that connects the Heart and Small Intestine channels. It is therefore useful in lower small bowel and urinary system conditions such as dysuria, haematuria and cystitis.

Special properties
This acupoint is especially useful in disorders of the tongue and speech including paralysis and stiffness of the tongue, stuttering, aphasia and other speech difficulties. It is often used as self-help pressure in actors and other orators who suddenly lose their voice. This, naturally, may be of psychosomatic origin, but the Heart channel is generally used in emotional conditions in any case, so the aetiology is not important.

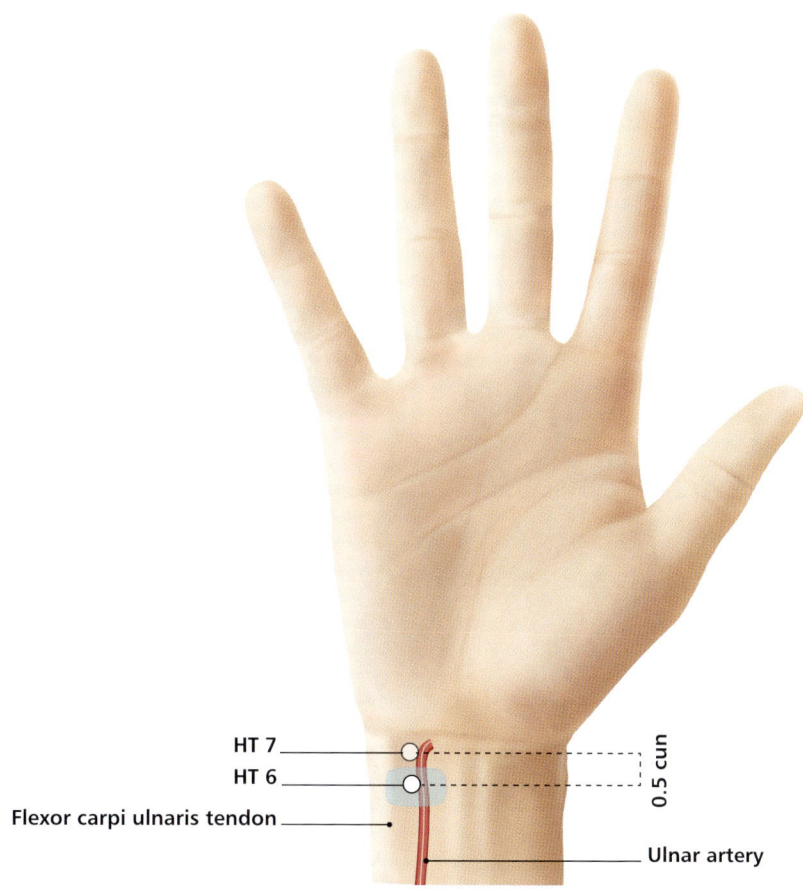

HT 7

HT 6

Flexor carpi ulnaris tendon

0.5 cun

Ulnar artery

Location

Situated on the radial side of the flexor carpi ulnaris tendon 0.5 cun proximal to the wrist crease.

Needle

Either shallow needle (up to 0.5 cun) perpendicular or obliquely to cover three other heart acupoints as discussed in the previous point.

Moxa and pressure

Mild moxa stimulation only but pressure techniques in combination with HT 5, HT 6 and HT 7 are very useful in many types of emotional conditions.

Indications

In common with other distal Heart meridian points, HT 6 is very good in clearing excess heat, inflammation and pain from the chest, upper arm and heart. They are paramountly used, though, in clearing the mind and obviously used in stress conditions. Symptoms would include excessive sweating, heat and fullness of the chest, angina pectoris, palpitations, tachycardia, insomnia, agitation and mental restlessness. It may also be used as a local point in wrist pain and inflammation.

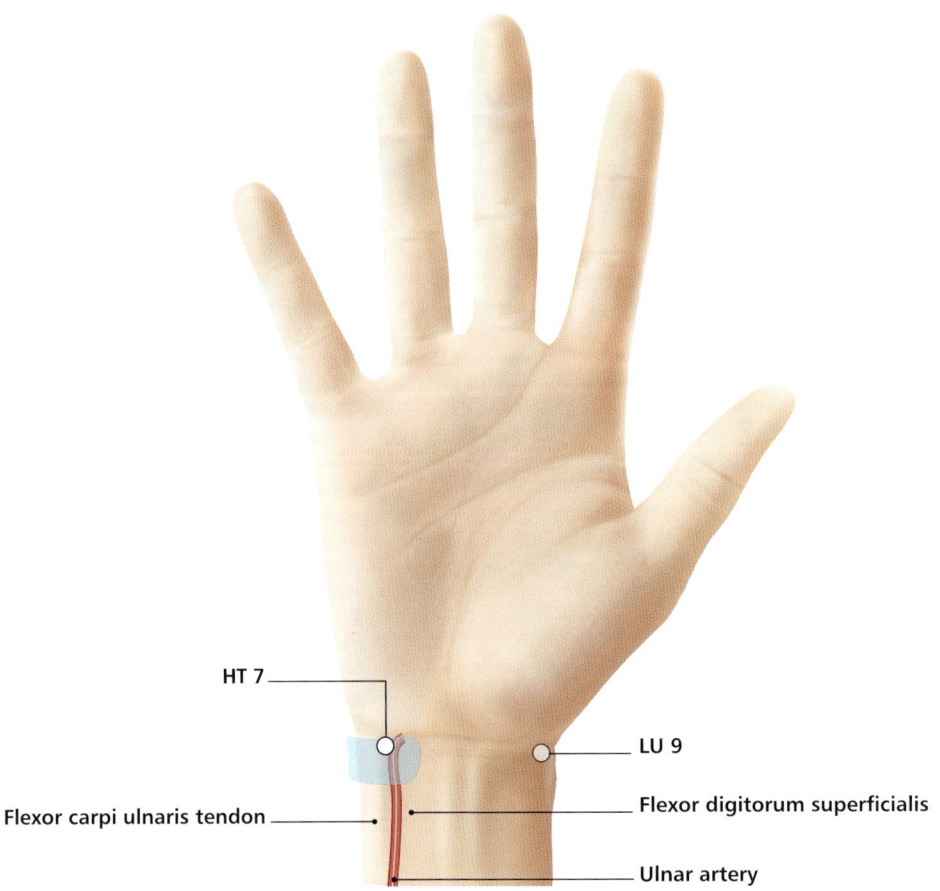

HT 7

LU 9

Flexor carpi ulnaris tendon

Flexor digitorum superficialis

Ulnar artery

Location

Situated at the proximal border of the pisiform bone on the radial side of the flexor carpi ulnaris tendon. It is best to slightly flex the patient's wrist to locate the point.

Needle

Shallow needling only up to 0.5 cun is sufficient to affect the point.

> The ulnar artery is only just lateral to the point and must be avoided.

Moxa and pressure

Use light stimulation only both directly and with a moxa stick. For pressure techniques, see 'special properties'.

Indications

HT 7 is one of the great points in acupuncture and the most popular acupoint on the Heart channel. It is the Source point and the Earth (sedation) point so it affects the heart directly and is the most important acupoint on the Heart channel in calming the mind. The common symptoms include palpitations, tachycardia, arrhythmia, angina pectoris, insomnia, worry, stress, anxiety, stage fright, poor memory and lethargy. It is also used in local wrist conditions. It has a major effect on the mouth (not as powerful as HT 5) and is useful in speech complications with stroke patients.

Special properties

When used with acupressure, HT 7 is the most influential acupoint in the treatment of insomnia. This is a wonderful point to teach the patient who is having trouble sleeping. A favourite technique of mine is to combine HT 7 with Yin Tang (between the eyes) – one calms the spirit and the other calms the mind. It is also influential as a self-help point in the treatment of anxiety, panic attacks and sheer dread such as stage fright.

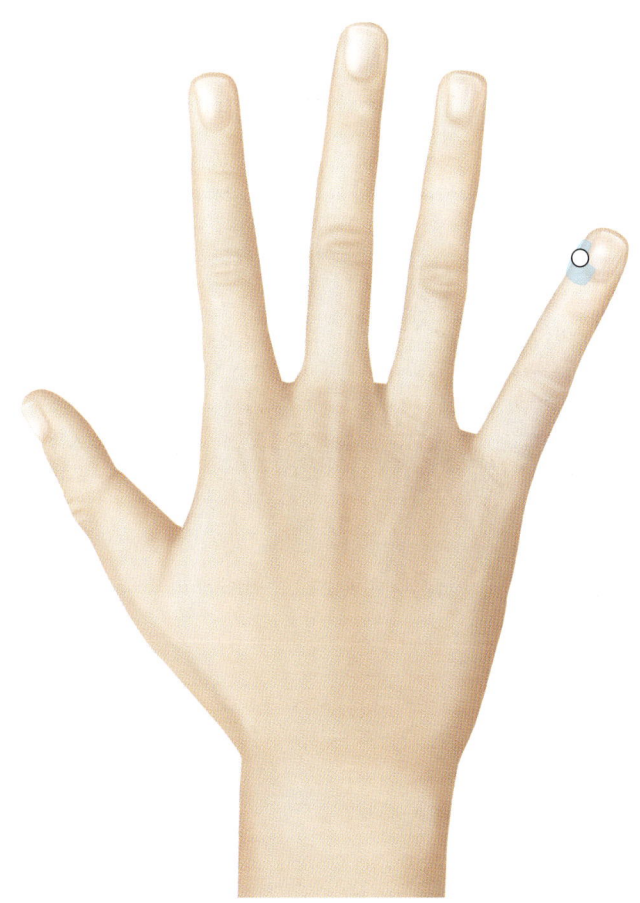

Location
Situated on the lateral side of the little finger at the Tsing (nail) point.

Needle
As it is a Tsing point, use the shallowest of needling (0.1 cun).

Moxa and pressure
Use very mild stimulation – some older texts consider this point to be forbidden to moxa. Acupressure is extremely useful as a first aid point in the treatment of fainting, shock and syncope. As it is a very superficial point, it may be easier to use a biro pen point to stimulate it.

Indications
In common with all Tsing points, HT 9 is used in stress conditions and in calming the mind and spirit. As mentioned previously, the point is useful in shock and fainting. In common with other Heart channel points, HT 9 is used in the treatment of arrhythmia, tachycardia, palpitations, angina pectoris, pain in the mouth and mental tiredness.

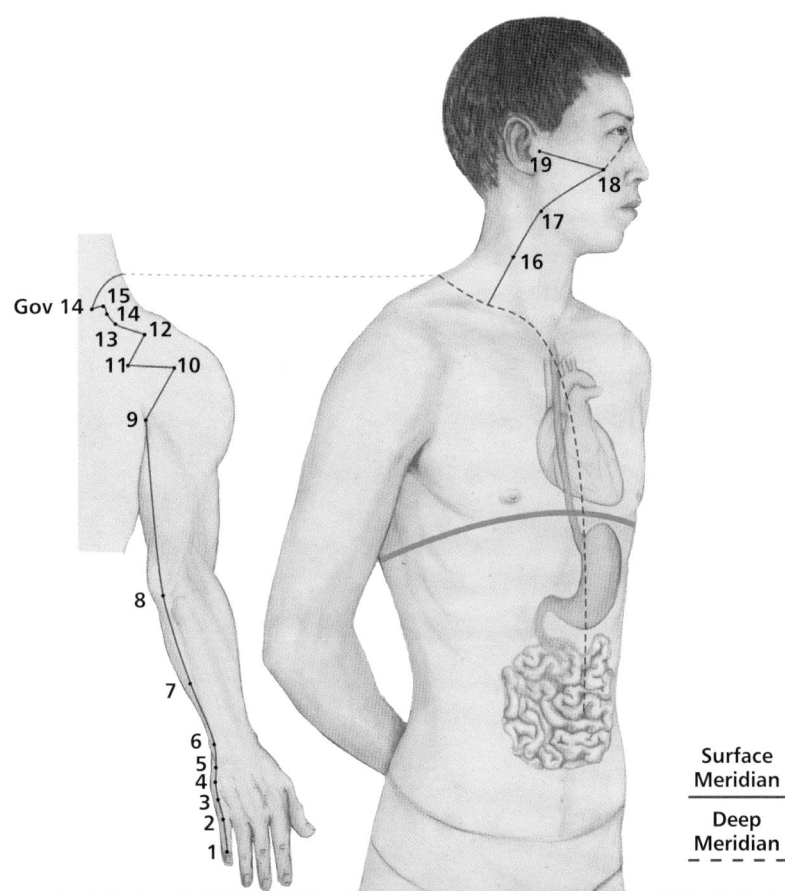

The Small Intestine meridian is one of the two Yang channels in the Fire element. There are nineteen (19) acupoints on its surface pathway. The meridian commences at the nail point on the ulnar surface of the little finger. It ascends the lateral aspect of the little finger to the posterior aspect of the elbow and posterior aspect of the shoulder. It zigzags over the scapula and connects to Gov 14 (C7–T1) before returning to the anterior aspect of the body at the root of the neck. The surface channel then ascends the lateral aspect of the neck to the cheek bone and ends at the front of the ear. There is an inner pathway that descends from the junction with Gov 14 that enters the heart, diaphragm and ends in the small bowel. Another inner pathway leaves SI 18 at the cheekbone towards the eye where it joins to the first point of the Bladder meridian. The meridian passes over the hand, wrist, elbow, shoulder and temporo-mandibular joints. The local points to these joints are used extensively to treat local conditions – some of these are not discussed in detail but this does not diminish their importance. We shall discuss the following acupoints: SI 1, SI 3, SI 4, SI 6, SI 9, SI 11, SI 18 and SI 19.

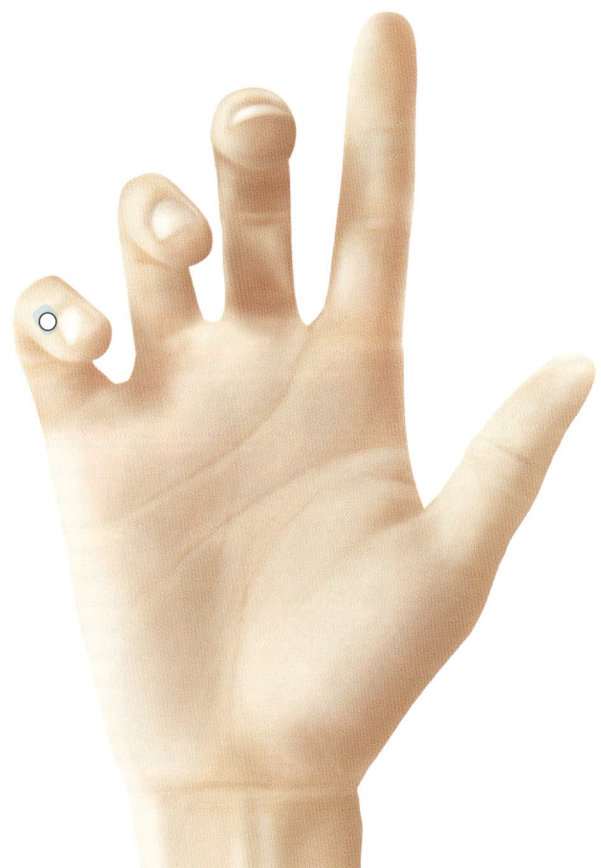

Location

This is the Tsing (nail) point on the ulnar side of the little finger.

Needle

Use very superficial needling (as with all Tsing points), copper or zinc small needles may be 'placed' on the points as opposed to using invasive techniques.

Moxa and pressure

Use mild moxa stimulation only. For pressure techniques, see 'special properties'.

Indications

In common with most Tsing points, SI 1 is used in calming the mind and releasing stress related tension. As per HT 9 (the other ring finger Tsing point) this point is used as an emergency one in fainting and syncope.

Special properties

SI 1 has a peculiarity of inducing and harmonizing bodily fluids, in particular, promoting lactation. This may obviously be done with needle but is much better with pressure. It remains an excellent self-help point with women who cannot produce breast milk naturally, for whatever reason.

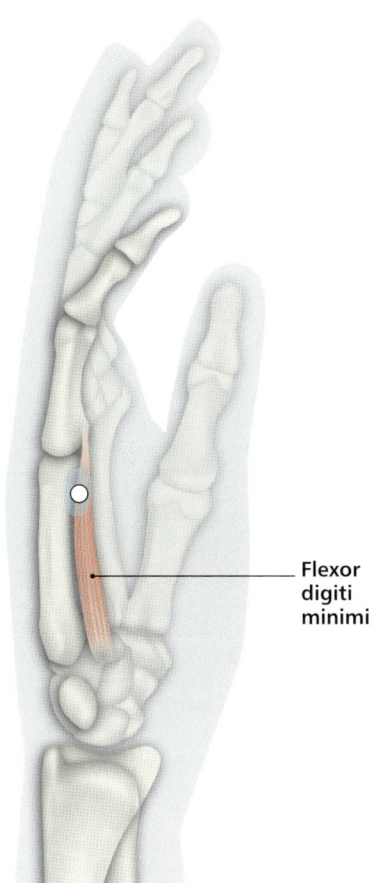

Flexor digiti minimi

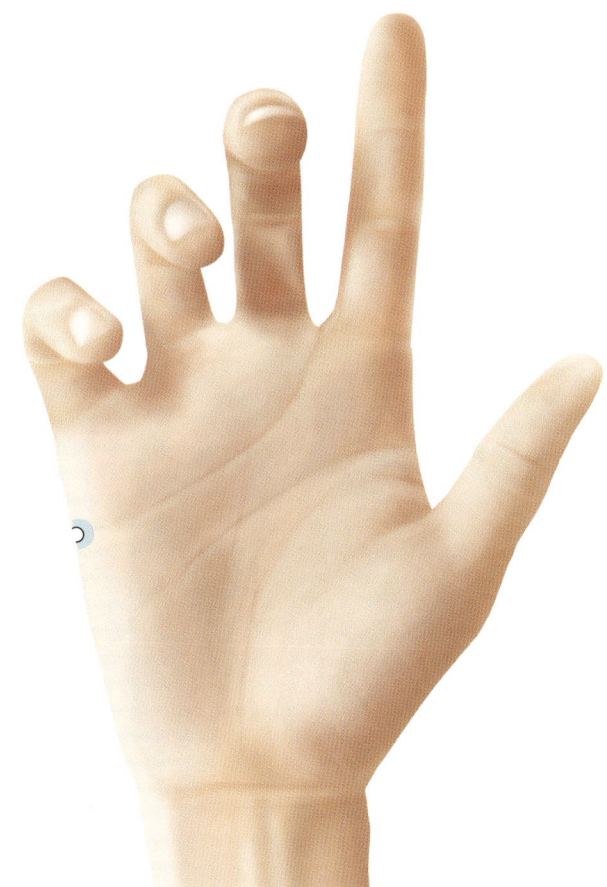

Location

Situated at the proximal end of the 5th metacarpal bone on the ulnar surface. It is easily found in a small depression when the patient makes a slight fist.

Needle

This point is quite superficial so the needle needs only a 0.7 cun penetration using perpendicular insertion. Oblique techniques may be tried but I have never found the need for these. This point has a very strong deqi sensation and the patient may jerk their hand away, so be aware of this.

Moxa and pressure

This point answers well to stimulating moxa either with a moxa stick or on the skin. If performing the latter technique, make sure the cone will stay on the point and ask the patient to keep the ulnar border of their hand uppermost. For a useful acupressure technique, see below.

Indications

This acupoint is far and away the most used on the Small Intestine channel and it has many uses. It is said to clear 'excess yang', especially from the posterior aspect of the body, i.e. neck and shoulders. Some of its many indications are in pain and stiffness of the neck and shoulders, occipital headaches, tinnitus, chills and fever, vertigo, mental restlessness and inflammation of the eye.

Special properties

*   SI 3 is the Key (Opening) point of the Governor (Du Mai) meridian and is particularly influential in treatment of lower cervical pain and stiffness but is often used to help treat all spinal conditions. This point, therefore, has to be used in all cases of cervical discomfort. It is a wonderful self-help point for patients to massage to control neck discomfort.
*   SI 3 is linked with BL 62 (just below the lateral malleolus) as a great couple of points to treat general spinal pain. This may be done with needle, pressure or with biomagnets. In the case of magnet therapy, the negative pole is placed on SI 3 and the positive pole on BL 62.

SI 4 *Wan Gu* (Wrist Bone)

腕骨 ⭐⭐

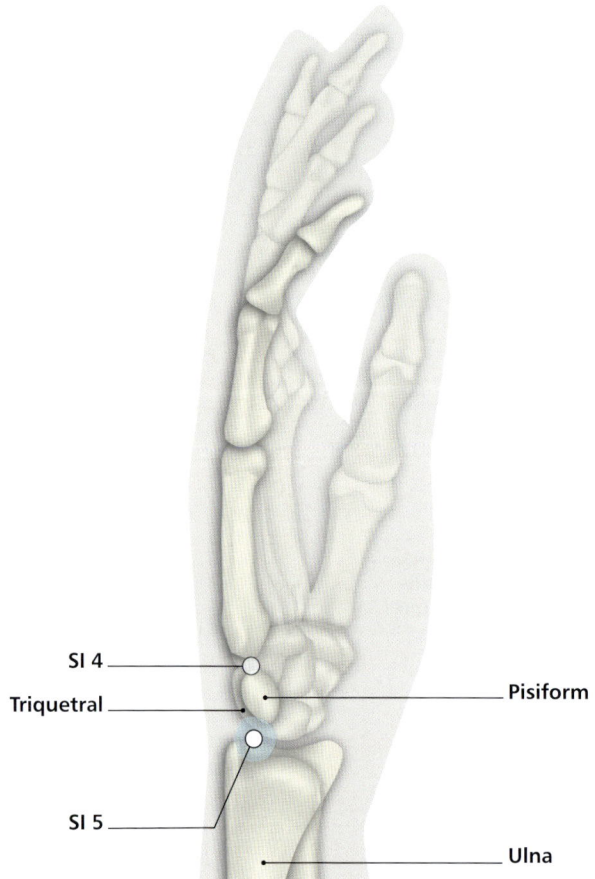

SI 4 — ○
Triquetral —
Pisiform
SI 5 —
Ulna

Location

Situated on the ulnar border of the hand between the base of the 5th metacarpal and the triquetral bone.

Needle

This point is very superficial so a 0.3 perpendicular insertion should affect it.

Moxa and pressure

Stimulating moxa may be used but this acupoint does not have many general properties so the moxa should be directed at wrist stiffness conditions. Tonifying acupressure is also useful in wrist conditions.

Indications

As stated before, this point is used mostly in localised wrist conditions where it is eminently effective. However, SI 4 is the Source (Yuan) point on this channel and therefore has a direct link with the small bowel. It is therefore used in gastritis and gastroenteritis. It may also be used in acupressure and magnet therapy as a parallel acupoint to treat pain and stiffness of the lateral aspect of the ankle.

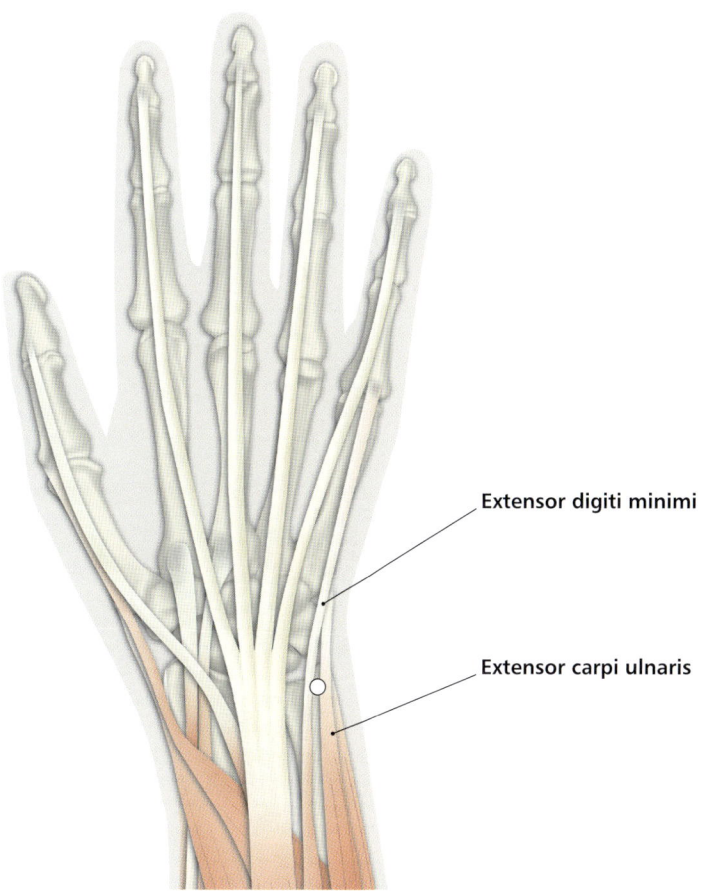

Extensor digiti minimi

Extensor carpi ulnaris

Location
This point is situated on the posterior aspect of the head of the ulna bone between the ulna and the tendon of extensor digiti minimi. Ask the patient to turn their palm towards their chest to aid location.

Needle
This can be a difficult point to locate and is best needled in an oblique fashion to 1.5 cun depth from a proximal direction.

Moxa and pressure
This point responds extremely well to quite a lot of moxa stimulation. Pressure techniques should also be stimulating as nothing will be achieved when used in sedation mode.

Indications
The principle action with this useful point is to treat painful conditions along the Small Intestine channel, particularly the wrist, elbow and shoulder. It also helps in painful hernias and appendix region.

Special properties
As the acupoint's name suggests it is quite often used in creating some vitality, especially in the elderly. I have used this on a number of occasions and been pleasantly surprised by its effectiveness.

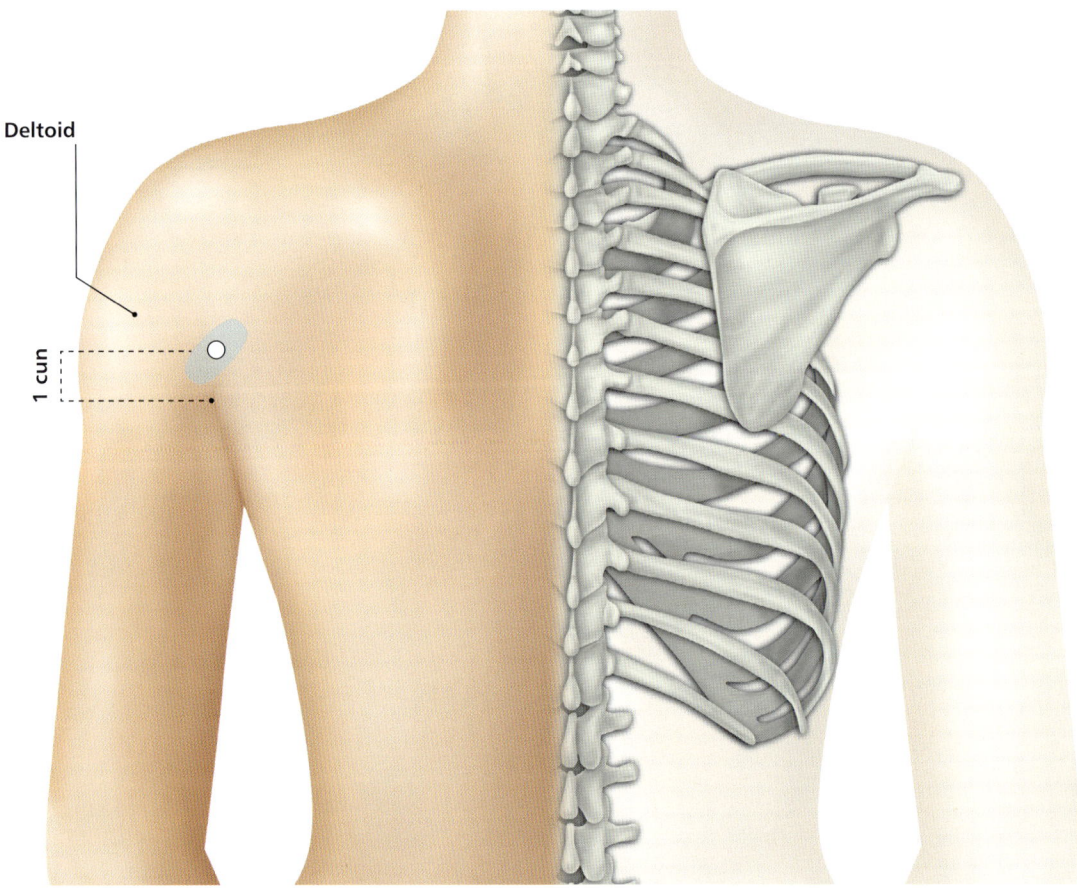

Deltoid

1 cun

Location
Situated on the posterior aspect of the shoulder 1 cun superior to the axillary crease when the arm is adducted.

Needle
Up to 1.5 cun using a perpendicular approach.

Do not needle any deeper as there is a danger of affecting the veins and arteries in the axilla.

Moxa and pressure
This point responds well to lots of stimulating moxa and pressure especially in the treatment of stiff shoulders.

Indications
SI 9 is one of four SI acupoints that are effective in treating shoulder conditions. Just this point and SI 11 are described but SI 10 and SI 12 locations are shown in the illustrations. This point helps in painful shoulder, frozen shoulder and lymphatic obstruction especially on the anterior aspect of the chest and breast tissue.

Special properties
This is a magnificent acupoint when used in parallel acupuncture/acupressure mode in the treatment of painful hips and sacro-iliac regions. The parallel point most used is BL 36 (just beneath the gluteal fold).

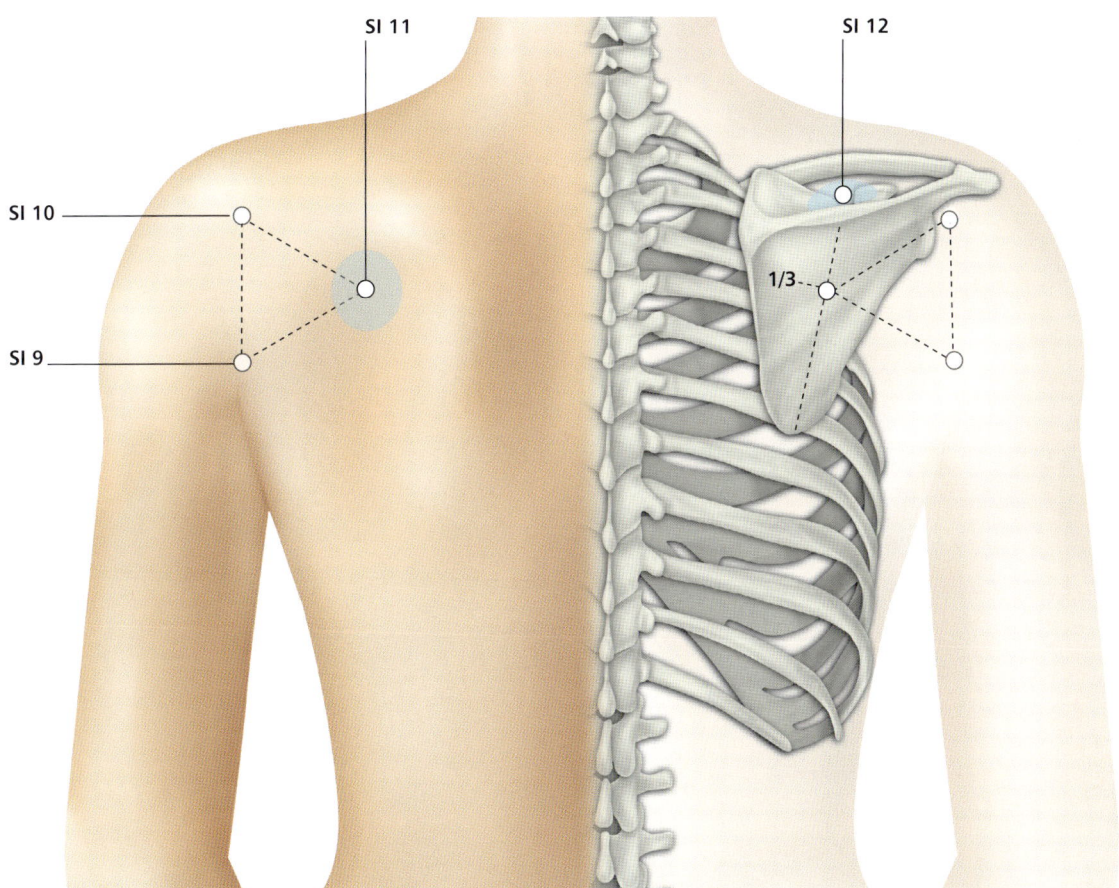

Location

Situated in the centre of the scapula where the spine of scapula is at its most pronounced. You will notice from the illustrations that an equilateral triangle exists between SI 9, SI 10 and SI 11 to aid location.

Needle

This point is fairly deep so use a 1.5 cun depth using a perpendicular approach.

Moxa and pressure

Heavy stimulating moxa and pressure are very useful in all the post scapula acupoints when treating stiff and painful shoulders.

Indications

Of the four post scapula Small Intestine acupoints, this point is the most powerful to ease shoulder and shoulder girdle pain and stiffness. It has general properties of calming the digestive system with acid reflux, irritable bowel and indigestion. It is also used in painful breast tissue and mastitis, especially when there is insufficient lactation.

SI 18 *Quan Liao* (Cheek Bone Crevice)

顴髎 ★★

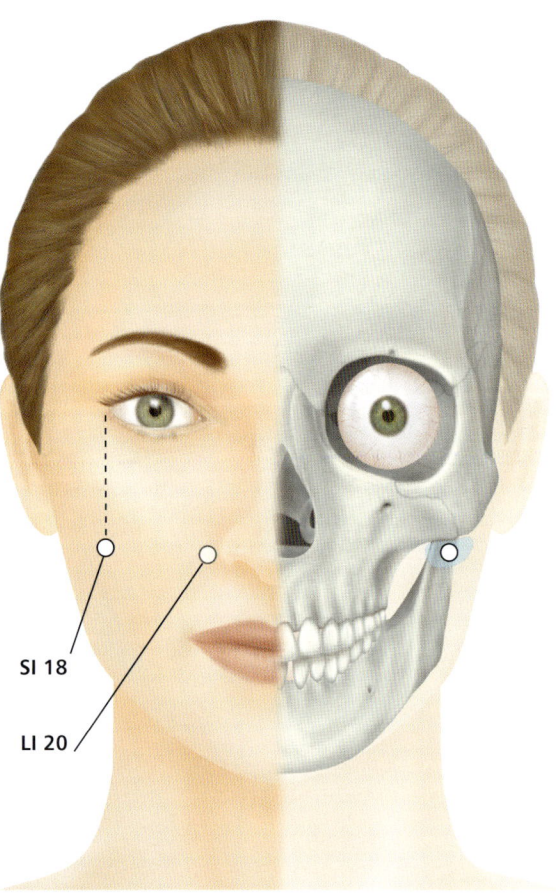

SI 18

LI 20

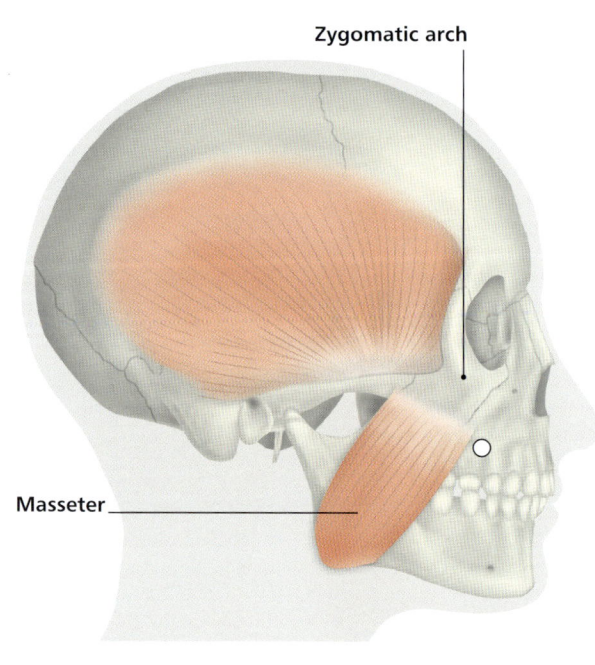

Zygomatic arch

Masseter

Location

This point is situated in the depression at the lower border of the zygomatic arch directly below the outer canthus of the eye and level with LI 20.

Needle

Up to 0.6 cun using a perpendicular approach although a needle can be 'threaded' along the inferior aspect of the zygoma to affect the point.

> Deeper needling may affect the parotid duct or the several circulatory vessels in the area.

Moxa and pressure

Use sedation pressure techniques only to aid eye or nasal conditions.

> Moxa is forbidden; except that mild stimulation using a moxa stick is allowed, although this is practically unsound as smoke will always go into the patient's eyes!

Indications

SI 18 is effective for problems of the cheek, eyes, teeth and nose. This includes facial paralysis, trigeminal neuralgia, sinusitis and eye inflammation. In recent years this acupoint has become one of the many on the face that is used in aesthetic and cosmetic situations. These would include thread veins and 'sagging' facial muscles.

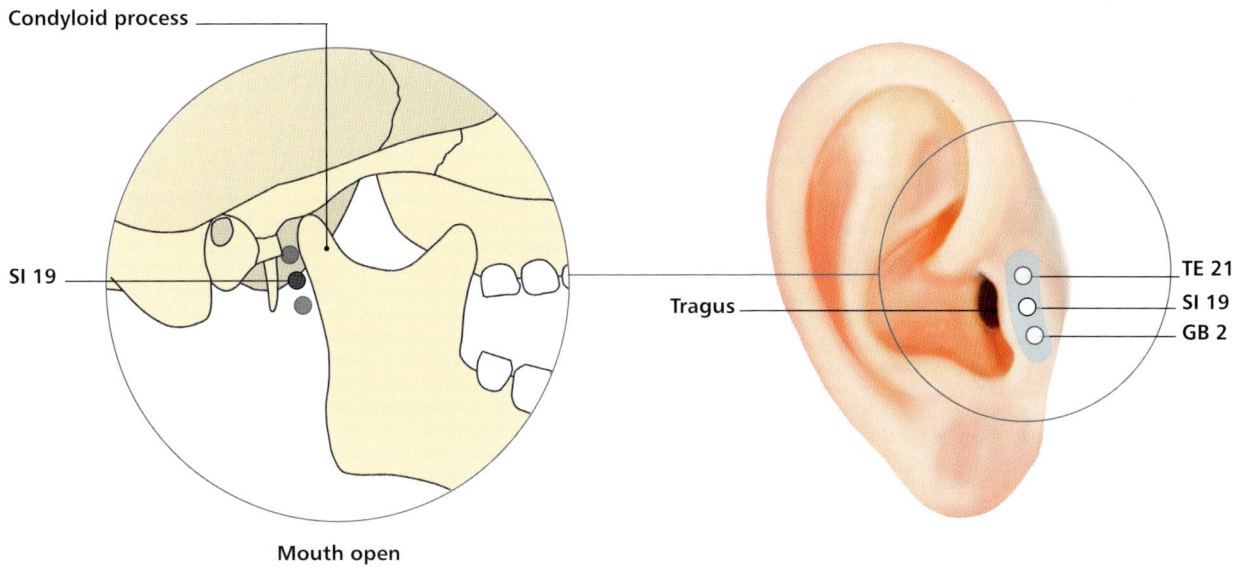

Condyloid process

SI 19

Mouth open

Tragus

TE 21

SI 19

GB 2

Location
Situated just anterior to the tragus in a depression formed when the mouth is just opened, between TE 21 and GB 2.

Needle
Up to 1 cun using a perpendicular approach.

Moxa and pressure
Although moxa is not forbidden, direct moxa is not recommended. Pressure techniques should be very light and gentle. The trio of points by the temporo-mandibular joint (TMJ) are favourite points of cranio-sacral therapists and therapists who use subtle touch techniques.

Indications
This point has two indications which are both important. Firstly it is used in many types of ear conditions including earache, tinnitus and mild deafness (if caused by mechanical irritation). Secondly it is one of a group of points around the head and face used in calming the mind and reducing tension. The TMJ is often in a state of tension and treating this point helps relax the joint. Pressure techniques seem more effective in calming the mind whereas needle seems better at relieving pain.

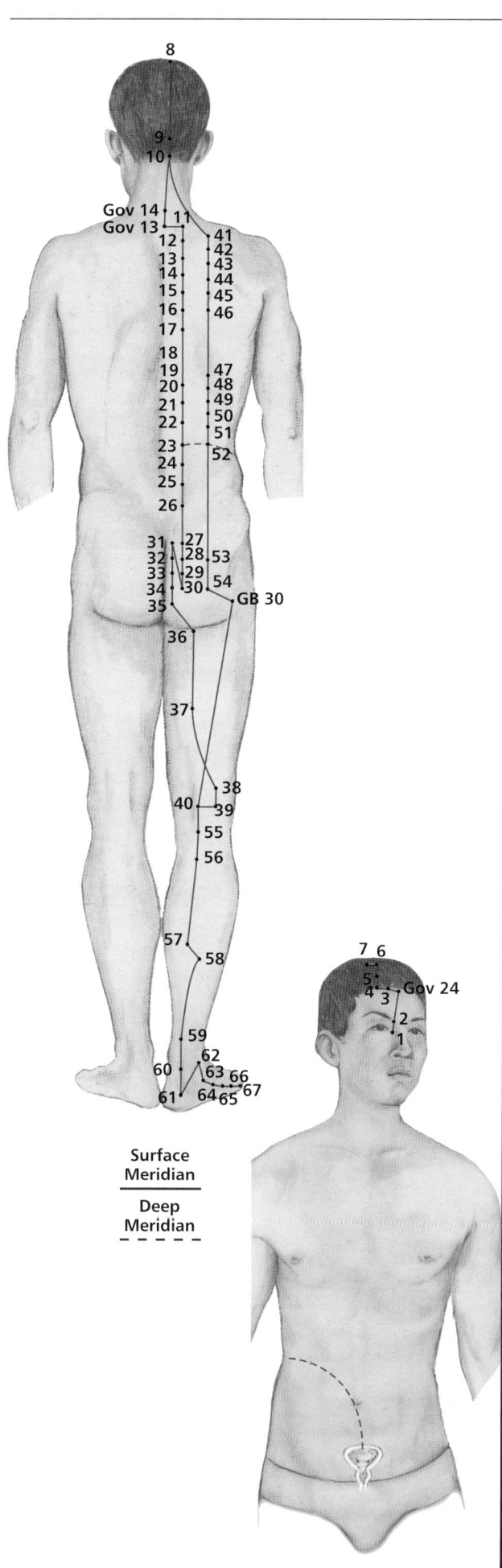

Surface
Meridian

Deep
Meridian
- - - - -

The Bladder meridian is the Yang channel of the Water element. It is the longest meridian in the body with sixty-seven (67) points. It has a huge range of influences which vary according to the position of its acupoints. The surface meridian commences at the inner canthus of the eye before ascending up and over the forehead to link with Gov 24 above the hairline. The channel then runs slightly laterally before going over the skull to BL 10 at the lateral aspect of the atlas. At BL 10 the meridian divides into two meridians that are relatively parallel to the spine and to each other. The 'inner bladder' channel firstly deviates to join with Gov 14 and Gov 13 before descending 1.5 cun laterally to the spine as far down as the lower end of the sacrum. Here it almost reverses its direction to ascend medially to BL 31 at the first sacral foramen where it reverses again to descend through the sacrum to the lower end of the buttock, down the posterior aspect of the thigh to the popliteal fossa where it joins the Outer Bladder channel at BL 40 in the centre of the popliteal fossa. Meanwhile the Outer Bladder channel leaves BL 10 at the occiput and descends roughly 3 cun parallel to the midline through the buttock and to the centre of the popliteal fossa at BL 40. At BL 52 a deep channel travels to the kidney and bladder. The surface pathway at BL 40 descends the calf to the lateral aspect of the lower leg towards the lateral malleolus where it finally travels along the outer aspect of the foot before ending at the nail point on the lateral aspect of the little toe. The acupoints will be discussed in five groups: head, the 'back transporting' points of the Inner Bladder channel, sacral region, the outer bladder channel and buttock/leg and foot.

BL 1 *Jing Ming* (Bright Eyes)

睛明 ★★★★★

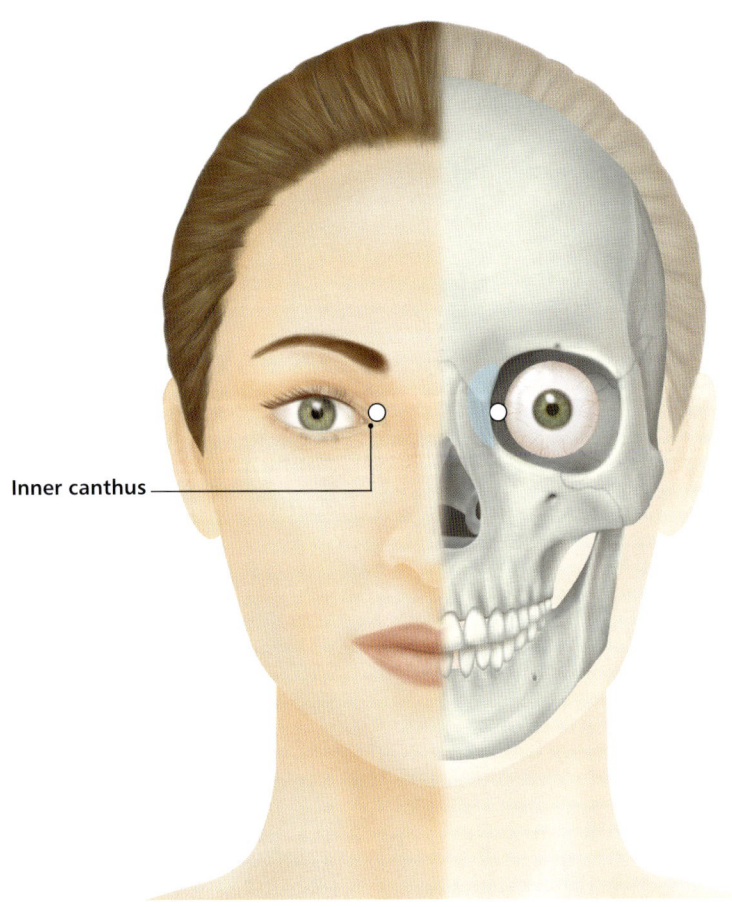

Inner canthus

Location
Situated just medially to the inner canthus of the eye.

Needle
Insert the needle slowly up to 1 cun whilst pushing the eyeball downwards and sidewards.

> Do not manipulate the needle once in situ. Needling this acupoint is potentially dangerous and should only be performed by highly skilled practitioners. Bruising often occurs even with perfect insertion.

Moxa and pressure

> This point is totally forbidden to any forms of moxa. Some texts permit the use of pressure. Experience has taught me that using pressure on BL 2 or Yin Tang (between the eyes) are excellent substitute points. Patients do not like your fingers being poked in their eyes!

Indications
The point's inaccessibility and awkwardness are compensated by its indications. It is mainly used as a local point for the eyes but has extensive general use. Local indications are tired and gritty eyes, inflammation and blurring. It also helps with excessive lacrimation, acute or chronic eye pain, poor or diminishing vision and some eye diseases.

Special properties
BL 1 is the meeting point of the Bladder, Small Intestine, Stomach, Gall Bladder, Triple Energizer and two of the eight extra meridians. It is therefore highly significant in balancing the patient's energies. It is particularly helpful in hormonal conditions in combination with other points and is said to be linked with the hypothalamus region of the brain.

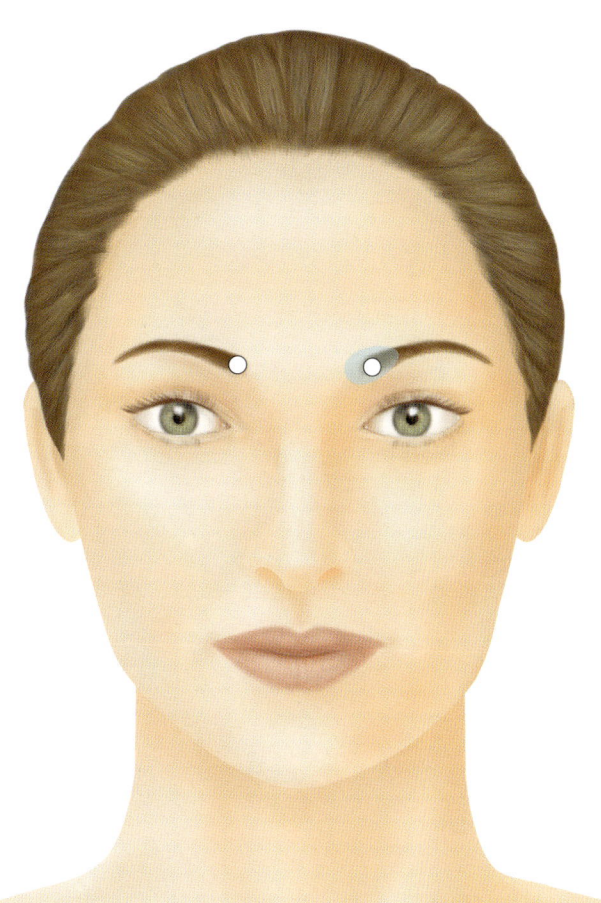

Location

Situated near the medial end of the eyebrow, in a small depression in a line directly above BL 1.

Needle

There are several ways to affect this point; 0.3 cun perpendicular insertion, 0.5 cun using a transverse insertion towards the base of the nose or up to 1 cun if positioned towards BL 1.

Moxa and pressure

Acupressure is very effective in the treatment of headaches, head pressure, frontal sinusitis. It is best to use sedation pressure. A very useful pressure technique is to 'energy balance' between BL 2 and BL 10 (by the atlas bone) to alleviate head pain and ease stress.

> Direct moxa is forbidden but moxa stick is permitted, although be careful that smoke does not enter the patient's eyes.

Indications

Apart from those already mentioned BL 2 is a useful point in frontal sinusitis, eye pain and strain, frontal headaches, eye inflammation and blurring. It remains an excellent point in the general balancing of a patient's heating mechanism (in conjunction with TE 5). As a self-help pressure point it has its uses in helping vertigo.

BL 10 *Tian Zhu* (Heavenly Column)

天柱 ★★★★

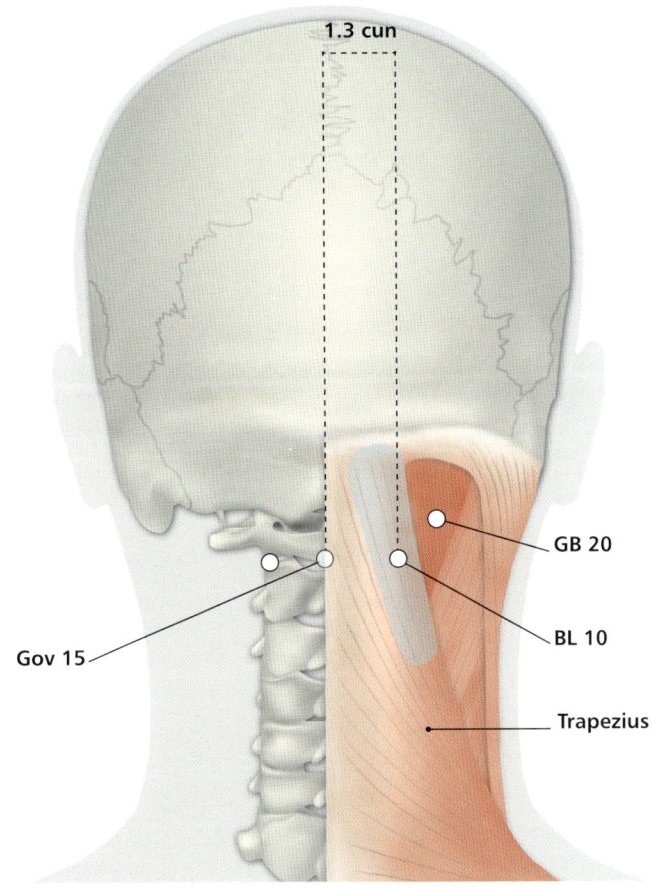

1.3 cun

GB 20

BL 10

Gov 15

Trapezius

Location

Situated 1.3 cun lateral to the midline at Gov 15 at the level of C1–C2 and on the lateral edge of the trapezius muscle.

Needle

Up to 1 cun with perpendicular insertion.

Moxa and pressure

Moxa is possible but not recommended due to hair being present. Acupressure techniques, both stimulating and sedatory can be very beneficial (see later).

Indications

BL 10 is an important acupoint in treating occipital, posterior and superior headaches as well as upper cervical pain and muscular spasm in the region. It is also useful in the treatment of nasal congestion, pain and inflammation of the eyes, lacrimation and blurred vision.

Special properties

BL 10 is situated at the outer margin of the atlanto-axial junction and is therefore an ideal point to use (with needle but mostly with pressure) in calming the mind and relaxing the whole body due to its influence on easing tension in the vagus nerve. Cranio-sacral therapists and cranial osteopaths make use of this point in their practices. Care must be taken though to use the point correctly and not to stimulate it too much. The upper cervical ganglion of the sympathetic nervous system is also anatomically adjacent and if stimulated would give the opposite effect of what is required.

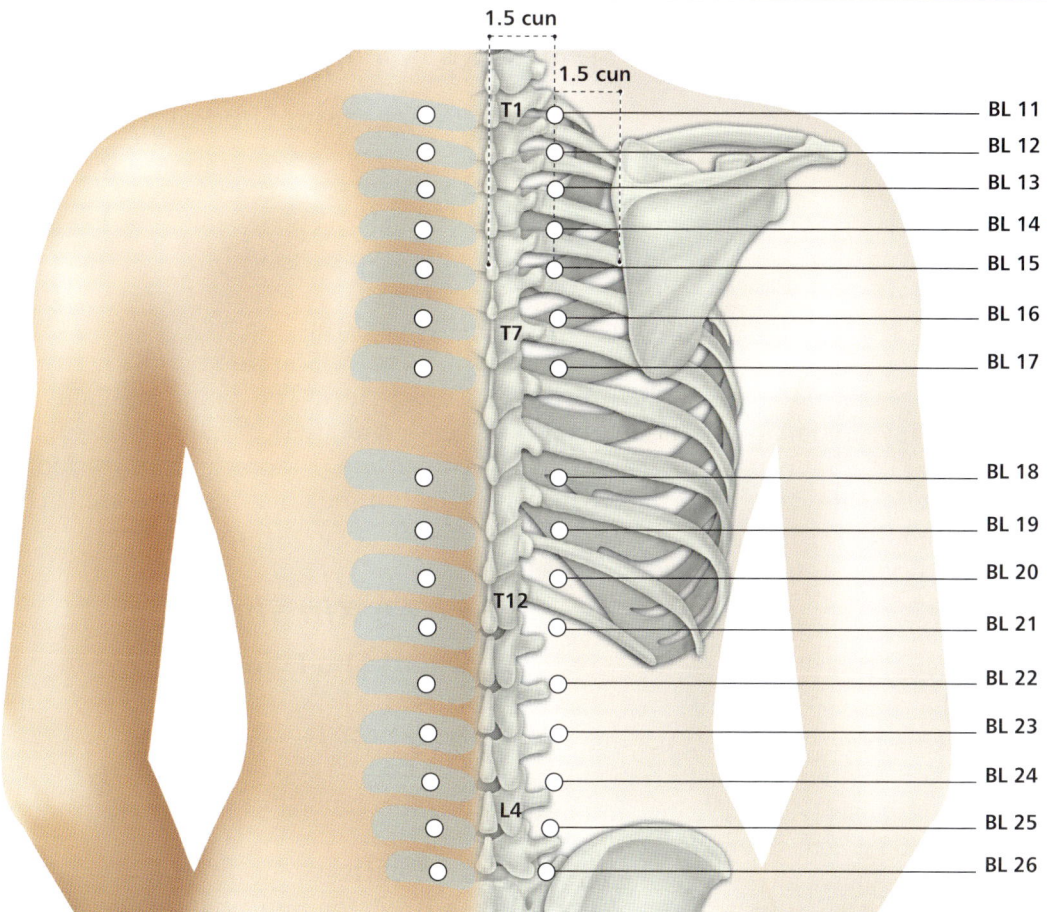

BL11 to BL 28 (only the most important will be discussed). The Back Transporting points (also known as Associated Effect or Back-Shu points) are extremely useful acupoints with needle, pressure, magnets, cupping, massage and any other therapy that treats spinal conditions. They lend themselves to diverse treatment protocols as they are easy to locate, can be treated all together (as in massage) or individually to affect the underlying organ or system. They can be considered as being reflected points of the underlying systems or organs with which they are associated.

Locations

All Inner Bladder channel points are situated 1.5 cun lateral to the midline, at the highest part of the erector spinae (longissimus) muscle. In TCM they are known as Shu points.

Needle

In general terms the thoracic points are needled slightly obliquely at 1.0 cun depth. The lumbar points may be needled to a depth of 1.5 cun and the sacral points up to 3 cun.

> Do not exceed the depth given when treating the thoracic points as there is a considerable risk of puncturing the lungs and other organs.

Moxa and pressure

Moxa may be used extensively either as a cone on the skin where the individual system or organ is energised or with a moxa stick where the treatment may be performed in spinal level sections. Moxa is particularly effective in the lumbo-sacral region dealing with chronic congested lumbar and sacral conditions where a moxa box is often employed. As stated before cupping and magnets may also be employed. Likewise, acupressure techniques may consist of stimulating pressure on a particular point or massaging using the index and middle finger pads all the length of the channel.

> Do not massage heavily in pregnancy or if there is any underlying swelling, contusions or ulcerations.

BL 11 *Da Zhu*
(Great Shuttle)

Location
Situated 1.5 cun lateral to the lower border of the spinous process of T1.

Indications
This is one of the more important Back Transporting points in that it has several indications and symptomatology. In combination with BL 12 and BL 13 it is used in conditions of the lungs to help with coughs and other upper respiratory conditions. It is also used to treat cervical and occipital stiffness and pain, sore throats and headaches.

Special properties
BL 11 is the master point of any disorder associated with bone and bony conditions. It should therefore be thought of in osteoporosis, kyphosis and scoliosis, osteo-arthritis, ankylosing spondylitis and where there is difficulty in fractures uniting. I have always assumed that the point stimulates the parathyroid glands (level with this point on the front of the neck) though have never read this anywhere; the anatomical juxtaposition is too much of a coincidence.

BL 13 *Fei Shu*
(Lung Shu Point)

Location
Situated 1.5 cun lateral to the lower border of the spinous process of T3.

Indications
BL 13 is the Shu point of the Lungs and is widely used in all manner of lung conditions. Symptoms include chronic or acute cough, sore throat, acute or chronic respiratory conditions, chronic tiredness, nasal congestion and night sweats. It is also used as a local point in painful upper thoracic conditions. Some texts consider it also useful in the treatment of grief and sadness (mental symptoms associated with the Metal element) but I would consider that points on the Outer Bladder channel are better suited in the treatment of emotional symptoms, although there are exceptions to this which will be annotated.

BL 14 *Jue Yin Shu*
(Pericardium Shu Point)

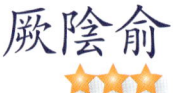

Location
Situated 1.5 cun lateral to the lower border of the spinous process of T4.

Indications
BL 14 is the Shu point of the Pericardium (Heart Constrictor). The point regulates pericardium, heart and liver chi and is used to treat chest congestion, thoracic oppression, dyspnoea, retching and vomiting. Also used in the treatment of stiffness in the upper spine.

BL 15 *Xin Shu*
(Heart Shu Point)

Location
Situated 1.5 cun lateral to the lower border of the spinous process of T5.

Indications
BL 15 is the Shu point of the Heart and as the point suggests, this acupoint is used to nourish, cool and soothe the heart and is therefore very useful in palpitations, arrhythmia, chest oppression, angina, retching and vomiting and general circulatory conditions.

Special properties
This is one of the most influential acupoints on the body to treat a range of psychosomatic disorders such as poor memory, amnesia, depression, anxiety, panic attacks and general phobias. It is associated with the posterior Heart chakra (based physically at T6–7) and, as such, deals with physical conditions that have emotional and mental aetiology.

BL 17 *Ge Shu*
(Diaphragm Shu Point)

Location
Situated 1.5 cun lateral to the lower border of the spinous process of T7.

Indications
BL 17 is the Shu point of the diaphragm. This, in some ways, is a misleading generalization as its

actions on the diaphragm are limited except there is an effect on abdominal tension, abdominal pain and distension. Its main thrust, though, is in the treatment of 'blood' related disorders. It is used to invigorate blood and dispel stasis as well as cooling blood and arresting bleeding. It is a well known first aid point with stimulating pressure techniques in the arrest of bleeding. Symptoms include anaemia, epistaxis, coughing blood, hiccoughs, dysmenorrhoea and tightness of the chest.

BL 18 *Gan Shu*
(Liver Shu Point)

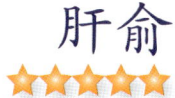

Location
Situated 1.5 cun lateral to the lower border of the spinous process of T9. Please note that no meridian acupoints exist on the midline or the Bladder channels at the level of T8.

Indications
BL 18 is the Shu point of the Liver and is extremely important in controlling chi to the organ and all that is associated with the organ. It is used extensively in decongestion of the liver due to blood conditions or excesses. It is therefore helpful in hepatitis, cholecystitis, heaviness and grittiness of the eyes, cramping of muscles and tightness in tendons anywhere in the body. It also has a significant effect in the treatment of emotional imbalance such as anger, irritability and general stress.

BL 19 *Dan Shu*
(Gall Bladder Shu Point)

Location
Situated 1.5 cun lateral to the lower border of the spinous process of T10.

Indications
BL 19 is the Shu point of the Gall Bladder. It is useful in treating disorders associated with the gall bladder and liver. Symptoms include bitter taste, nausea, cholecystitis, hepatitis, jaundice, shoulder pain and conditions associated with the eyes and tendons. It is also a significant acupoint in the treatment of emotional disorders such as mental restlessness, anxiety, fright, panic attacks, timidity and shyness. It is also useful as a local point in thoracic spinal spasm and scoliosis.

N.B. Constant irritation of the sympathetic nerve chain due to scoliosis or other physical conditions affecting both T9 and T10 are, in my opinion, a common cause of such emotional problems.

BL 20 *Pi Shu*
(Spleen Shu Point)

Location
Situated 1.5 cun lateral to the lower border of the spinous process of T11.

Indications
BL 20 is the Shu point of the Spleen. It is used widely in all cases of spleen chi deficiency. Symptoms are tiredness and weakness of the limbs, sweating, flaccidity, water retention and a tendency to gain weight, abdominal distension, loose stools, infertility and amenorrhoea. It is also useful in treating urinary conditions such as cystitis and urethritis.

BL 21 *Wei Shu*
(Stomach Shu Point)

Location
Situated 1.5 cun lateral to the lower border of the spinous process of T12.

Indications
BL 21 is the Shu point of the Stomach and is widely used in most stomach related conditions. These include stomach distension and pain, gastritis, indigestion, burping, poor appetite, nausea, vomiting, jaundice, abdominal distension, loose stools and diarrhoea.

BL 23 *Shen Shu*
(Kidney Shu Point)

Location
Situated 1.5 cun lateral to the lower border of the spinous process of L2.

Indications
BL 23 is the Shu point of the Kidney and is widely used to tonify the kidney and its related conditions. It is a major point for many disorders of the lumbo-sacral spine, legs and bones. Symptoms and conditions include lumbar pain and weakness, low back pain, chronic weakness

or paralysis of the legs, coldness in the lower back, sciatica and restless legs. It is also used to treat conditions of the genito-urinary system including frequent urination, impotence and infertility among others.

Special properties

It is one of the most important acupoints in the body dealing with lethargy, tiredness and chronic weakness. It answers superbly to moxa, needle tonification and stimulating pressure techniques to improve the general energy levels and well being. It is an excellent self-help point and is used with other local points in all manner of chronic conditions by vigorously massaging the area with the clenched fists several times a day.

BL 25 *Da Chang Shu*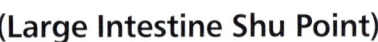
(Large Intestine Shu Point)

Location

Situated 1.5 cun lateral to the lower border of the spinous process of L4.

Indications

BL 25 is the Shu point of the Large Intestine and is a major player in the treatment of many large bowel conditions including constipation and diarrhoea, ileo-caecal valve syndrome, abdominal rumbling, pain and distension. It is also very useful, alongside other local points in lumbar conditions such as pain, sciatica and spasm.

> Do not stimulate in pregnancy.

BL 27 *Xia Chang Shu* 小腸俞
(Small Intestine Shu Point)

Location

Situated 1.5 cun lateral to the posterior midline, level with the first sacral foramen.

Indications

BL 27 is the Shu point of the Small Intestine. It is used in both urinary conditions and small bowel imbalance. Symptoms and conditions include intestinal pain, enteritis, difficulty in urination, incontinence and haematuria. As a local point it is used in sacral pain, sacroiliitis and sciatica.

> Do not stimulate in pregnancy.

BL 28 *Pang Guang Shu* 膀胱俞
(Bladder Shu Point)

Location

Situated 1.5 cun lateral to the midline at the level of the second sacral foramen.

Indications

BL 28 is the Shu point of the Bladder and is a very influential point in treating bladder conditions. Symptoms and conditions include urinary tract infections, urine incontinence, impotence and genital pain and inflammation. It is also used as a local point in sacroiliitis, sacral pain and discomfort in the buttocks.

> Do not stimulate in pregnancy.

BL 28 is the last of the Back Transporting points and we shall now discuss the Sacral points before returning to the Outer Bladder channel that commences at BL 42 level with T3.

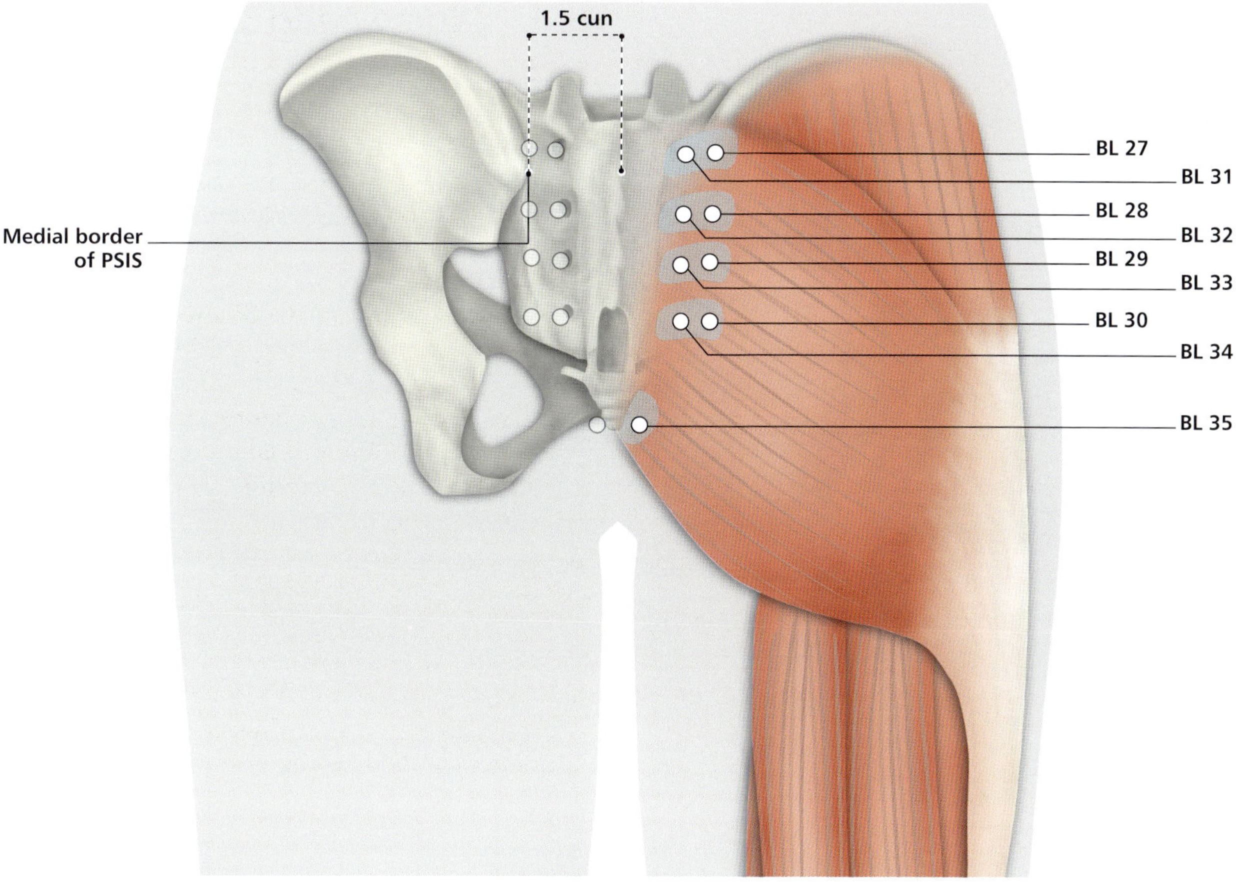

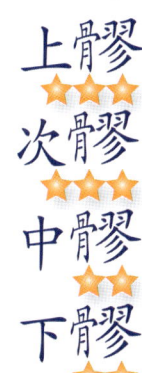

1.5 cun

Medial border of PSIS

BL 27
BL 31
BL 28
BL 32
BL 29
BL 33
BL 30
BL 34
BL 35

BL 31 *Shang Liao*
(Upper Crevice)
上髎
⭐⭐⭐

BL 32 *Ci Liao*
(Second Crevice)
次髎
⭐⭐⭐

BL 33 *Zhong Liao*
(Middle Crevice)
中髎
⭐⭐

BL 34 *Xia Liao*
(Lower Crevice)
下髎
⭐⭐

These four acupoints are discussed together as they all have similar indications and, in practice, are usually treated together.

Location
Situated in the 1st, 2nd, 3rd and 4th sacral foramen respectively.

Needle
These four points are usually needled with a perpendicular insertion to 1.0 cun in depth.

> Do not stimulate in pregnancy.

Moxa and pressure
These points answer very well to stimulating moxa and massage (see below BL 35 description) as well as cupping and magnets.

Indications
Although the four Sacral Foramen points are usually needled (or otherwise treated) together, the upper two seem to be more powerful when it comes to the treatment of conditions. Symptoms and conditions include lumbo-sacral pain and stiffness, irregular menstruation, vaginal prolapse, impotence and difficulty in urinating.

BL 35 *Hui Yang* (Meeting of Yang)

會陽 ★★★★

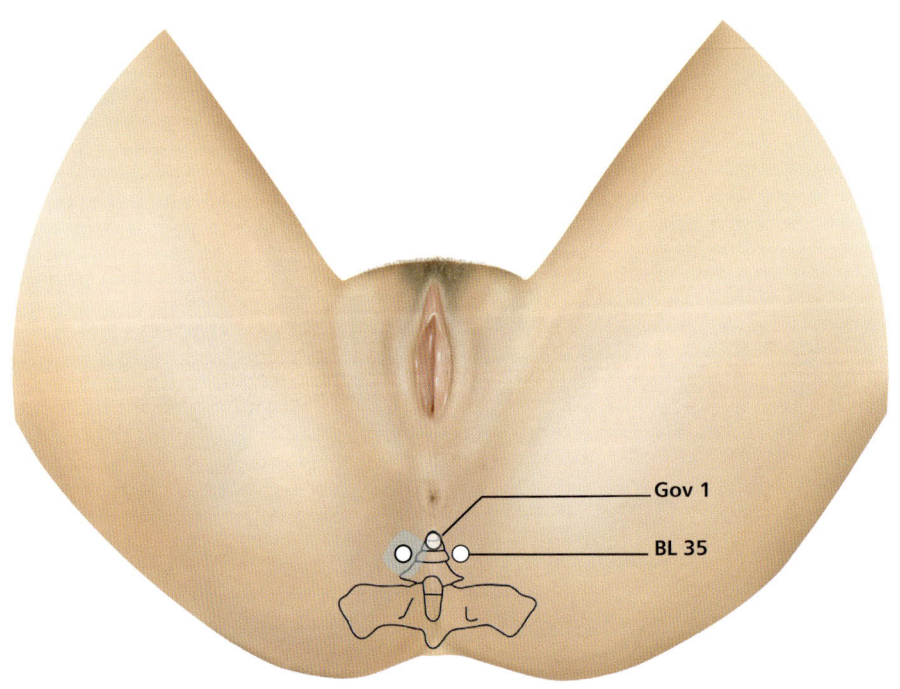

Gov 1

BL 35

Location
Situated 0.5 cun lateral to the midline level with the tip of the coccyx, just adjacent to Gov 1.

Needle
Up to 1.0 cun with a perpendicular insertion.

Do not stimulate in pregnancy.

Moxa and pressure
Although it is not forbidden to moxa, direct moxa is almost impossible due to its anatomy. For pressure, see 'special properties'.

Indications
As its anatomical position would suggest this point is an important one in the treatment of coccyx, anal and genital conditions. Symptoms include painful haemorrhoids, coccyx pain, genital pain and dysmenorrhoea.

Special properties of all the 'sacral' acupoints: BL 27 to BL 35
This whole area, combined with the lower lumbar spinal points answers extremely well to stimulating massage (not in pregnancy) in all cases of sluggishness of the muscles and chronic conditions of the kidneys, bladder, uterus, testes, sacrum and coccyx. One of the very best ways to incorporate all the points is with connective tissue massage (CTM). This is a stimulating type of massage that uses the medial aspect of the middle finger, with or without oil, in deep and controlled strokes. (For more information on this excellent massage method, see 'resources'.)

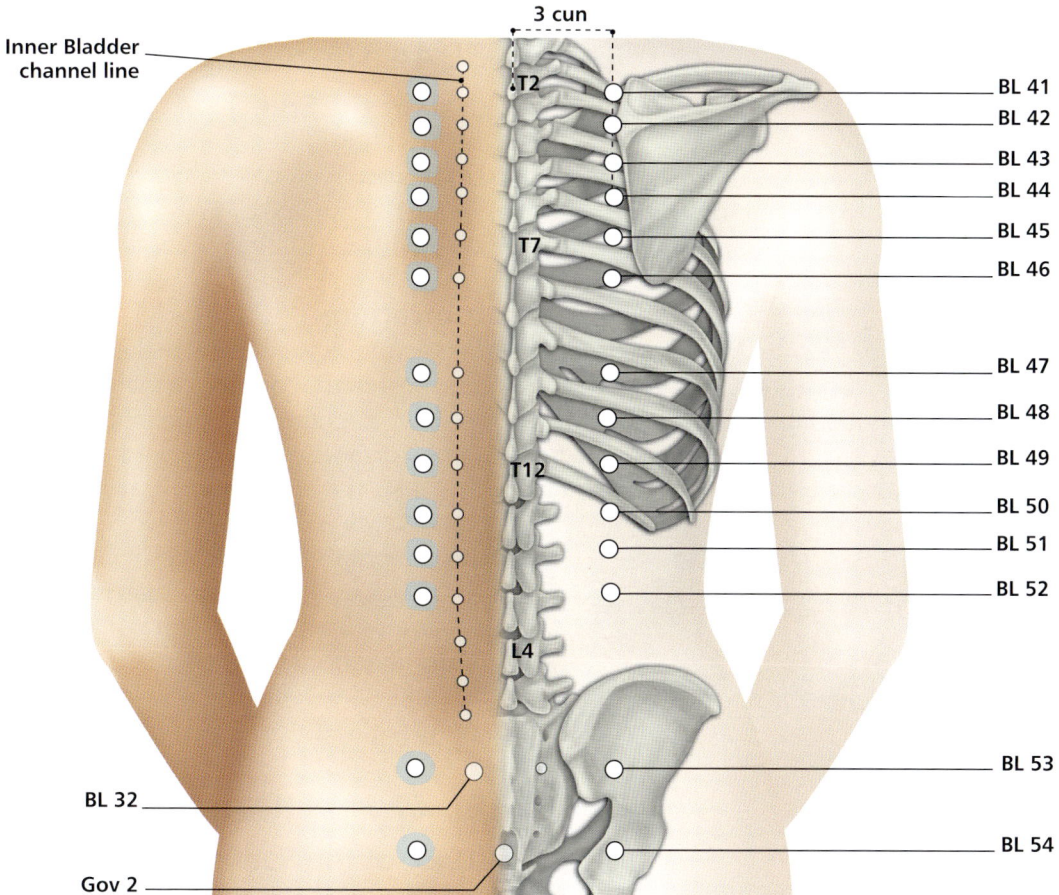

Inner Bladder channel line

3 cun

T2

BL 41
BL 42
BL 43
BL 44
BL 45
BL 46

T7

BL 47

BL 48

BL 49

T12

BL 50

BL 51

BL 52

L4

BL 53

BL 54

BL 32

Gov 2

We shall now return to discussing the Outer Bladder channel commencing at BL 42 and ending at BL 54. Each of the main Outer Bladder channel points relates to a point on the Inner Bladder channel that is at the same anatomical level and 1.5 cun medially. This important line of acupoints contains some of the least understood in acupuncture as to their purpose and indications. Tradition dictates that each one is the 'emotional' equivalent of its Inner channel partner and you would not be far wrong in this assumption. They are, though, more important than the traditional texts give them credit for. Some of them are related to the endocrine system of the body via the sympathetic nervous system, thus having influence on hormonal balance.

Needle

Each of the Outer Bladder points should be needled with a slight oblique insertion medially towards its partner to a depth of up to 0.8 cun. The lumbar point may be needled slightly deeper to 1.5 cun.

Do not needle any deeper in the thoracic points for fear of pneumothorax or puncturing the underlying organ.

Moxa and pressure

Once again, these points answer very well to much stimulating moxa depending on the individual condition. Acupressure of single points or massage of the line can be very effective in helping emotional and stress induced conditions. Have tissues to hand as therapy on these points can induce some emotional release such as crying. These points may also be treated with biomagnets and cupping.

BL 42 *Po Hu*
(Door of the Soul)

Location
Situated 3 cun lateral to the spinous process of T3 level with BL 13.

Indications
It has similar properties to BL 13 in treating many respiratory conditions. In addition it helps with the emotional aspect of the Metal element imbalance, i.e. the treatment of acute or long standing grief, sadness, melancholy and depression due to grief.

BL 43 *Gao Huang Shu*

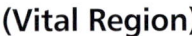

(Vital Region)

Location
Situated 3 cun lateral to the spinous process of T4 level with BL 14.

Indications
Symptoms include chronic cough, shortness of breath and asthma, bronchitis and haemoptysis.

Special properties
This is a remarkable acupoint in that it helps boost energy in very chronic disease. Moxa and tonifying acupuncture are required here but stimulating acupressure is also effective. If patients have chronic respiratory, cardiac or throat conditions, treatment on this point will help boost their chi (vital force) sufficiently so as to use other points in addressing the symptoms. Practitioners of the manipulative and soft tissue arts know the value of mobilizing the fourth thoracic vertebra in chronic spinal and organic conditions in order to enable the patient to gain more general energy. The point is extensively used in conjunction with BL 14.

BL 44 *Shen Tang*
(Hall of the Spirit)

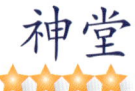

Location
Situated 3 cun lateral to the spinous process of T5 level with BL 15.

Indications
This acupoint is excellent in the treatment of many psychosomatic conditions including restlessness, anxiety, nightmares, panic attacks, insomnia, some forms of epilepsy and stress in general. It is also useful in many cardiac conditions in conjunction with BL 15. In esoteric medicine this acupoint is directly associated with both BL 15 and Gov 10 (T6–7) in that they comprise the posterior Heart chakra (Anahata) that deals with many emotional symptoms. In children under the age of seven, this point also relates to the thymus gland.

BL 47 *Hun Men*
(Door of the Soul)

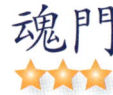

Location
Situated 3 cun lateral to the spinous process of T9 level with BL 18.

Indications
Physical symptoms include epigastric and thoracic pain, hepatitis and diarrhoea. Emotional symptoms include those associated with the liver and Wood element, i.e. anger, rage, irritability, frustration, anxiety, boredom and lack of inspiration.

BL 49 *Yi She*
(Abode of Thought)

Location
Situated 3 cun lateral to the spinous process of T11 level with BL 20.

Indications
This is a very influential acupoint in that it is used to treat physical and emotional conditions connected with the spleen and stomach. Physical symptoms include abdominal distension, nausea, vomiting, jaundice, indigestion and the symptoms of diabetes. Emotional symptoms are those associated with the Earth element and include depression, worry, poor concentration, diminishing memory and in people who have to do much thinking and pondering (making decisions).

Special properties
BL 49 and BL 20 are both associated with Gov 6 (T12–L1) and in turn are part of the physical counterpart of the Solar Plexus chakra. This chakra deals with the treatment of depression and worry and the symptoms it causes (ulcers etc.) if negative thought is habitually practiced! These three points are also linked to the solar plexus sympathetic ganglion which in turn is linked to the pancreas. It therefore is used to regulate insulin in patients with some types of diabetes.

> Please note that it is not ethical for practitioners to claim to treat diabetes; just to help the patient who happens to be suffering from the disease.

BL 52 *Zhi Shi*
(Residence of the Will)

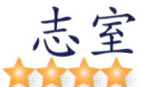

Location
Situated 3 cun lateral to the spinous process of L2 level with BL 23.

Indications
As with all the Outer Bladder channel acupoints, BL 52 has both physical and emotional properties. It helps regulate urination and strengthens the lumbar region as well as treating with kidney symptoms. Its emotional properties are paramount however, in that it helps the patient to deal with situations of fear, anxiety and lack of willpower. If the patient's will is in low ebb, treatment of this point helps to address the situation in strengthening their resolve.

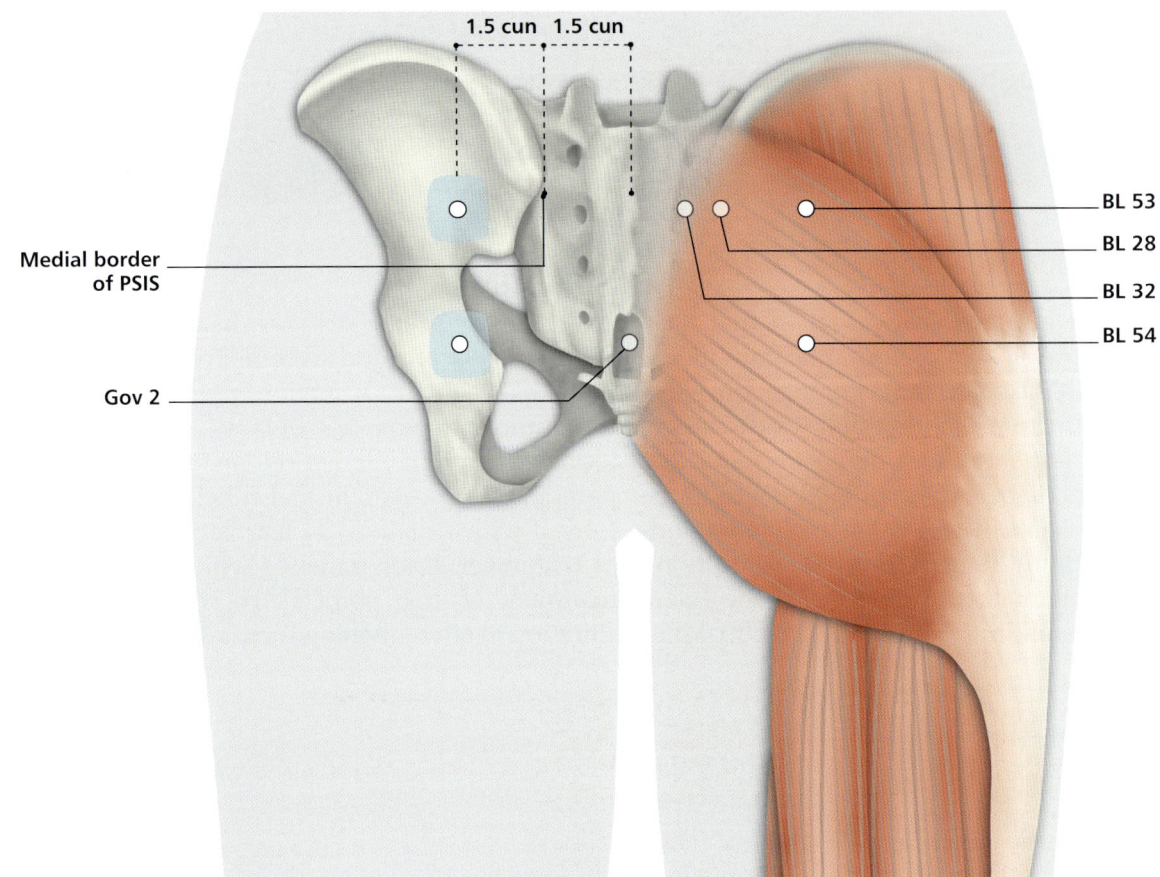

BL 54 *Zhi Bian*
(Order's Limit)

秩邊
★★★

Location
Situated at the level of the 4th sacral foramen, 3 cun lateral to the midline, at the highest part of the buttock.

Needle
This is a very deep acupoint so needle up to 2.5 cun using a perpendicular approach or up to 3 cun, using an oblique insertion towards the anus.

Moxa and pressure
Moxa is very effective in chronic hip, sacral, lumbar and gluteal conditions. Similarly, acupressure if administered correctly (using heavy techniques with the thumb or knuckle) can work wonders in helping chronic soft tissue congestion around the region.

Indications
This is a very useful point in treating localised pain and inflammation including sciatica. It also helps with haemorrhoids, prostate conditions and chronic gluteal or piriformis spasm.

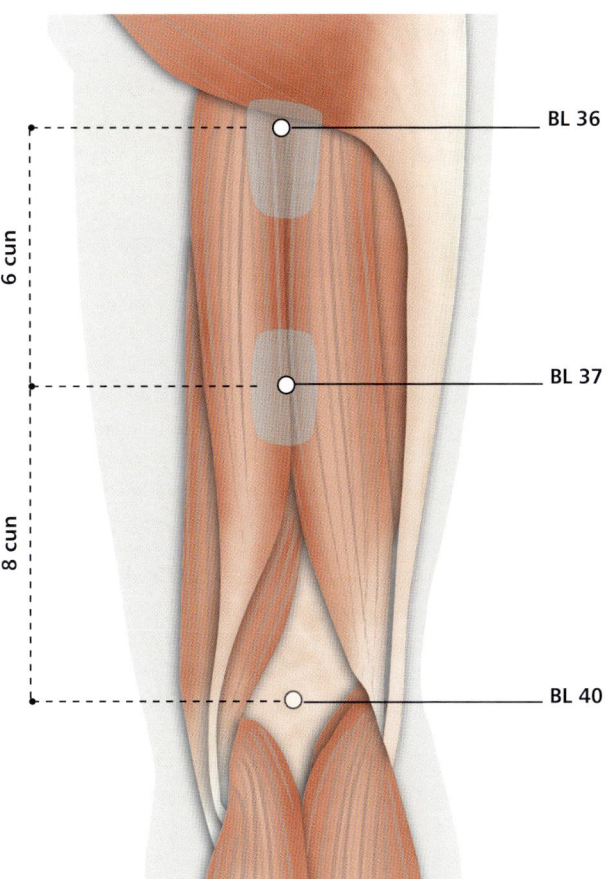

Location

Situated at the centre of the transverse gluteal crease, inferior to the gluteus maximus between the biceps femoris and the semitendinosus muscles.

Needle

Up to 1.5 cun using a perpendicular insertion.

Moxa and pressure

This point answers very well to stimulating moxa in chronic hip, sacral and buttock conditions. Do not moxa though in acute sciatica. Deep frictions are also indicated for posterior hip, sacral and gluteal pain and soft tissue congestion. It is pointless using any 'subtle' acupressure techniques at this point.

Indications

As with BL 54, this point is used in alleviating pain in localised conditions such as haemorrhoids, posterior hip pain, sciatica, dysuria and weakness of the legs.

BL 39 *Wei Yang* (Outside of the Crease)

委陽 ★★★

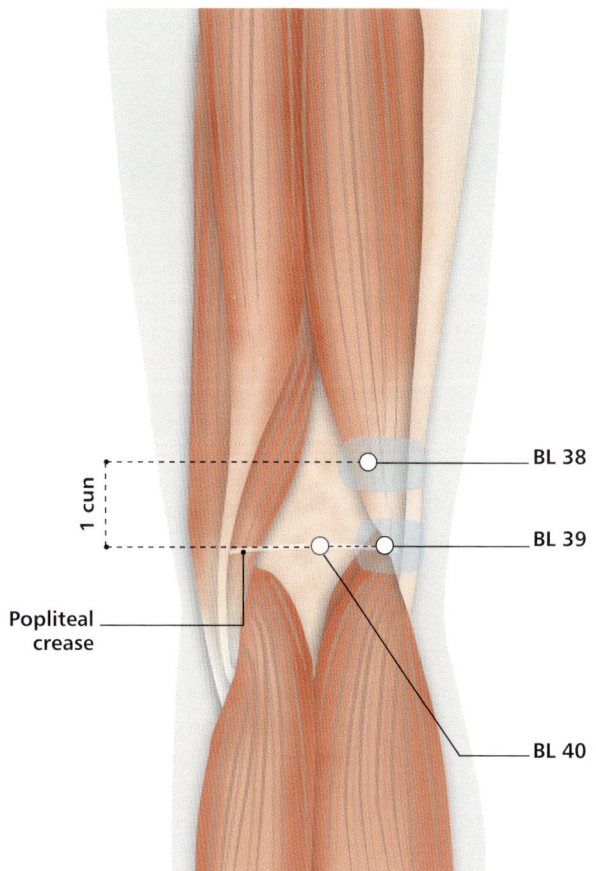

1 cun

BL 38

BL 39

BL 40

Popliteal crease

Location
Situated at the lateral end of the popliteal crease on the medial side of the biceps femoris tendon.

Needle
Up to 1 cun using a perpendicular insertion.

> Deeper needling may puncture the common peroneal nerve.

Moxa and pressure
Use light moxa only due to the underlying vessels. Frictions of the biceps femoris tendon may be indicated in postero-lateral knee pain.

Indications
This acupoint has two main properties. Firstly it may be used in the regulation of urine and is particularly effective with urine retention. Its main attribute, though, is as a local point in the treatment of chronic knee pain and inflammation. It is particularly effective in the treatment of osteo-arthritis (if the patient can lie prone) by using a heated needle (burning punk moxa wrapped around the end of a long copper needle).

BL 40 *Wei Zhong* (Perfect Equilibrium or Middle of the Crease)

委中

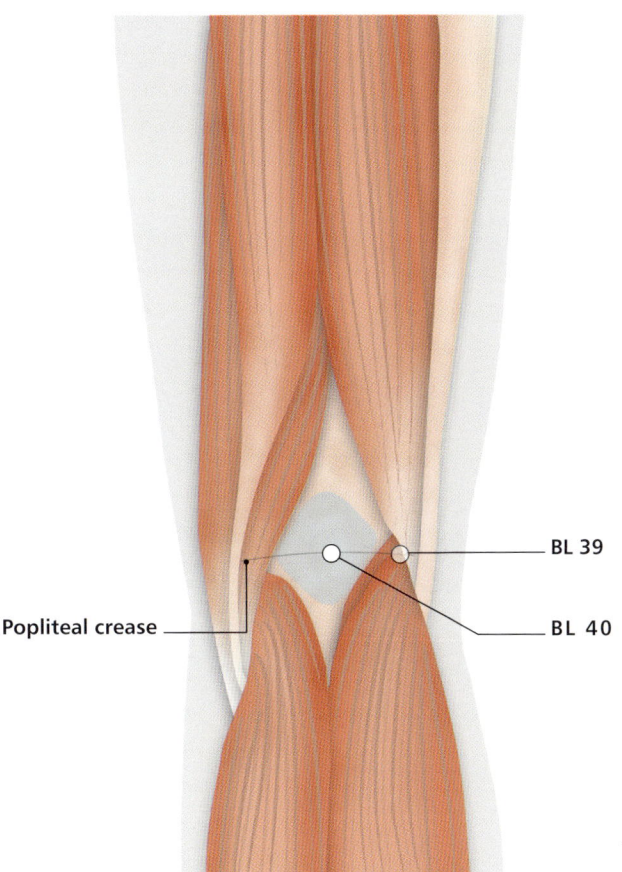

Popliteal crease

BL 39

BL 40

Location
Situated in the very centre of the popliteal fossa.

Needle
Up to 1.0 cun with perpendicular approach.

> Deeper needling could affect the many nerves and veins in the popliteal region.

Moxa and pressure
Some old texts indicate that this useful point is forbidden to moxa although I have never seen this as a useful guide. Use light stimulation only, though, because of the nerves and veins in the vicinity. It is useful as a self-help one to help the patient with their lower back pain. Also see 'special properties' below.

Indications
BL 40 is a major acupoint on the body and is used in several ways:
- It is firstly known as the Command point of the back and may be used in the treatment of any low back condition, osteo-arthritic and pain syndromes. It is particularly excellent if this point is combined with localised lumbo-sacral points in the treatment of low back pain and sciatica.
- It is also a good point in clearing heat in the system, especially the skin, throat and stomach. Symptoms and conditions would be epistaxis, sore throat, night sweats, skin rash, itching, eczema, vomiting and gastritis.
- It is also used in urinary conditions such as frequent or painful urination, haematuria, water retention, oedema and incontinence.
- It is also a major point in the treatment of localised knee conditions such as osteo-arthritis (heated needle as per BL 39) and popliteus muscle strain.

Special properties
- BL 40 is considered to be the physical acupoint of the Knee chakra. This is a minor chakra point and is associated with both the Base chakra (major) and the Elbow chakra (minor). This triad of acupoints may be used in many chronic conditions.
- This point is also widely used in reflextherapy as being the parallel acupoint to PC 3 which is in the centre of the cubital fossa of the elbow joint.

BL 57 *Cheng Shan* (Mountain Support)

承山 ★★★

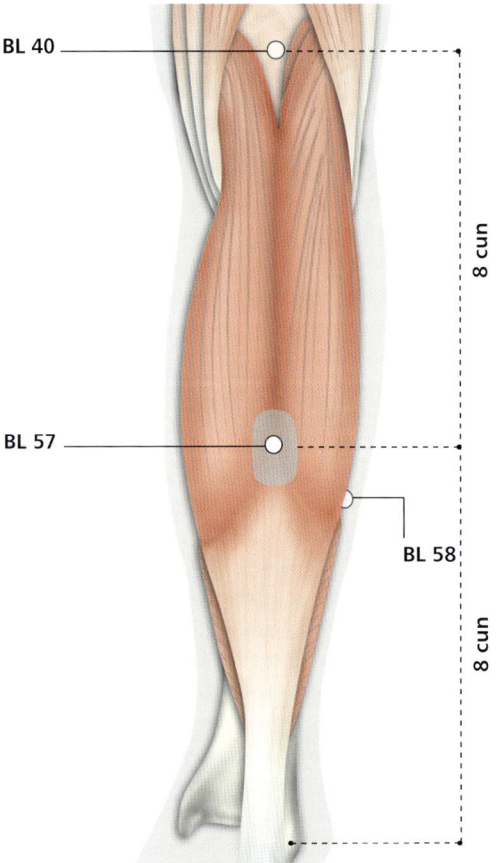

BL 40

8 cun

BL 57

BL 58

8 cun

Location

Situated at the centre of the depression below the two bellies of the gastrocnemius muscle, approximately 8 cun inferior to BL 40 or midway between BL 40 and the insertion of the Achilles tendon on the heel.

Needle

Up to 1 cun using a perpendicular approach.

Moxa and pressure

Use mild moxa only due to underlying vessels.

Pressure is contraindicated if there are any localised blood vessel inflammation or any underlying complication such as deep venous thrombosis.

If there are no complications, acupressure can be very effective in treating calf spasm.

Indications

BL 57 is a useful distal point in the treatment of the anal and genital regions and conditions associated such as haemorrhoids, rectal prolapse, pain in the perineum or scrotum. It is also used in bladder conditions such as cystitis. Localised pain and spasm may also be treated with this point.

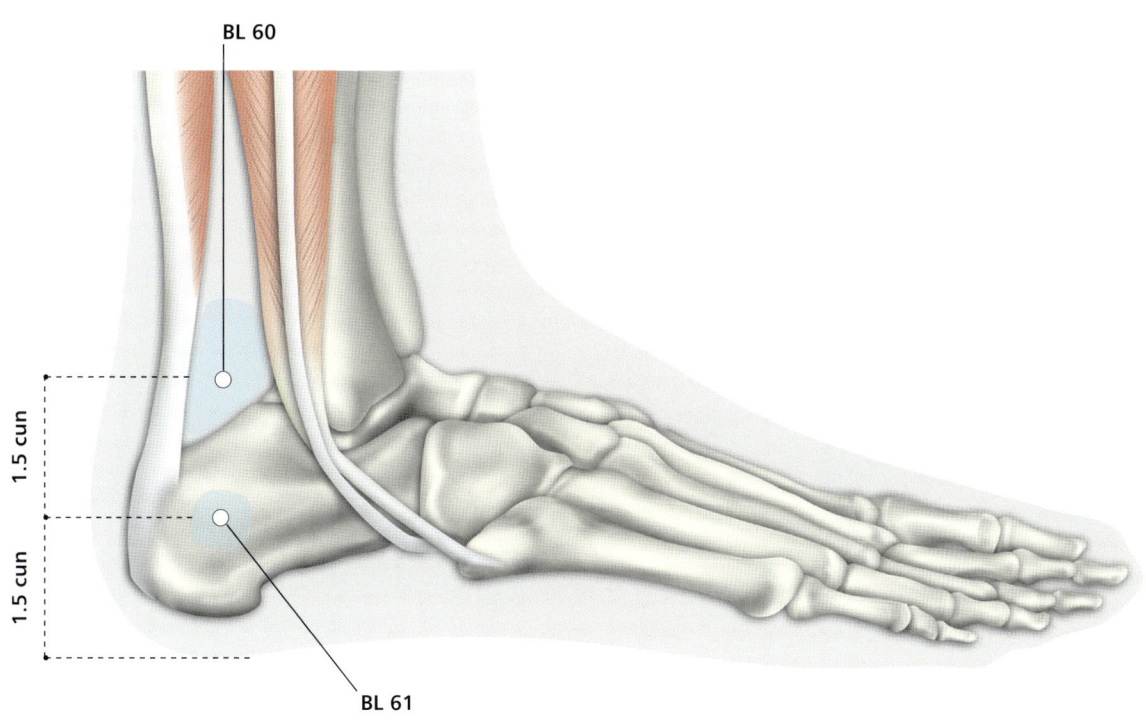

Location
Situated at the midpoint between the prominence of the lateral malleolus and the Achilles tendon.

Needle
Up to 0.5 cun with perpendicular insertion. There is a technique where a needle may be inserted into BL 60 to emerge at KI 6 via the front of the Achilles tendon.

> Only attempt this technique if you are an experienced acupuncturist.

Moxa and pressure
BL 60 is a very useful point for moxa as both a local acupoint in Achilles tendonitis and a distal point in Bladder channel imbalance. For pressure techniques, see 'special properties' below.

Indications
BL 60 is a major acupoint and is used in a variety of symptoms and conditions. It has a direct influence on the whole of the Bladder channel and reduces heat and inflammation from the whole length of the channel including the eye, head, spine, bladder and leg. Symptoms and conditions include headache, stiff neck, eye inflammation, acute and chronic back pain, and sciatica and Achilles tendonitis. It is also used extensively on conditions of the uterus such as alleviating pain and inflammation. It is one of the acupoints used in the final stages of labour to help with easing the birth process (experienced practitioners only).

Special properties
As mentioned in the needle section, this point may be joined with its 'partner' on the medial aspect of the Achilles, KI 6. This couple has a major effect on pain syndromes of the lower spine, uterus, testicles, groin and leg. When used with acupressure, the practitioner simply uses the thumb and forefinger either side of the Achilles. This is also an excellent (if slightly inaccessible) technique in self-help.

BL 62 *Shen Mai* (Extending Vessel)

申脈 ★★★★★

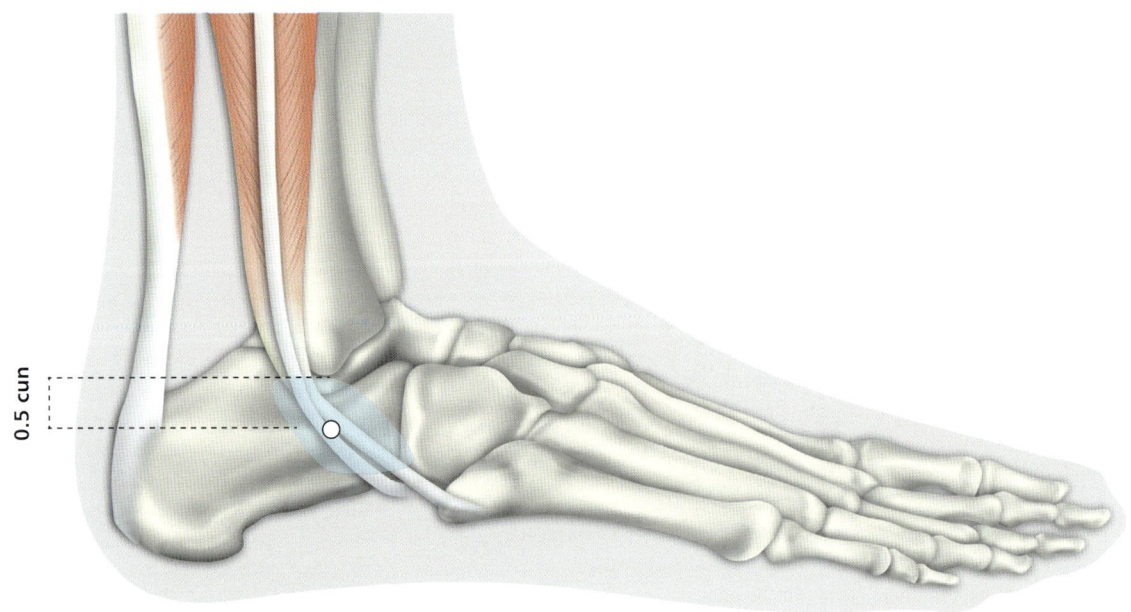

0.5 cun

Location
Situated directly inferior to the lateral malleolus in a slight depression.

Needle
Up to 0.5 cun using a perpendicular insertion.

Moxa and pressure
Stimulating moxa helps with localised ankle ligament sprains but does not seem to be as effective in generalised conditions. Acupressure is also helpful in localised ankle sprains or by 'energy balancing' with SI 3, see 'special properties'.

Indications
BL 62 is a major player in acupuncture and is used for many conditions. Conditions and symptoms include headache, neck stiffness, tinnitus, facial paralysis, hemiplegia, epilepsy, epistaxis, eye inflammation, depression, irritability and insomnia. It is also one of the Great points in treating low back pain and sciatica.

Special properties
BL 62 is the Opening or Key point of the Yang Wei Mai meridian (one of the eight extraordinary channels). It is often used in connection with the key point of the Governor channel, SI 3 in such conditions as acute arthritis and pain amongst others. One of the best ways to treat these points is with biomagnets, although pressure and needle are also effective.

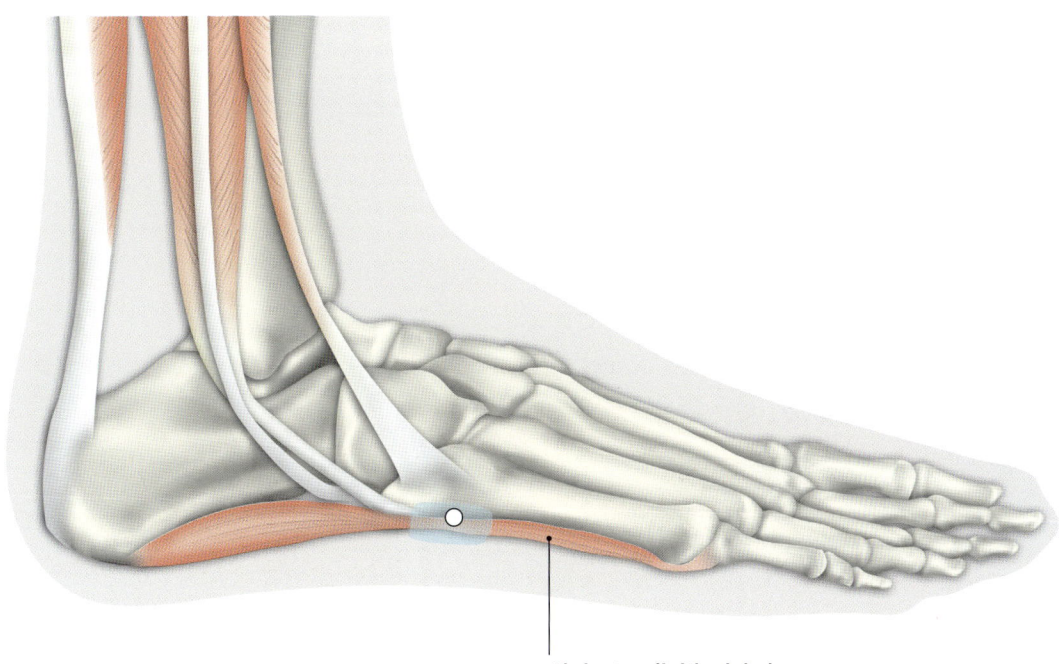

Abductor digiti minimi

Location
This point is situated on the lateral aspect of the foot, in the depression anterior and inferior to the tuberosity of the 5th metatarsal bone.

Needle
Up to 0.5 with a perpendicular insertion.

Moxa and pressure
Moxa is useful in chronic urinary conditions and acupressure is best to treat acute cystitis when the finger is just held on the point.

Indications
BL 64 is the Source (Yuan) point of the Bladder channel and, as such, has a direct communication with the organ. It is therefore used in bladder irritation and cystitis as well as incontinence. It has many general indications such as neck stiffness, chills, eye inflammation, epilepsy, low back pain and stiffness along with pain along the course of the meridian.

BL 67 *Zhi Yin* (Arrival of Yin)

至陰 ★★★★★

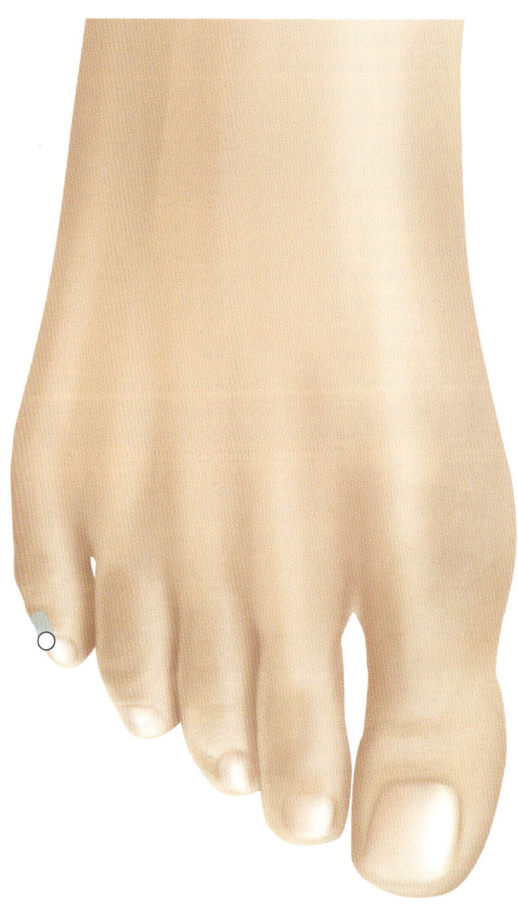

Location
This point is situated on the lateral aspect of the nail of the little toe (Tsing point).

Needle
0.1 cun using a perpendicular insertion. Please note that this point is very sensitive and the needle should be inserted with an applicator otherwise the patient will suddenly move the foot.

This point is also contraindicated in the first six months of pregnancy.

Moxa and pressure
See 'special properties' below.

Indications
BL 67 is a seemingly ineffectual acupoint but has some remarkable actions. It may be used in general Bladder channel obstruction and discomfort along the course of the meridian. Symptoms and conditions include chills and fever, headache, stiff neck, eye inflammation, rhinitis and epistaxis.

Special properties
BL 67 has a powerful effect on the uterus so is contraindicated in early pregnancy. In the case of breach presentation, moxa or stimulating acupressure may be applied during the 7th and 8th month. Once full term has arrived this point is used to induce labour (in combination with other points) and expedite delivery of the baby and placenta.

Only use this technique if you have been properly trained and preferably as a 'team' member.

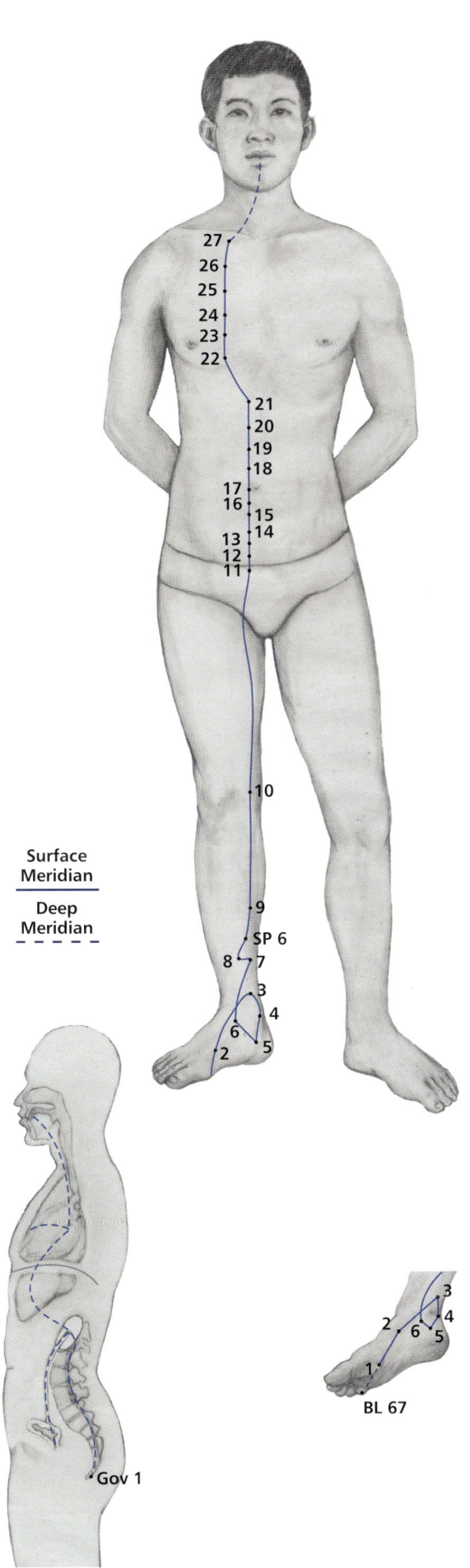

Surface
Meridian

Deep
Meridian

SP 6

BL 67

Gov 1

The Kidney meridian represents the Yin aspect of the Water element. The surface channel has twenty-seven (27) acupoints from the foot to the upper aspect of the chest. Although point KI 1 is on the sole of the foot, the Kidney channel actually commences on the underside of the little toe as a direct continuation link with the Bladder channel. KI 1 is unique amongst acupoints in that it is the only one on the sole of the foot – although a strong argument can be made that an acupoint is merely a reflected energy point and is on a par with all the reflex areas on the foot. The surface meridian leaves the medial aspect of the foot and loops back on itself before ascending the medial aspect of the leg and anterior aspect of the abdomen and chest to end on the medial aspect of the clavicle. An internal channel leaves KI 11 at the groin and supplies the kidney, bladder, lower spine, stomach, diaphragm and mouth cavity with a further internal channel leaving KI 27 towards the throat.

We shall discuss the following acupoints: KI 1, KI 2, KI 3, KI 4, KI 6, KI 7, KI 9, KI 16 and KI 27.

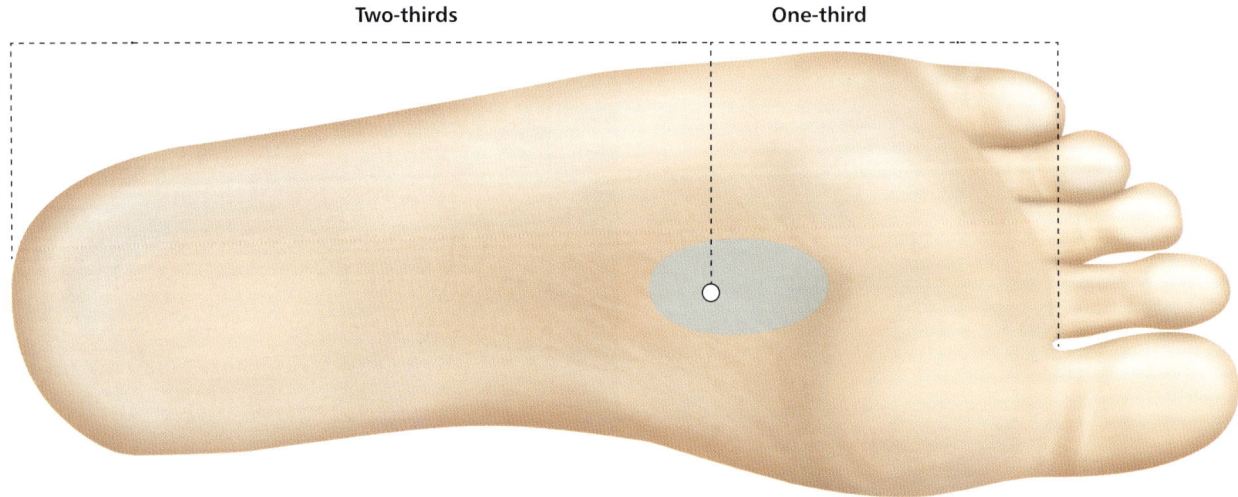

Location

As previously stated, this is the only acupoint on the sole of the foot in the depression formed when the foot is plantar flexed, between the 2nd and 3rd metatarsals, approximately one-third of the distance from the base of the 2nd toe to the heel.

Needle

The point is approximately 0.5 to 1 cun deep and needs to be approached with perpendicular insertion.

> This point is extremely painful to needle and should only be used if there is overwhelming evidence for its use. When it is inserted, it must be performed quickly and with a guide tube or the patient's reflex action is to pull the foot away with great rapidity.

Moxa and pressure

Moxa can be quite useful in conditions that show depletion of energy. Use a moxa roll but be aware that some patients are very sensitive on the soles of the feet. For its use with pressure, see 'special properties'.

Indications

If used correctly, KI 1 can be a wonderful acupoint to use. It is, though, a little bit of an enigma in that it may be used in cases of energy depletion but also to help the upper region of the body where there is excess – seemingly using the same techniques. Symptoms and conditions include headache (usually at the top of the head), dizziness, vertigo, hypertension, insomnia, mental agitation, anxiety and panic attacks, fear, shock, urination difficulties, weakness of the lower limbs, abdominal pain and localised foot pain and tension.

Special properties

KI 1 is said to be the Foot chakra point and is associated with the Hand chakra at PC 8 (minor) and the Crown at Gov 20 (major). This powerful triad may be used in conditions of mental agitation, fear, hypertension, panic and generally relaxing and calming the whole body. It is particularly responsive to gentle pressure techniques with the therapist holding both KI 1 points with the pads of the middle fingers or by combining the three points of the chakra combination. It is an easy acupoint to use when giving a reflexology treatment and (in my opinion) is superior to the solar plexus reflex in general relaxation of the patient.

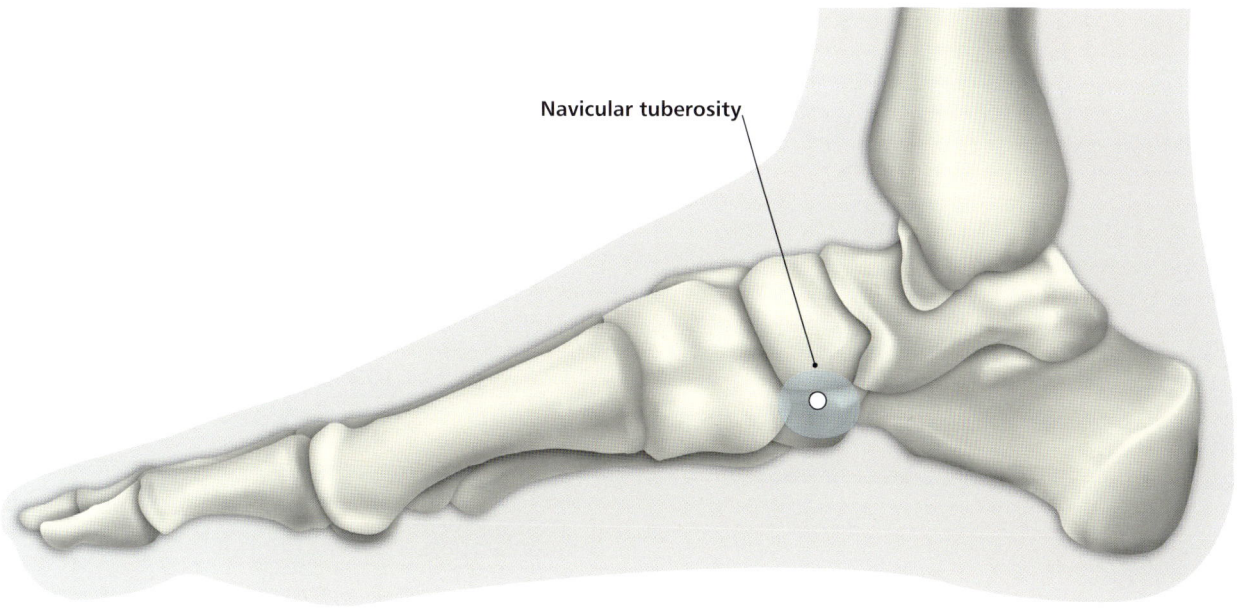

Navicular tuberosity

Location

Situated on the medial aspect of the foot, in the depression inferior and slightly anterior to the navicular tuberosity.

Needle

Only needle up to 0.5 cun with a perpendicular approach.

Deeper needling may pierce the medial crural nerve or the medial tarsal artery.

Moxa and pressure

This point answers well to moxa in energy depletion. Pressure techniques should be stimulating but initially may be quite painful.

Indications

KI 2 is primarily used in conditions of kidney energy depletion and covers such conditions and symptoms such as uterine prolapse, leucorrhoea, infertility, irregular menstruation and excessive menstrual bleeding. It is also used for urethritis, cystitis, prostatitis, impotence and premature ejaculation. It is also handy in localised medial foot pain.

KI 3 *Tai Xi* (Supreme Stream) 太谿 ★★★★

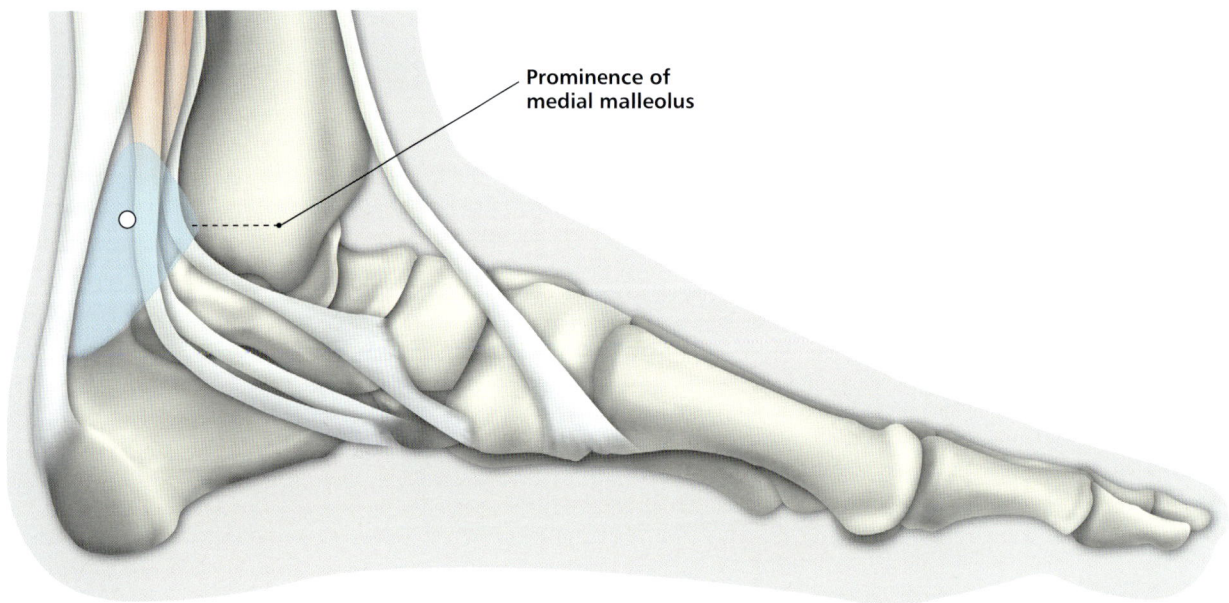

Prominence of medial malleolus

Location

Situated in the depression between the prominence of the medial malleolus and the Achilles tendon.

Needle

Up to 1.0 cun towards BL 60 using a perpendicular insertion. See description of BL 60 for another possible needle technique.

Moxa and pressure

Moxa is useful in kidney energy deficiency but is contraindicated if there are any thread veins in the area. Acupressure is suitable, especially in tandem with BL 60 with thumb and forefinger frictions.

Indications

KI 3 is both the Earth point and the Source point; therefore it may be used in symptoms and conditions the whole length of the Kidney channel but concentrating on organic kidney imbalance. Symptoms and conditions include exhaustion and tiredness, diminished hearing, tinnitus, dizziness, hypertension, disturbed sleep, infertility, premature ejaculation, irregular menstruation, frequent urination, oedema, abdominal pain and weakness of the groin and leg muscles.

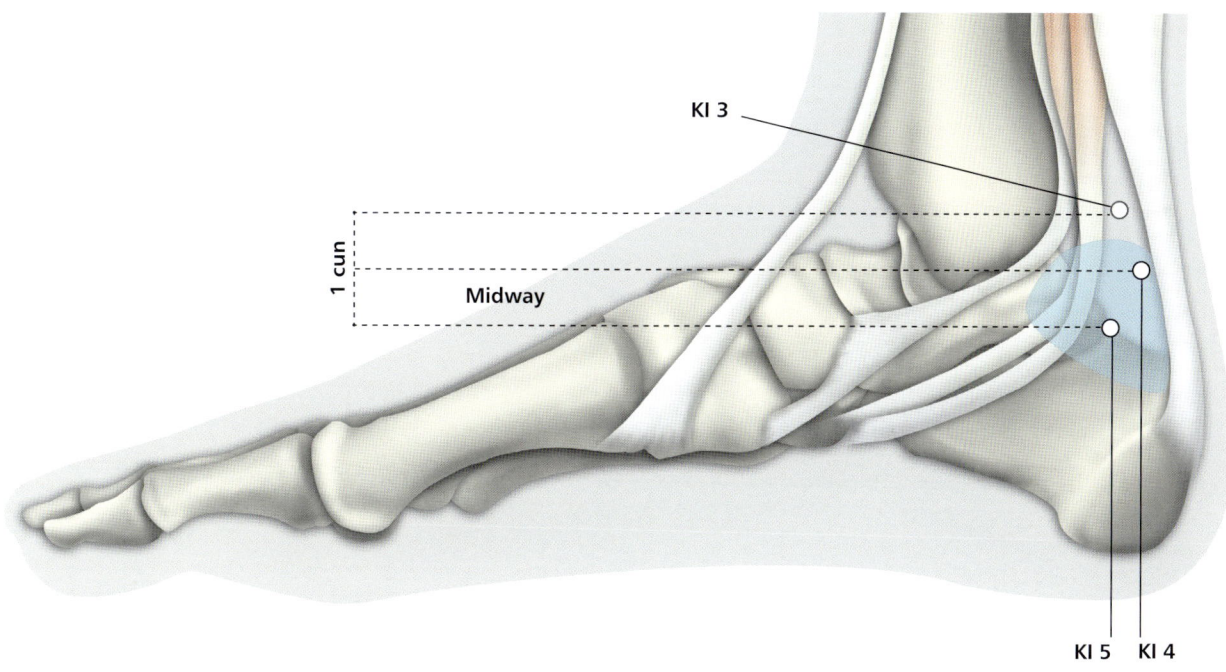

Location
This point is situated in a small depression 0.5 cun distal and posterior to KI 3 at the anterior border of the Achilles tendon.

Needle
This point may be treated to 0.5 cun depth using perpendicular or oblique insertion.

Moxa and pressure
Stimulating moxabustion is indicated in kidney energy deficiency. Acupressure is effective either by stimulating the point or by balancing it with its 'reflex' point of LU 9 on the wrist.

Indications
KI 4 is the Luo point and is connected with BL 58 on the Bladder channel. This point, therefore, strengthens the kidneys and bladder in both physical and psychosomatic conditions. (See 'special properties'.) Symptoms and conditions include shallow breathing, asthma, cough, sore and dry mouth and sore throat. It is also indicated in lumbar pain and weakness of the spine, abdominal distension, urinary retention, exhaustion, chronic constipation, impotence, infertility and irregular menstruation.

Special properties
KI 4 is one of the very best acupoints on the body in the treatment (and to a certain extent prevention) of psychosomatic disorders. The predominant emotion is fear, sometimes explained but often is unexplained. It is also helpful in chronic phobias, psychological insecurity and introversion, lack of willpower, anxiety, panic attacks and insomnia.

KI 6 *Zhao Hai* (Shining Sea)

照海 ★★★★★

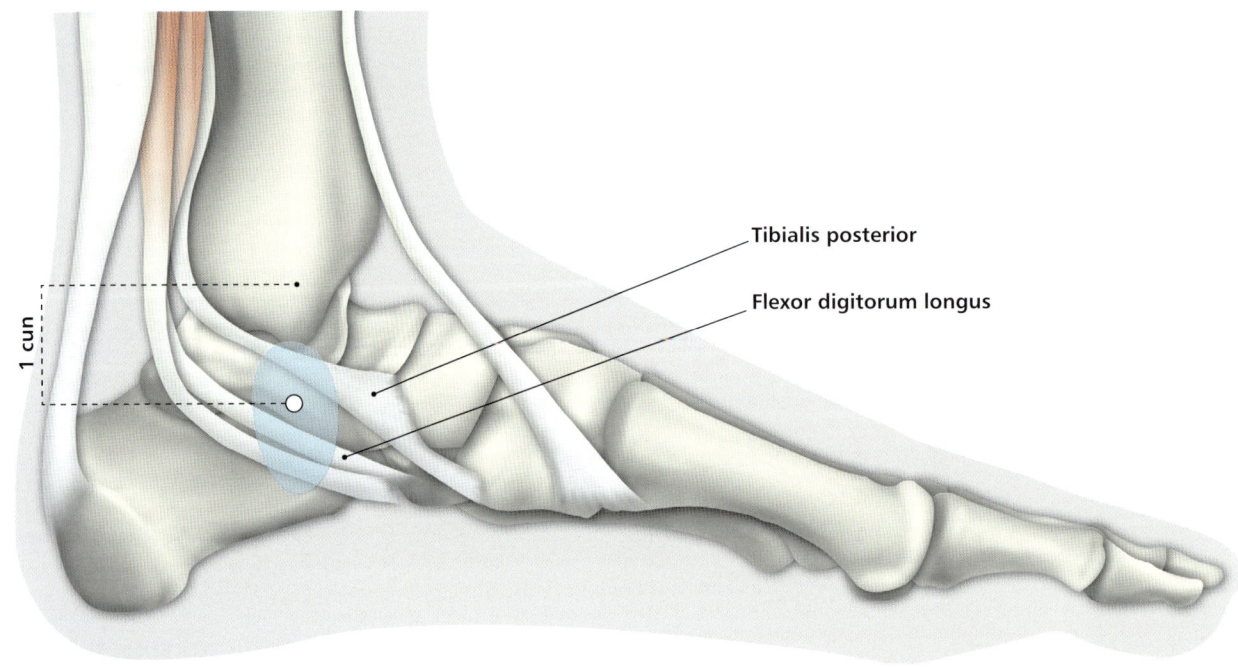

1 cun

Tibialis posterior

Flexor digitorum longus

Location
Situated in the depression 1 cun below the prominence of the medial malleolus between the tendons of tibialis posterior and flexor digitorum longus.

Needle
Needle to 0.5 cun with a perpendicular approach and slightly superior direction.

Moxa and pressure
Both moxa and pressure are effective on this point, especially in energy depletion of the Yin Chiao Mai and Conception meridians. (See 'special properties'.)

Indications
KI 6 has many actions that affect the whole length of the meridian as far as symptoms and conditions are related. One of its main effects is to help clear heat and inflammation along the channel. It is therefore indicated in night sweats, low grade fever, dry mouth and thirst, headache, dizziness, sore throat, hot flushes, dryness and pain in the eyes, tinnitus, pain and inflammation in the joints.

It is also indicated in many gynaecological conditions such as infertility, irregular menstruation, excessive bleeding, genital itching and dryness. KI 6 is also a useful point in calming the mind and treating stress.

Special properties
KI 6 is the Key (Opening) point of the Yinchiao Mai – one of the eight extraordinary meridians (Yin Motility channel) that flows from KI 6 to BL 1 in the eye. It is often coupled with LU 7 (key point of the Conception channel) to form a very powerful duo in the treatment of many chronic conditions. One of the very best ways of treating these two points is with biomagnets – positive pole on LU 7 and negative pole on KI 6.

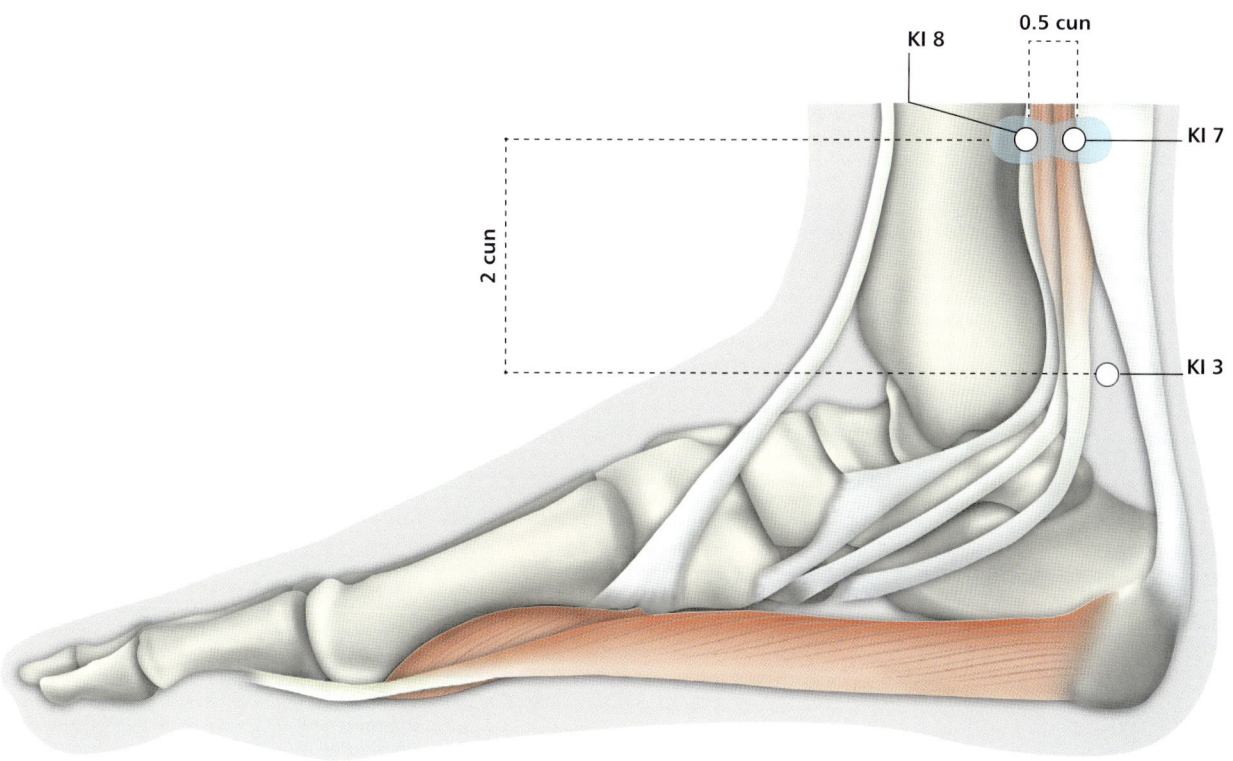

Location
Situated 2 cun proximal to KI 3 in the depression anterior to the border of the Achilles tendon and inferior to the soleus muscle.

Needle
Up to 1 cun using perpendicular insertion.

Moxa and pressure
KI 7 is similar to many of the other points on the medial aspect of the ankle region in that it is used in chronic conditions and, as such, answers well to stimulating moxa. It is an excellent self-help acupoint in the treatment of water imbalance and excess sweating.

Indications
This point helps balance kidney energy in that it helps promote the body's water metabolism. It is therefore indicated in the following symptoms and conditions – oedema, frequent urination, excessive or lack of sweating – even excessive dribbling.

It is also indicated in night sweats, leucorrhoea, diarrhoea and haemorrhoids. Similar to other Kidney channel command points, it is useful in the treatment of tiredness, exhaustion and many emotional imbalances.

Special properties
KI 7 is also the Tonification point of the Kidney channel and is therefore used to 'feed' energy to the liver via the Sheng cycle of the Law of Five Elements.

KI 9 *Zhu Bin* (Guest House or Building on the Beach)

築賓 ★★★★

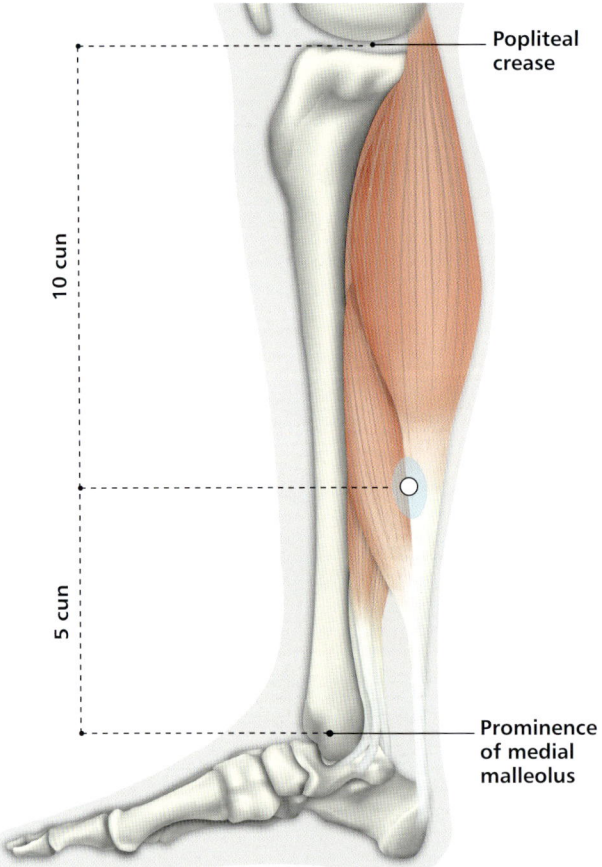

Popliteal crease

10 cun

5 cun

Prominence of medial malleolus

Location
Situated 5 cun superior to KI 3 on a line joining KI 3 and KI 10.

Needle
This is a deep point and requires up to 1.5 cun insertion using a perpendicular approach.

> Deeper needling may puncture the medial crural nerves, veins or arteries.

Moxa and pressure
Moxa is very useful at this point with the exception of the presence of varicosities when it is contraindicated. Acupressure may be used as a general point or locally in upper Achilles tendonitis.

Indications
This acupoint is one of the great points in the body to treat mental and psychosomatic disorders. Symptoms and conditions include insomnia, stress, anger, rage, fear, anxiety, panic attacks and even insanity (or the sensation that the patient feels 'out of this world').

Special properties
This is a very useful point in the treatment of abdominal or inguinal hernia.

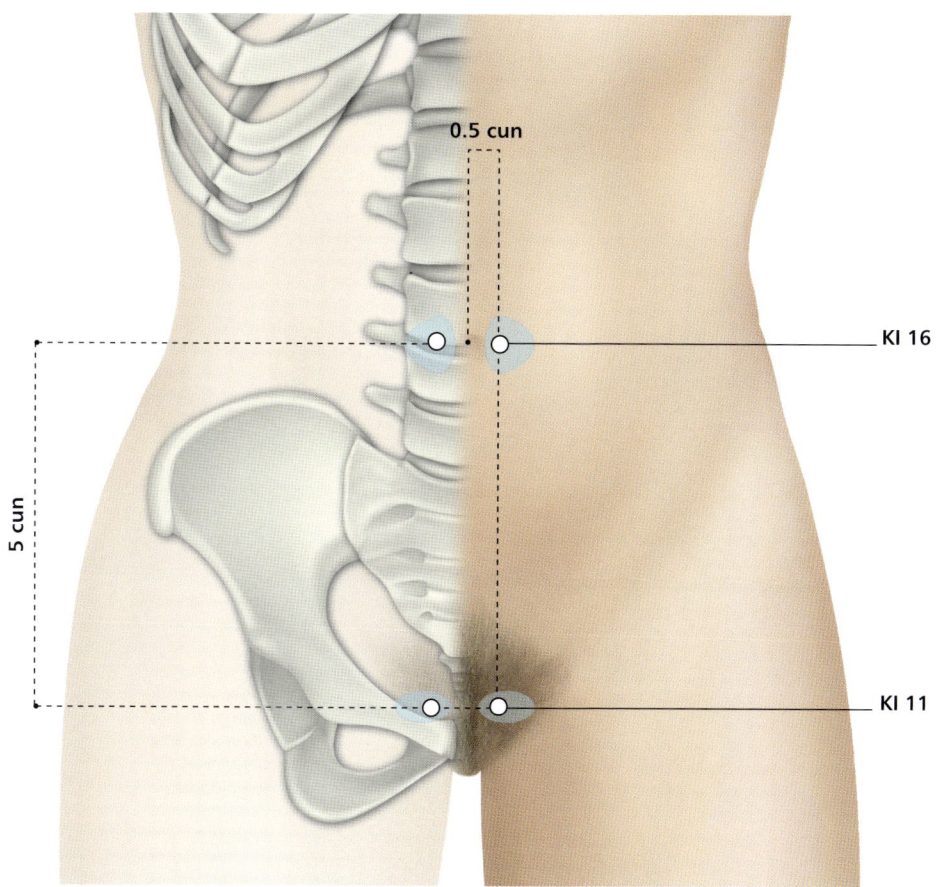

Location
Situated 0.5 cun lateral to the centre of the umbilicus at Con 8.

Needle
Up to 1.5 cun using a perpendicular insertion.

All treatment is contraindicated in pregnancy.

Moxa and pressure
Moxa is predominantly used here in cases of severe energy depletion. Stimulating acupressure may be performed by the patient as a useful self-help procedure in energy depletion.

Not to be used in pregnancy or in emaciated patients.

Indications
KI 16 acts in a similar way to ST 25, Con 8 and SP 15 (all points adjacent to the umbilicus) in that it helps with overall energy depletion. It is also specifically indicated in constipation, dry stools, abdominal pain, distension and vomiting.

Special properties
KI 16 is the Navel minor chakra acupoint and is associated with the Shoulder chakra at LI 15 (minor) and the Throat chakra at Con 22 (major). This triad of points helps in all cases of inability to excrete or express.

KI 27 *Shu Fu* (Shu Mansion)

俞府 ★★★★★

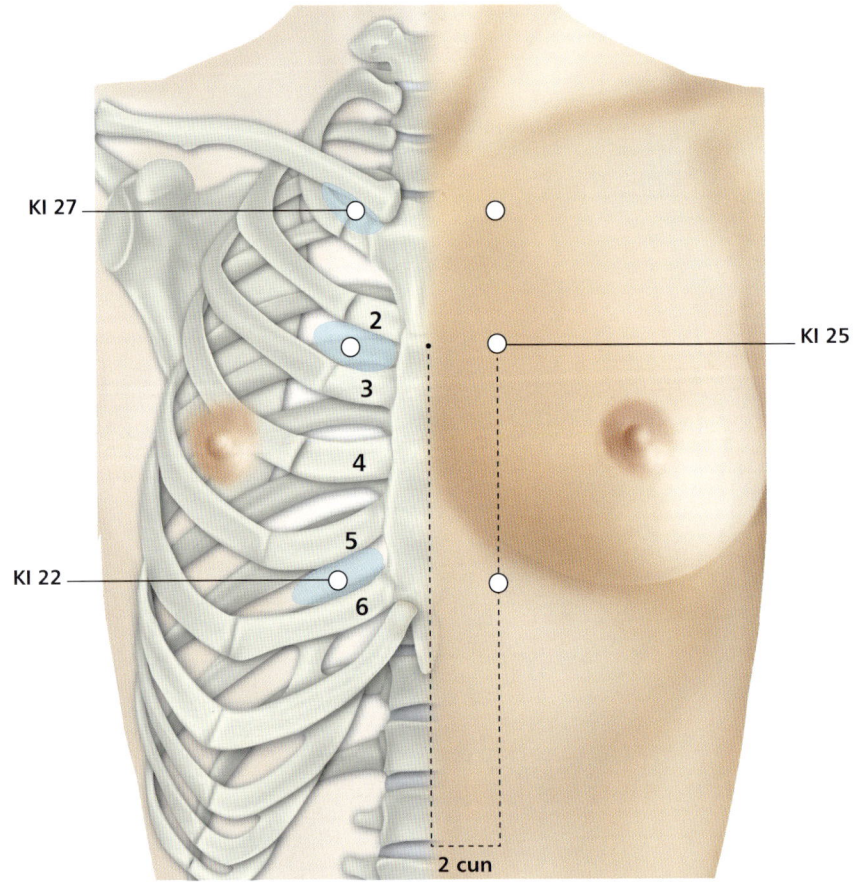

Location

Situated in the depression inferior to the medial end of the clavicle, 2 cun lateral to the midline.

Needle

Only needle 0.4 cun using a perpendicular insertion as deeper needling may pierce the lung tissue.

Moxa and pressure

Moxa could be useful in localised lung conditions such as dyspnoea. For pressure, see 'special properties'.

Indications

KI 27 is a deceptively important point and has many uses. Its main action is with symptoms and conditions associated with its position, namely conditions of the respiratory tract and thorax, throat, goitre, cough, dyspnoea and asthma. It is also an excellent local point in sterno-clavicular conditions, neck pain and thyroid imbalance. General symptomatology includes nausea, abdominal distension, and lack of appetite, groin pain and discomfort along the course of the channel.

Special properties

KI 27 is said to be the Clavicular chakra. This is a minor chakra that is associated with both the Groin chakra at ST 30 (minor) and the Brow chakra at Extra 1 (major). It is therefore indicated in many psychosomatic disorders, low blood pressure and general stress conditions.

KI 27 is also related to BL 11 (almost the equivalent acupoint on the posterior aspect) and is indicated in tandem with BL 11 in the treatment of 'bone' conditions in that it stimulates the parathyroid glands. Stimulating needle or moxa is indicated in this case. The patient may be instructed to massage the point if there is thyroid deficiency.

KI 27 is also one of the acupoints that is used in 'acupressure tapping' in many modern philosophies of combining acupressure and self-hypnotherapy in helping stress and phobias.

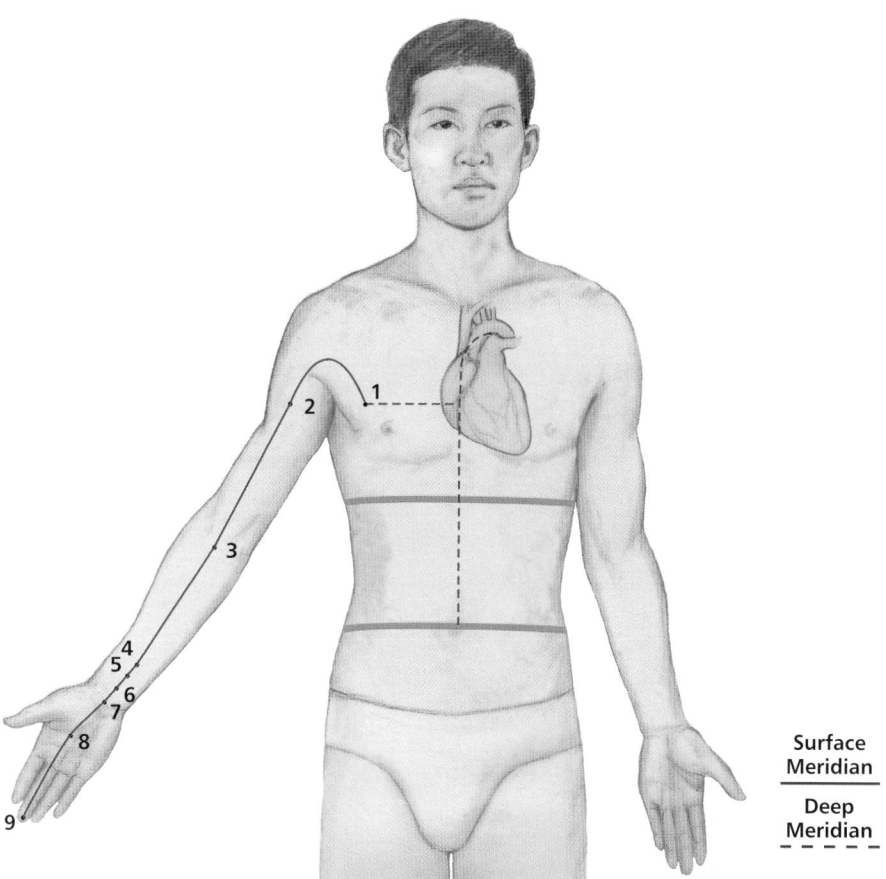

Surface
Meridian

Deep
Meridian

The Pericardium channel represents one of the yin aspects of the Fire element and is the second shortest channel in the body, having only nine (9) surface points. It used to be called Heart Constrictor and is still known as Circulation-Sex in some modern kinesiology interpretations. It commences as a deep channel below the diaphragm where it ascends through the chest, heart, pericardium and emerges to form the first surface channel point just lateral to the nipple. It ascends to the axilla and follows the antero-medial aspect of the upper arm to the cubital fossa. The meridian then descends the anterior aspect of the forearm to the wrist crease then to the palm of the hand and ending on the tip of the middle finger. A deeper branch leads away from PC 8 to the tip of the ring finger where it connects with the Triple Energizer meridian. We shall discuss PC 1, PC 3, PC 6, PC 7, PC 8 and PC 9.

PC 1 *Tian Chi* (Heavenly Pool)

天池 ⭐⭐

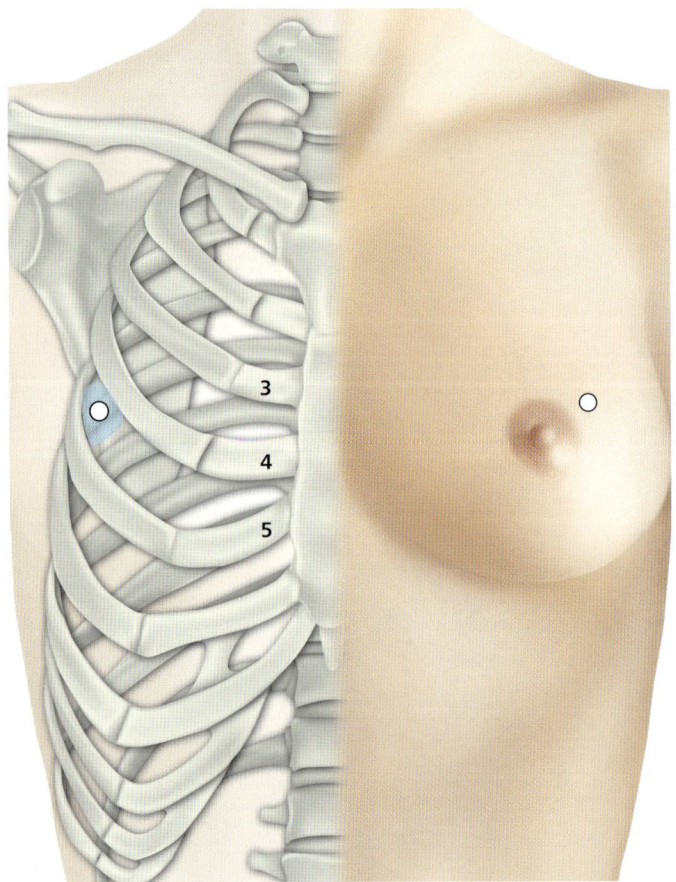

Location
Situated approximately 1 cun lateral and superior to the nipple in the 4th intercostal space.

Needle
Up to 0.5 only with a perpendicular approach.

> Be careful that the mammary gland is not punctured.

Moxa and pressure

> Direct moxa is contraindicated.

Pressure techniques may be useful with localised pain and stagnation.

> Do not use any stimulating techniques if there is any evidence of swelling or lumps of any kind within the breast tissue.

Indications
This point is limited in its use and is mainly used to treat local conditions of the breast and chest due to stagnation. Symptoms and conditions include pain and swelling in the breast tissue, insufficient lactation, axillary swelling and shoulder pain and stiffness.

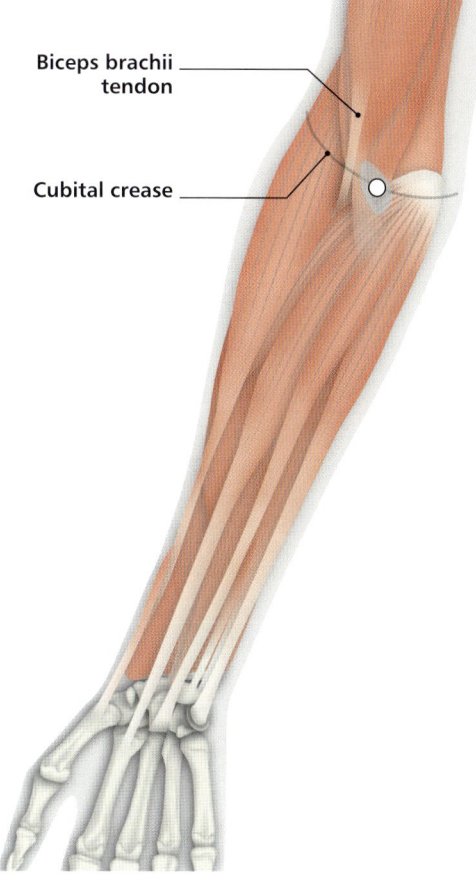

Biceps brachii tendon

Cubital crease

Location
Situated on the transverse cubital crease in the depression on the medial side of the biceps brachii muscle.

Needle
0.5 to 0.8 cun insertion using a perpendicular approach.

Do not needle any deeper for fear of piercing the basilic vein or medial cutaneous nerve.

Moxa and pressure
Use very light moxa only due to underlying vessels. For pressure techniques, see under 'special properties'.

Indications
PC 3 is indicated in two areas: circulatory and miscellaneous. Circulatory symptoms and conditions include pectoral angina, palpitations and fullness of the chest, arrhythmia, tachycardia and dyspnoea. Other symptoms include nausea, gastritis, insomnia, headaches, convulsions and heat stroke. It may be also used as a local point in anterior elbow pain.

Special properties
PC 3 is the Water point of the channel and is therefore used to dampen down heat in many conditions. It has two very useful functions when used with pressure and reflextherapy. Firstly it is the parallel point to BL 40 in the middle of the popliteal fossa of the knee so may be used as an adjunct point in knee pain. It is also the Elbow chakra point. This is a minor chakra that is associated with the Knee chakra at BL 40 (minor) and the Base chakra at Con 1 or Gov 1 (major). This triad of points is used in the treatment of many chronic conditions.

PC 6 *Nei Guan* (Inner Barrier or Inner Gate)

內關 ★★★★★

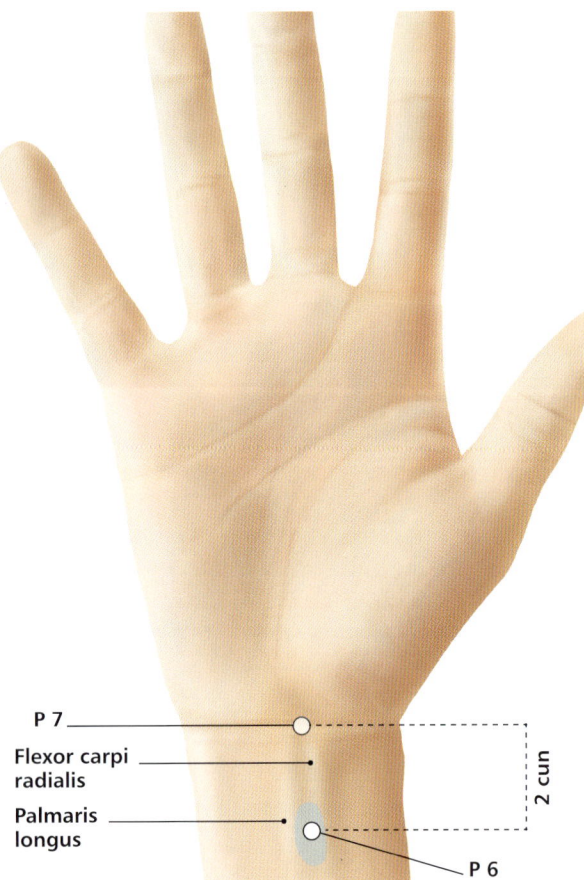

P 7

Flexor carpi radialis

Palmaris longus

2 cun

P 6

Location

Situated 2 cun proximal to the anterior wrist crease between the tendons of palmaris longus and flexor carpi radialis muscles.

Needle

Only needle up to 0.5 cun if using a perpendicular approach or up to 1.5 cun if there is an oblique insertion along the channel. Another technique is to needle all the way through the arm to emerge at TE 5 on the posterior aspect of the forearm.

> This technique should only be performed by experienced practitioners.

Please note that this point often gives an 'electric' sensation of deqi which mimics hitting a nerve!

Moxa and pressure

Use light moxa only due to underlying vessels being present. For pressure, see 'special properties'.

Indications

PC 6 is one of the very great acupoints on the body and has several indications and actions. It regulates the circulation of chi, restores clarity to the brain, eases pain, strengthens the spleen and stomach and relaxes the chest. It is used in the following symptoms and conditions:

- Angina, heaviness in the chest, goitre, palpitations and arrhythmia, fever, headache and migraine. It is a first aid point in the discomfort of myocardial infarction.
- Epigastric pain, acid reflux, heartburn, gastritis, nausea, morning sickness in pregnancy and vomiting.
- It calms the mind and is used in many emotional imbalances such as insomnia, anxiety, irritability, mood swings, depression and grief.
- Premenstrual tension, mastitis, dysmenorrhoea, irregular menstruation and infertility.
- It is used as a local point in anterior wrist conditions such as carpal tunnel syndrome.
- Miscellaneous symptoms include fever, malaria, jaundice, epilepsy, coma and blood in the stool.

Special properties

- PC 6 is the Luo (Connecting) point with TE 5. This may be done with pressure, needles or magnets. This is an excellent duo in the treatment of lower cervical pain, hormonal imbalance, shoulder pain and many others.
- It is also the Key point of the Yinwei Mai (Regulating channel) and is used in conjunction with the Chong Mai (Key point SP 4) in helping many conditions.
- PC 6 is one of the best points for motion sickness or morning sickness in pregnancy. This may be achieved by needle, magnets, pressure or the so-called 'Sea Bands'. Using PC 6 for this symptom has been the subject of hundreds of research projects!

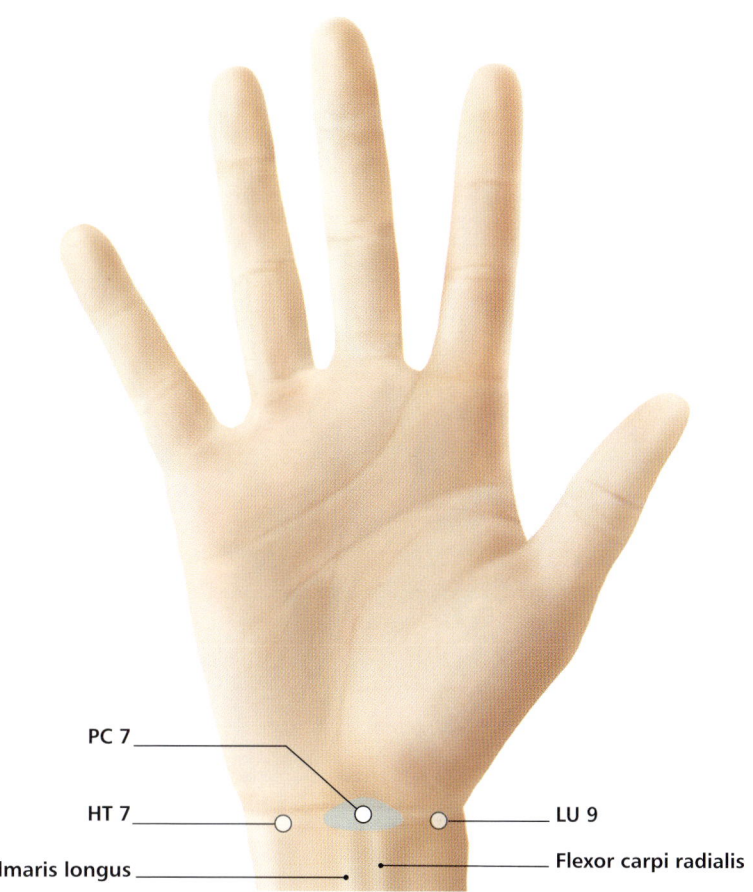

PC 7 _____
HT 7 _____ ○   ○ _____ LU 9
Palmaris longus _____   _____ Flexor carpi radialis

Location
Situated in the middle of the anterior wrist crease between the tendons of palmaris longus and flexor carpi radialis.

Needle
Needle up to 0.5 cun using a perpendicular approach.

> Deeper needling may affect the median nerve; this acupoint is a naturally 'painful' point to needle and the patient should be warned in advance.

Moxa and pressure
Use mild to moderate moxa due to underlying vessels. Acupressure is extremely effective when used as a local point in the treatment of carpal tunnel syndrome. It is also a major point when used in parallel reflextherapy to treat ankle joint imbalance.

Indications
PC 7 is the Source (Yuan) point of the Pericardium channel, and is therefore influential in cooling down conditions with heat and calming the mind. Symptoms and conditions include pain and tightness in the chest, angina pectoris, palpitations and arrhythmia, fever, epilepsy, depression and anxiety. It is also very effective as a local point in treating carpal tunnel syndrome (if of a local aetiology and not caused by a lower cervical problem).

PC 8 *Lao Gong* (Palace of Labour) 勞宮 ★★ Needle ★★★★★ Pressure

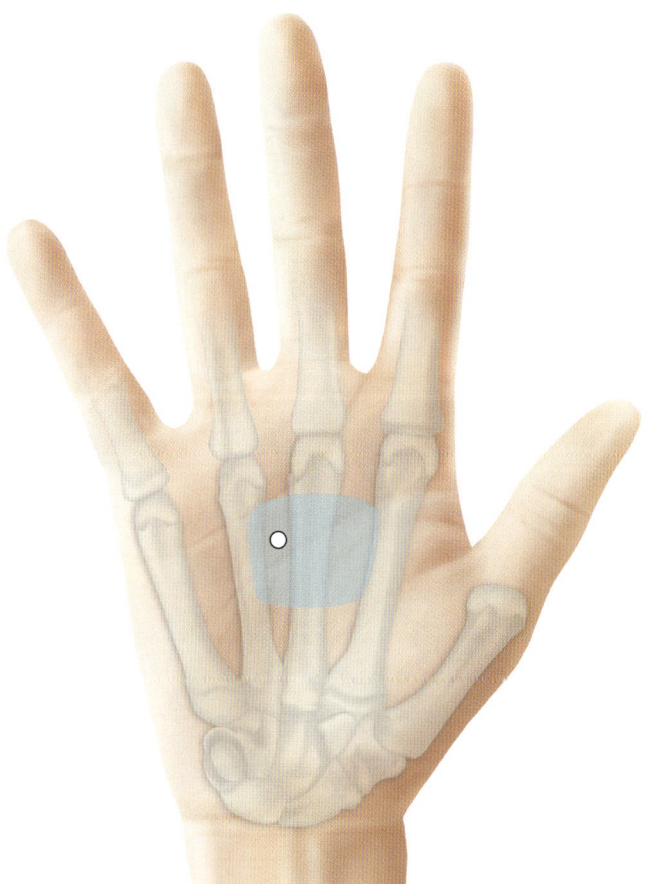

Location

Situated in the centre of the palm where the middle finger of a clenched fist touches the palm.

Needle

Only needle up to 0.5 cun using a perpendicular approach. Please note that this point can be painful to needle and the patient should be warned.

Moxa and pressure

PC 8 answers well to stimulating moxa in general energy depletion. Acupressure is extremely powerful, see 'special properties'.

Indications

The great asset of PC 8 is in calming the mind and clearing 'heat' from the head, throat and chest areas. It is colloquially called the 'stigmata' point. Symptoms and conditions include sweating, angina pectoris and chest heaviness, epilepsy, mouth and throat inflammation and halitosis. It is also used as a local point in soft tissue lesions of the hand.

Special properties

PC 8 is the Hand chakra (minor) and is linked with the Foot chakra at KI 1 (minor) and the Crown chakra at Gov 20 (major) to give a triad of points that are used in stress release and calming of the mind. It is one of the most useful self-help points on the body to help patients relax, calm the mind, ease tension headaches and dizziness and help reduce hypertension. It is much easier for the patient to access than KI 1. The point is used extensively in qigong and other Eastern body work and martial arts as a point of focus and to strengthen a person's chi.

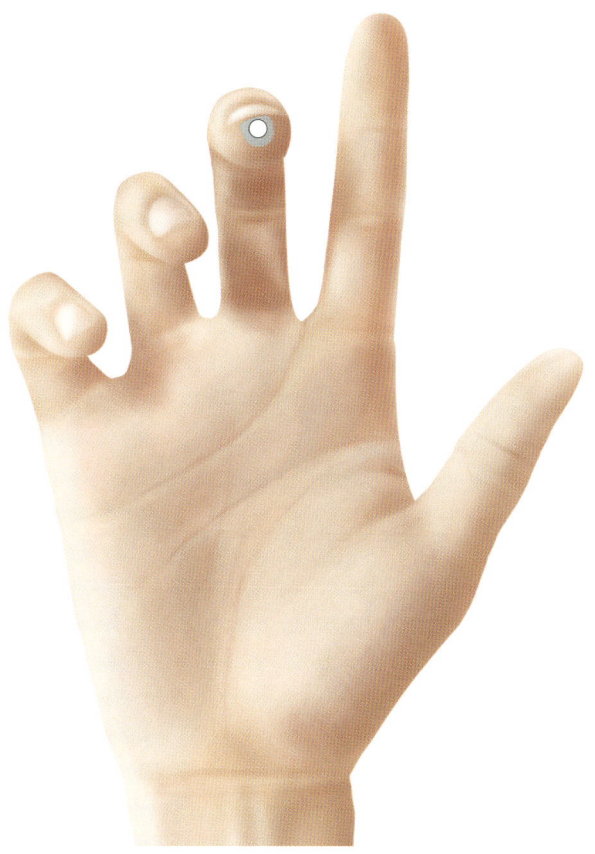

Location

There is much disagreement in the texts as to exactly where this acupoint lies! The recognised position is in the centre of the tip of the middle finger – this makes it the only Tsing point that is not officially a 'nail' point. The usual alternative is the nail point on the radial (lateral) aspect of the middle finger. It has even been placed on the ulnar side of the finger.

Needle

Only needle up to 0.2 cun with a perpendicular insertion.

Moxa and pressure

Moxa may be used in cases of sudden collapse or fainting but stimulating acupressure is the better option in this case.

Indications

PC 9 is one of best first aid acupoints to restore consciousness in fainting, syncope, coma and shock. It may also be used in fever cases, especially in children. Because of its powerful effect as a 'heart tonic', the point is used extensively in qigong and similar therapies and disciplines to project chi in healing or martial arts.

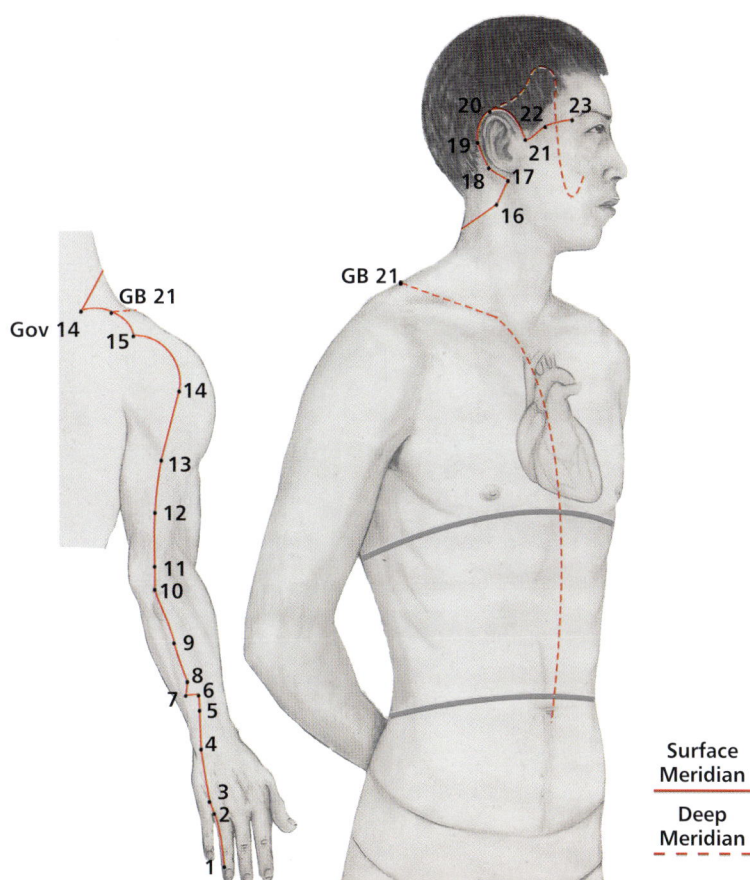

GB 21

GB 21

Gov 14

Surface
Meridian

Deep
Meridian

This meridian is one of the least understood by practitioners of Western medicine, simply because it does not relate to an internal organ. In TCM it is considered to be the central body cavity. It pertains to the transformation, purification and distribution of air, food and water. The upper TE regulates respiration and circulation of blood, the middle TE governs the digestive system, and the lower TE controls the absorption of fluids and nutrients, excretion and sexuality. The channel was originally just called by its TCM name Sanjiao and it has been called Triple Heater, Triple Burner, Three Heater and Triple Warmer. The name Triple Energizer was standardised in the late 1990s.

It represents one of the two Yang channels in the Fire element and is associated with the Pericardium as its Yin counterpart. It has twenty-three (23) acupoints along its surface pathway that originates in the ring finger and ends at the lateral aspect of the eye. It commences at the ulnar side of the ring finger and ascends the dorsal aspect of the hand to the posterior aspect of the forearm to the tip of the elbow. From here it ascends the posterior aspect of the arm to the back of the shoulder at TE 15. From here it links to GB 21 on the anterior aspect of the chest and back across to the dorsal aspect to link with Gov 14 before it returns to the side of the neck to the lower aspect of the ear. It travels around the ear to the side of the TMJ before travelling to the outer aspect of the eye at TE 23. From its link with GB 21 it descends through the heart, pleura and diaphragm towards the umbilicus region via a deeper channel. We shall discuss TE 3, TE 4, TE 5, TE 6, TE 10, TE 14, TE 16, TE 17 and TE 21.

TE 3 *Zhong Zu* (Middle of the Sea)

中渚 ★★★

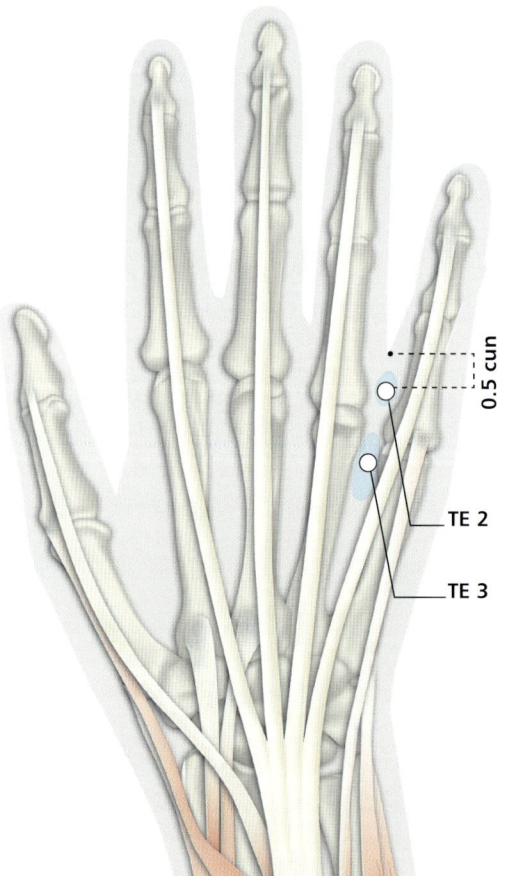

0.5 cun

TE 2

TE 3

Location
Situated on the dorsum of the hand in the depression proximal to the metacarpo-phalangeal joints between the 4th and 5th metacarpal bones.

Needle
This acupoint may be needled up to 0.5 cun using a perpendicular approach or 1.5 cun using an oblique insertion threading the needle towards the wrist.

Moxa and pressure
Mild moxabustion is useful on this point in chronic ear and localised hand conditions. In acupressure, TE 3 is used to draw pain and heat down from the ear and side of the face.

Indications
Symptoms and conditions include ear inflammation, tinnitus, and mild hard of hearing, eye inflammation and headache. Some authorities insist that this point is better suited to draw heat and inflammation away from the side of the head than its more illustrious cousin TE 5.

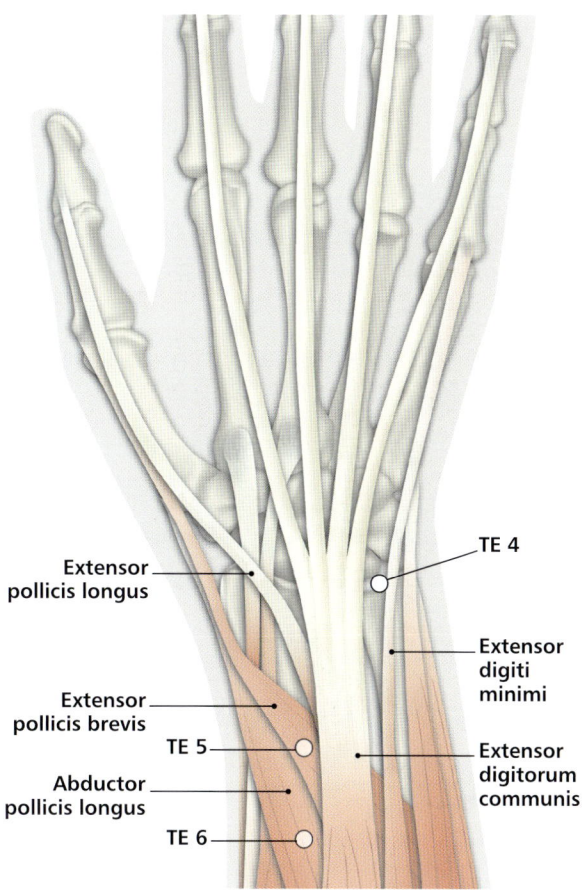

Location

Situated on the dorsum of the wrist crease in the depression between the tendons of extensor digitorum and extensor digiti minimi.

Needle

Up to 0.5 cun using a perpendicular insertion.

> Be careful not to affect the cutaneous veins or the dorsal branch of the ulnar nerve.

Moxa and pressure

Some authorities suggest that this point is forbidden to moxa, but in practice it does not warrant this. Pressure techniques are useful using the point as a local one in dorsal wrist conditions and as a general point to affect the channel.

Indications

This is a very useful point in treating channel conditions, e.g. eye, ear, shoulder, elbow and wrist conditions. It is classically used to ease sore throats.

Special properties

TE 4 is the reflected acupoint to GB 40 and may be used with either pressure or needle to treat ankle conditions. TE 4 is also the Key point of the Ear chakra at TE 17 and is used to 'open up' the energies associated with this chakra.

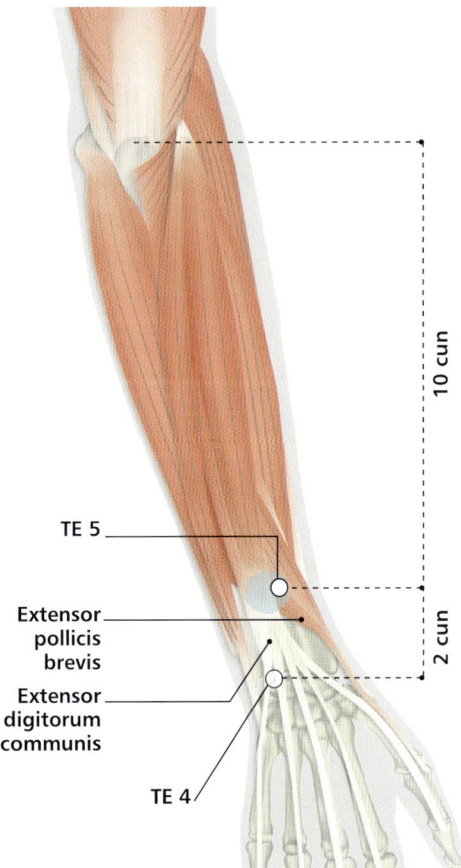

TE 5

Extensor
pollicis
brevis

Extensor
digitorum
communis

TE 4

10 cun

2 cun

Location

Situated centrally between the radius and ulna, 2 cun above the posterior wrist crease.

Needle

TE 5 is a relatively deep point so needling up to 1 cun using a perpendicular insertion is the usual way to affect it. TE 5 is directly opposite PC 6 on the anterior aspect of the wrist and it is possible to effect both acupoints with one needle.

> This should not be attempted unless you are an experienced practitioner.

Moxa and pressure

Moxa is very effective here in conditions associated with the channel and localised wrist conditions. Pressure techniques are numerous and may be used locally in wrist sprains, to draw heat and inflammation away from the ear and head, in conjunction with PC 6 (they are both Luo points) and in conjunction with GB 41 (see 'special properties').

Indications

This acupoint is one of the Great points on the body and is useful either in isolation or in tandem with other points to treat many conditions. It is one of the best points to clear heat and inflammation away from the head (eyes, ears and throat) so is used to improve eyesight and hearing and to ease sore throats. It is also indicated in tinnitus, upper respiratory tract conditions, colds and flu, toothache, hypertension and headaches.

Special properties

As well as being the Luo (Connecting) point, TE 5 is also the Key point of the Yangwei Mai (Regulating channel) which is one of the eight extraordinary meridians. In conjunction with GB 41 (Dai Mai Key point) it is used extensively in hemi-cranial headaches, detoxification of the gall bladder and liver, vomiting, epigastric pain, irritability and depression. Another aspect of this point is in self-help to help patients suffering from depression. I have found that if the patient stimulates this and the surrounding region of the upper wrist region, it can help with mood swings and depression.

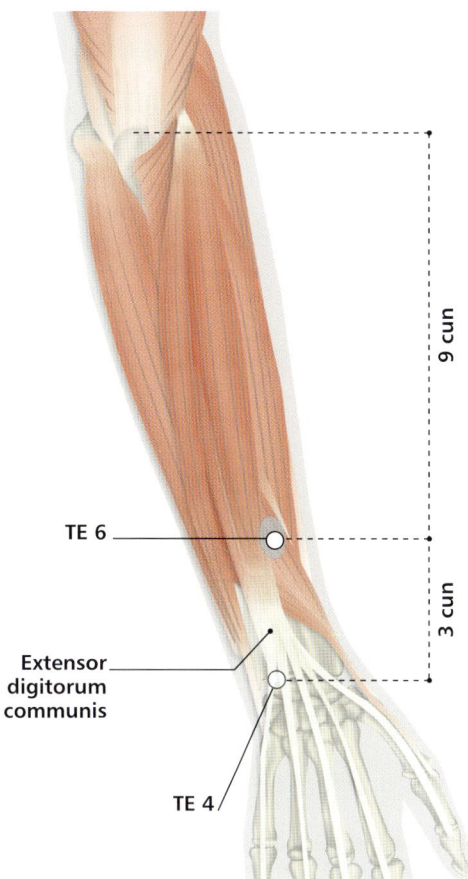

TE 6

Extensor digitorum communis

TE 4

9 cun

3 cun

Location
Situated 3 cun proximal to the dorsal wrist crease, between the radius and the extensor digitorum muscle.

Needle
Up to 1.2 cun using a perpendicular insertion.

Moxa and pressure
Use moderate moxa. It is useful when used as a local pressure point in wrist and posterior arm discomfort. It has limited application in channel conditions unless it is combined with TE points around the head to dissipate heat from the head.

Indications
TE 6 is an effective point in any condition that has heat and inflammation associated with it. It is therefore effective in helping all three Jiao (Energizer) areas. Symptoms and conditions include pain and inflammation of the ear, tinnitus, deafness, throat inflammation, intercostal neuralgia, some 'hot' skin conditions, fullness and bloating of the abdomen, oppression of the chest, chronic constipation and gynaecological pain.

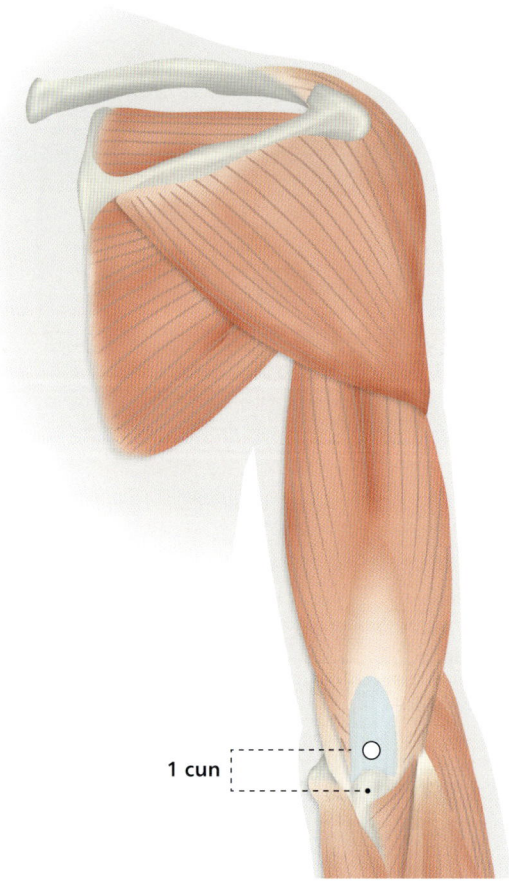

1 cun

Location

Situated in the depression 1 cun proximal to the tip of the olecranon process when the elbow is flexed.

Needle

Up to 0.8 cun using a perpendicular insertion.

Moxa and pressure

Moxa is indicated in the treatment of chronic elbow 'congestion' and swelling. Acupressure is useful used as a local point in the treatment of triceps tightness. See 'special properties' for other pressure indications.

Indications

TE 10 is used to treat channel conditions but is particularly effective in treating localised elbow pain and stiffness, shoulder pain and cervical discomfort. It is also useful in helping lymphatic obstruction in the neck and shoulder regions.

Special properties

TE 10 is the reflected acupoint of the superior aspect of the knee, especially the quadriceps tendon. It is therefore helpful in treating knee pain and stiffness.

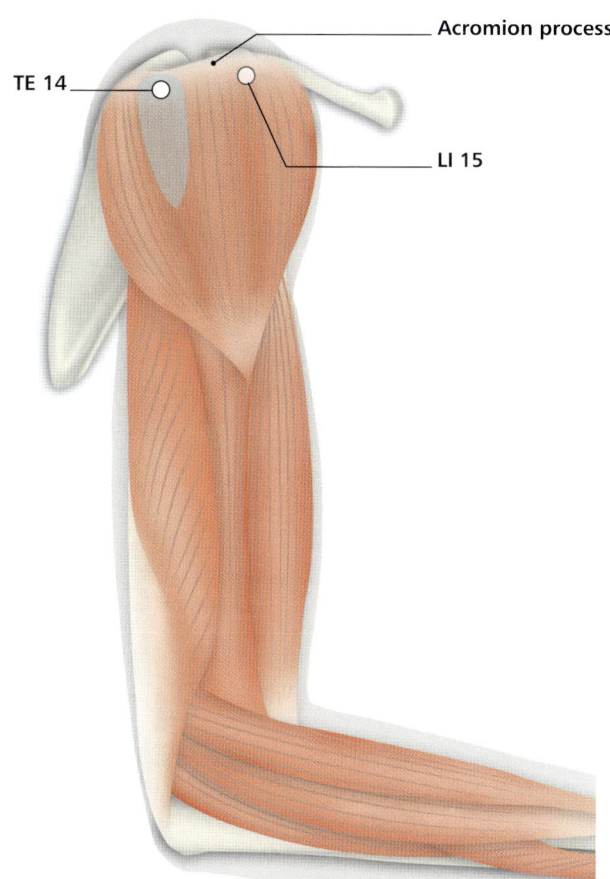

Location

Situated on the postero-lateral aspect of the shoulder in the depression between the acromion process and the greater tubercle of the humerus, distal to LI 15.

Needle

This point is usually approached by perpendicular insertion at 1 cun depth.

Moxa and pressure

This point is very effective when used with moxa for chronic shoulder pain and stiffness. It is usually used in conjunction with other local shoulder acupoints including LI 15, LI 16, GB 21, SI 12 and SI 11. Acupressure is equally effective either in isolation or combined with the other stated points in shoulder pain and stiffness. It may also be used as a parallel acupoint to the hip in easing hip pain.

Indications

This is a super point when used in conjunction with the others stated in the treatment of frozen shoulder (adhesive capsulitis of the gleno-humeral joint), atrophy or paralysis of the upper limb. This point has limited actions on channel symptoms.

TE 16 *Tian You* (Heavenly Window)

天牖 ★★★★

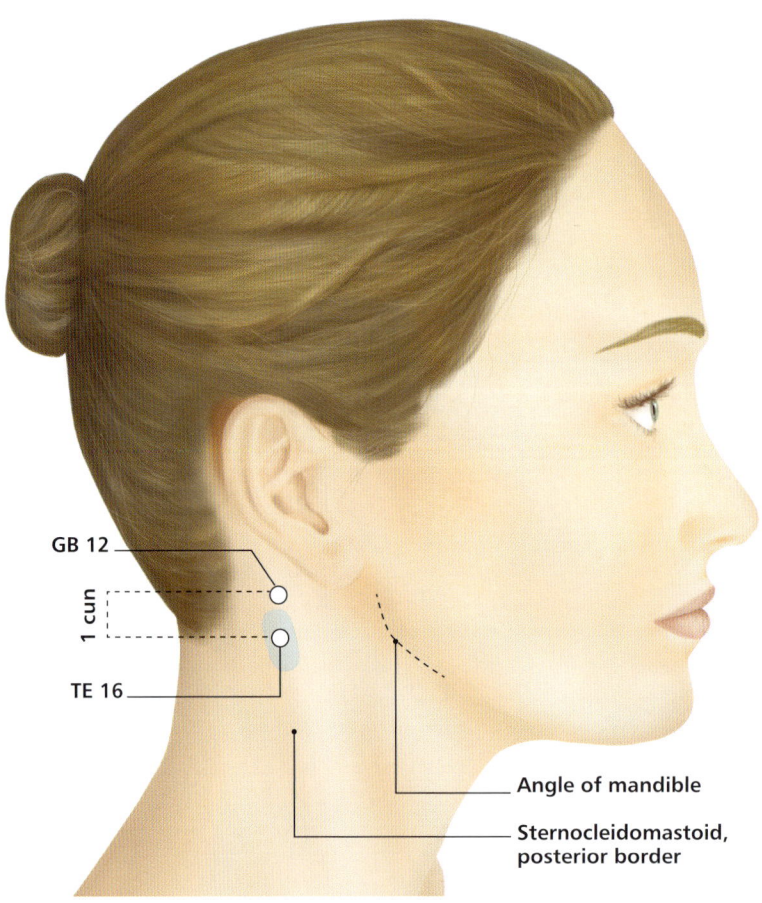

GB 12

1 cun

TE 16

Angle of mandible

Sternocleidomastoid, posterior border

Location
Situated on the posterior border of the sternocleidomastoid muscle, level with the angle of the mandible, posterior and approximately 1 cun inferior to the tip of the mastoid process.

Needle
In spite of its awkward anatomical position, this point is worth getting acquainted with. Needle up to 0.8 cun using a perpendicular approach.

> Do not insert any deeper in case the auricular nerve, cervical artery and vein are pierced.

Moxa and pressure
The point can be useful in sedation acupressure for localised spasm; do not stimulate this point!

> Direct moxa is contraindicated, but a moxa roll is permissible though hardly ever used.

Indications
Symptoms and conditions include pain and inflammation of the ears and eyes, impaired hearing, tinnitus, catarrh, headache (hemi-cranial), dizziness, neck stiffness, torticollis and some aspects of mastitis if caused by lymphatic obstruction.

TE 17 *Yi Feng* (Wind Screen)

翳風 ★★★★★

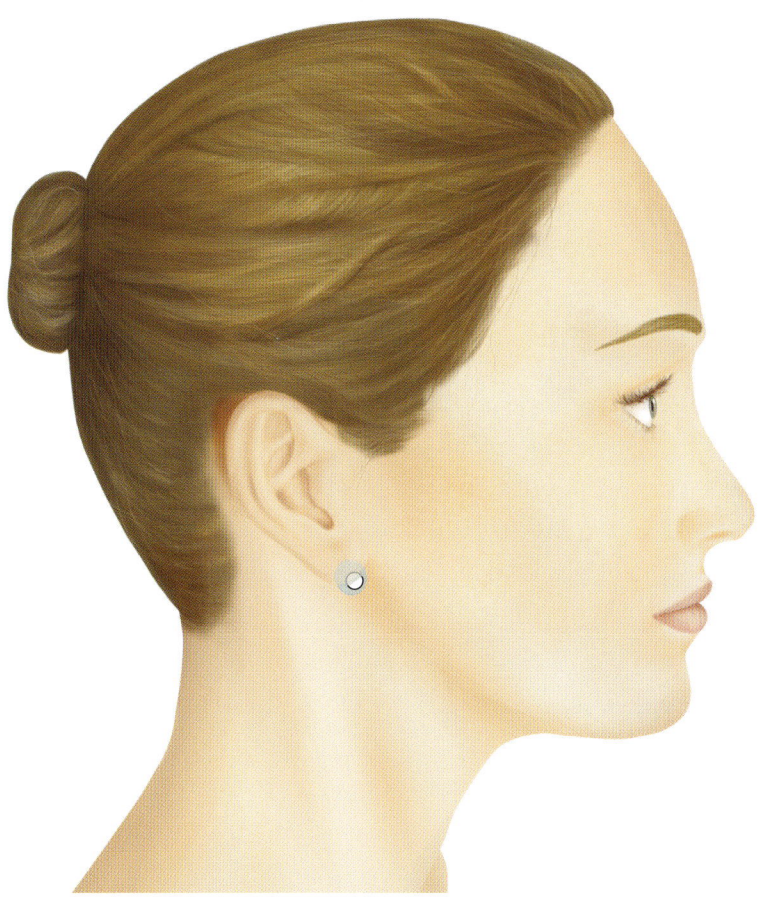

Location

Situated directly behind the ear lobe at the centre of the depression formed between the mastoid process and the lower jaw.

Needle

This acupoint is surprisingly deep, so needle up to 1 cun with a perpendicular insertion.

> Do not attempt to needle any deeper as there may be danger of puncturing the jugular vein, carotid artery or facial nerve.

Moxa and pressure

Direct moxabustion is almost impossible unless the patient is in side-lying and the ear lobe is moved to one side. Do not use any stimulating acupressure, this point reacts wonderfully to chi balancing using stationary fingers, see 'special properties'.

Indications

TE 17 is probably the most influential point in many conditions of the ear. Symptoms and conditions include tinnitus, diminished hearing, earache, acute or chronic otitis, discharge and general ear inflammation. It is also an excellent point in treating Ménière's syndrome, dizziness, vertigo, TMJ stiffness, headache, nausea, and facial nerve disorders such as eye, mouth and tongue paralysis.

Special properties

TE 17 is regarded as being the Ear chakra (minor). It is associated with the Intercostal chakra at SP 21 (minor) and the Heart chakra at Con 17 (major). It is therefore very influential with needle, or better still with pressure, in treating stress-related conditions, clearing the mind and treating old emotional 'blockages' such as grief, worry and anxiety.

TE 21 *Er Men* (Ear Gate)

耳門 ★★★★

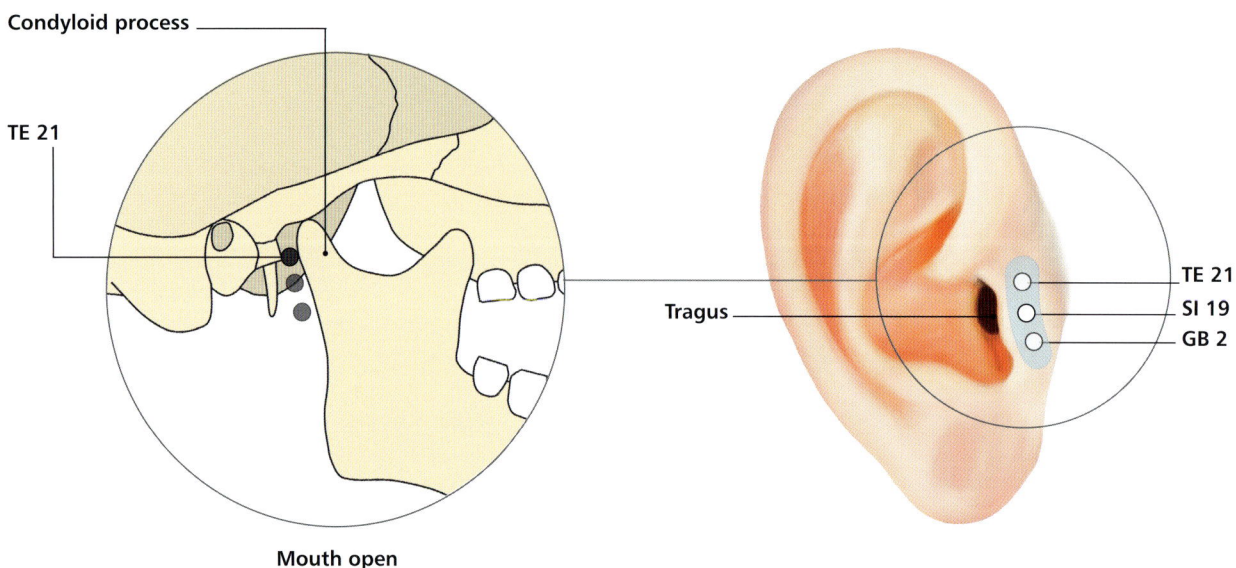

Condyloid process

TE 21

Mouth open

Tragus

TE 21
SI 19
GB 2

Location
Situated in the depression anterior to the supratragic notch and slightly superior to the condyloid process of the mandible in line with SI 19 and GB 2.

Needle
This acupoint should be needled up to 1 cun using a perpendicular approach or using a superficial thread needle where all three points mentioned may be linked.

Deeper needling may pierce the temporal artery and vein.

Moxa and pressure
Some authorities indicate that this point is contraindicated to moxa, but I see no reason why a moxa stick cannot be utilised in deep-seated ear conditions, e.g. glue ear. Acupressure can be very useful in TMJ conditions as well as general stress release.

Indications
TE 21 is used mostly with ear conditions such as otitis, Ménière's syndrome, tinnitus and deafness plus facial nerve palsy, toothache and temporal headache. This point is also very good, in conjunction with SI 19 and GB 2, in the treatment of TMJ disorders and many stress issues.

Gall Bladder Meridian (GB)

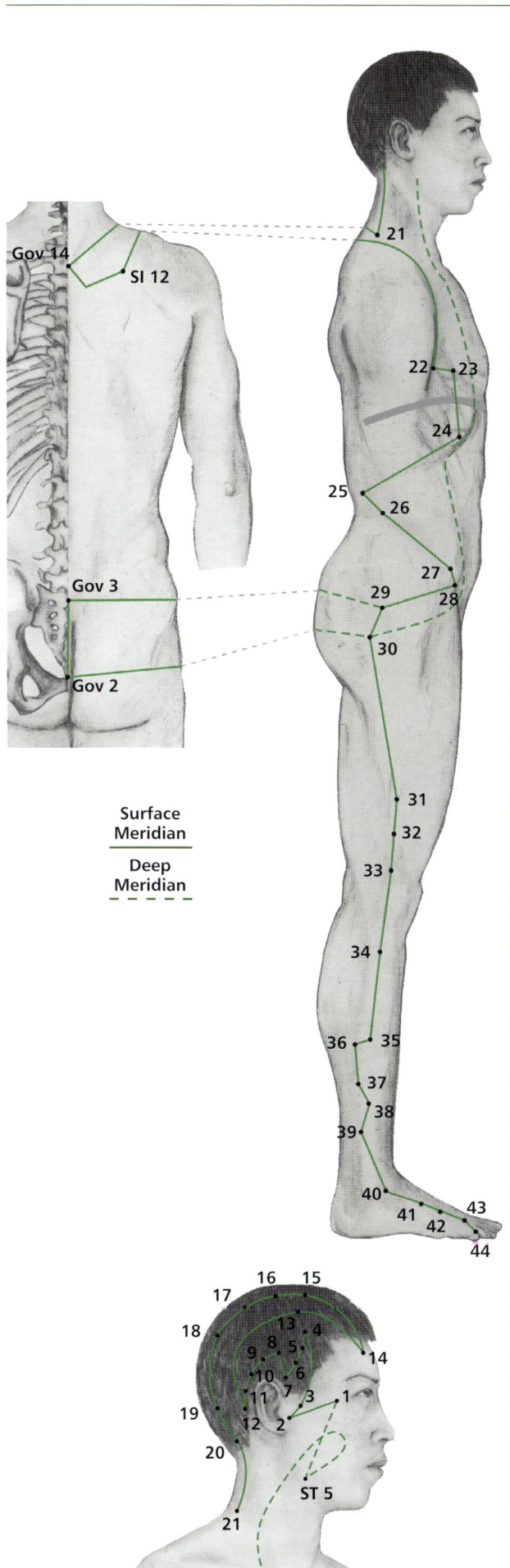

Surface
Meridian

Deep
Meridian
- - - - - -

The Gall Bladder (sometimes called Gallbladder) channel represents the Yang aspect of the Wood element. The surface Gall Bladder meridian contains forty-four (44) acupoints, commencing at the eye and ending on the 4th toe. It has a most unusual journey, linking with the Bladder, Stomach, Liver, Small Intestine and Governor along its course. Its winding and zigzag trajectory along the side of the head is the curse of every poor acupuncture student due to its complexity. It is the only channel to innervate the lateral side of the body and the hips. Because of its unions and complicated course, it is instrumental in being used in many different types of symptoms and conditions. We shall discuss: GB 1, GB 2, GB 3–19 as a whole, GB 14, GB 20, GB 21, GB 24, GB 26, GB 29, GB 30, GB 34, GB 37, GB 39, GB 40 and GB 41.

GB 1 *Tong Zi Liao* (Bone of the Eye or Pupil Crevice) 瞳子髎 ★★★

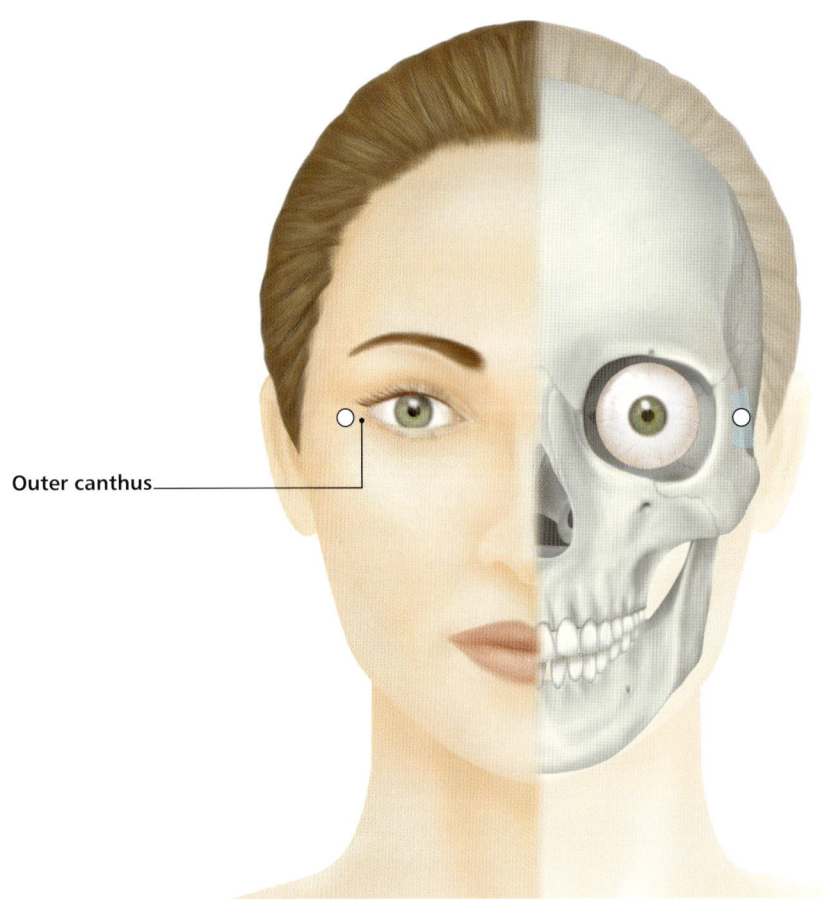

Outer canthus

Location
Situated 0.5 cun lateral to the outer canthus of the eye, in the depression at the lateral end of the border.

Needle
Needle only to 0.4 cun using a transverse insertion directed to the back of the head.

> Do not manipulate the needle as this area will bruise easily.

Moxa and pressure
Moxa is not contraindicated but due to its proximity to the eye it is hardly ever used. Use only stationary or gentle pressure with the finger pads and be careful not to use oil on the fingers or any substance that may irritate the patient's eyes.

Indications
This point, naturally, is used mainly for localised complaints. Symptoms and conditions include; pain, inflammation, itching and redness in the eye, conjunctivitis, trigeminal neuralgia, facial paralysis, eye deviation and diminished vision.

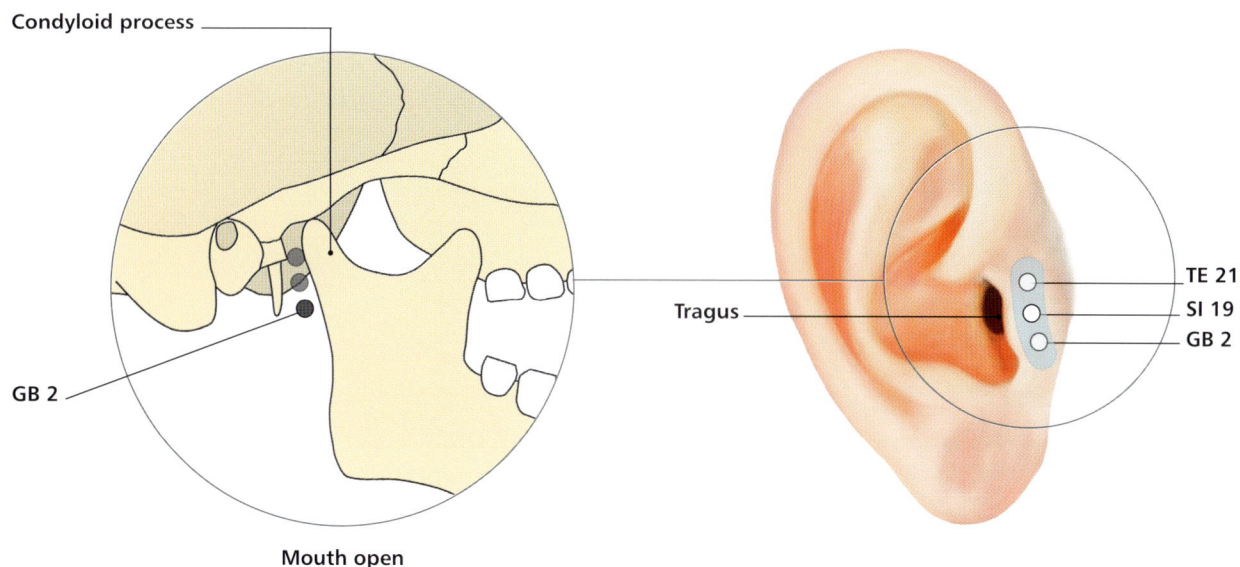

Location
Situated in the depression anterior to the supratragic notch, directly below SI 19, posterior to the mandible.

Needle
Needle up to 1 cun with a perpendicular insertion directed posteriorly, or TE 21, SI 19 and GB 2 may be treated together by threading through subcutaneously.

Moxa and pressure
Direct moxa is contraindicated but a moxa stick is permissible using mild stimulation only. Acupressure can be very useful in TMJ conditions and general stress.

Indications
Either in isolation or combined with SI 19 and TE 21, GB 2, may be used in most symptoms and conditions associated with the ear and TMJ as well as generalised stress symptoms. Symptoms and conditions include; pain, inflammation, itching and congestion of the ear, tinnitus, deafness, facial pain and paralysis, facial and trigeminal neuralgia, headache, migraine, TMJ syndrome and stress release.

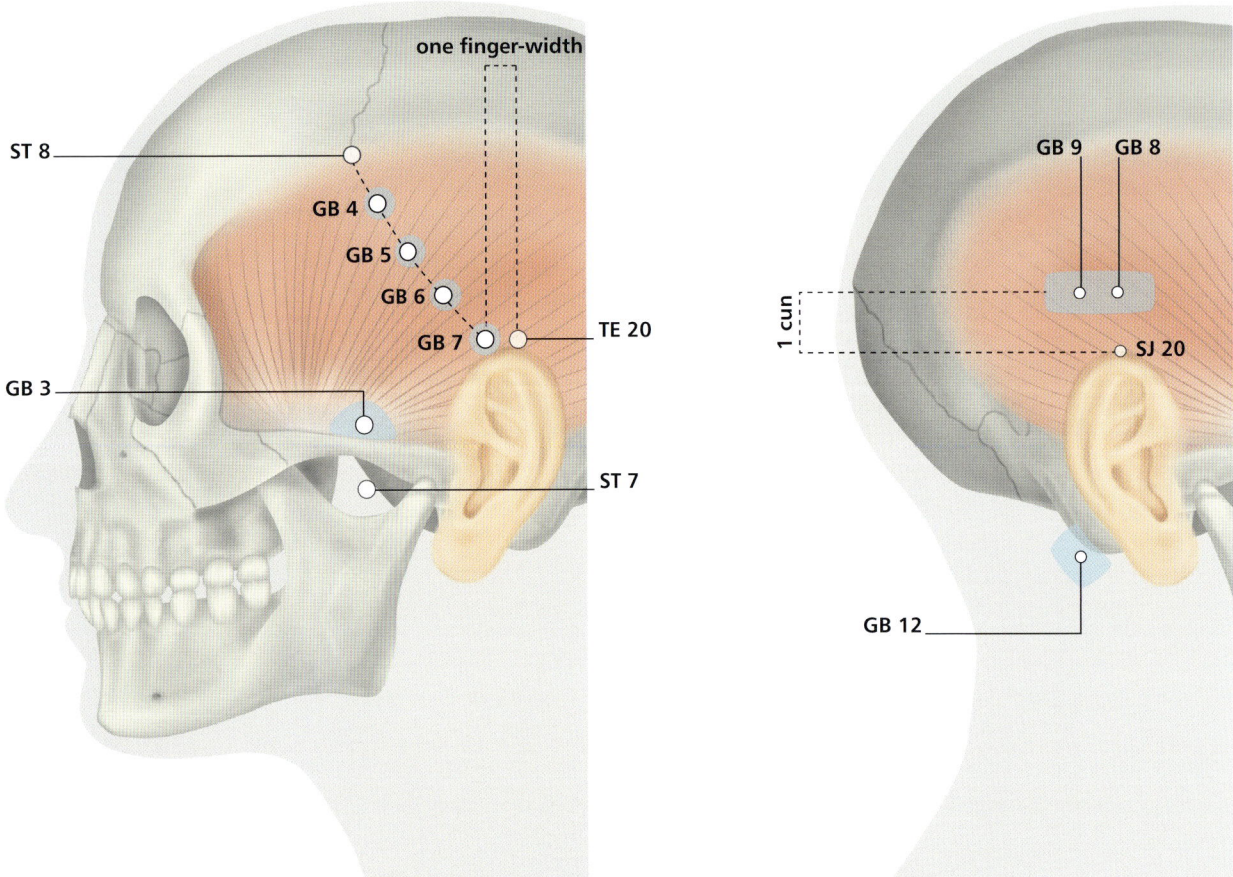

Location

This group of acupoints are situated on the lateral aspect of the skull and form a complicated zigzag line over the temporal, parietal, occipital and frontal bones. (See diagram above and the meridian diagram on previous page for individual locations.)

Needle

Needling in all cases is superficial – up to 0.4 cun and with a perpendicular insertion.

Moxa and pressure

With a few exceptions, moxa is impossible because of the presence of hair. Even when the patient has no hair, these points do not usually require moxa. Pressure techniques are paramount and form the basis of such therapies as cranio-sacral therapy, indian head massage as well as many other forms of traditional pressure and massage philosophies.

Indications

They are wonderful acupoints in the treatment of stress-related conditions such as depression, worry, anxiety, hypertension, palpitations, digestive imbalance, diaphragmatic tension, headache and migraine. Some philosophies indicate that stimulating pressure is indicated whilst others promote stationary pressure.

GB 14 *Yang Bai* (Yang White)

陽白 ★★★ Needle ★★★★ Pressure

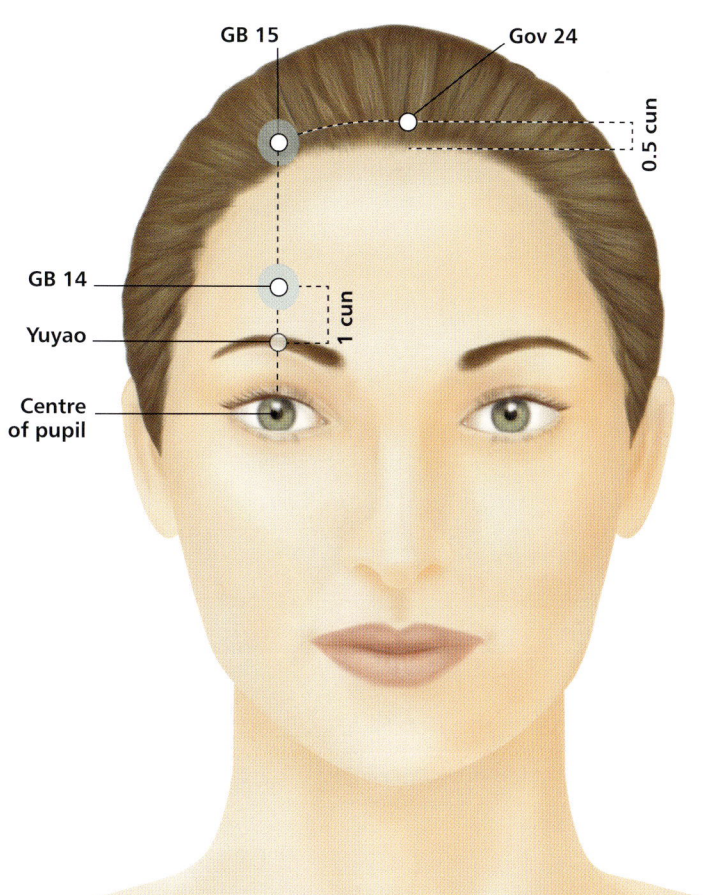

GB 15   Gov 24

0.5 cun

GB 14

1 cun

Yuyao

Centre
of pupil

Location
Situated on the forehead, in a shallow depression 1 cun above the midpoint of the eyebrow.

Needle
Needle up to 0.5 cun in an inferior direction having pinched the skin to needle subcutaneously.

Moxa and pressure

Direct moxa is forbidden but a moxa stick is acceptable; use mild moxa only and be careful that smoke does not enter the patient's eyes. Acupressure is very useful at the point, see 'special properties'.

Indications
GB 14 is a very important point to relax the forehead, brighten the eyes and calm the mind. Symptoms and conditions include headache, dizziness, forehead pain, excessive lacrimation, deviation of the eye and facial paralysis, twitching or spasm of the eyelids.

Special properties
GB 14 is colloquially called the 'hypnotherapy' point. In another of my books, *Acupressure and Reflextherapy in the Treatment of Medical Conditions*, I coined this term after describing it as one of the Listening Posts on the skull. This point is used to assess 'emotional energy' of the patient prior to treatment.

GB 20 *Feng Chi* (Wind Pool)

風池 ★★★★★

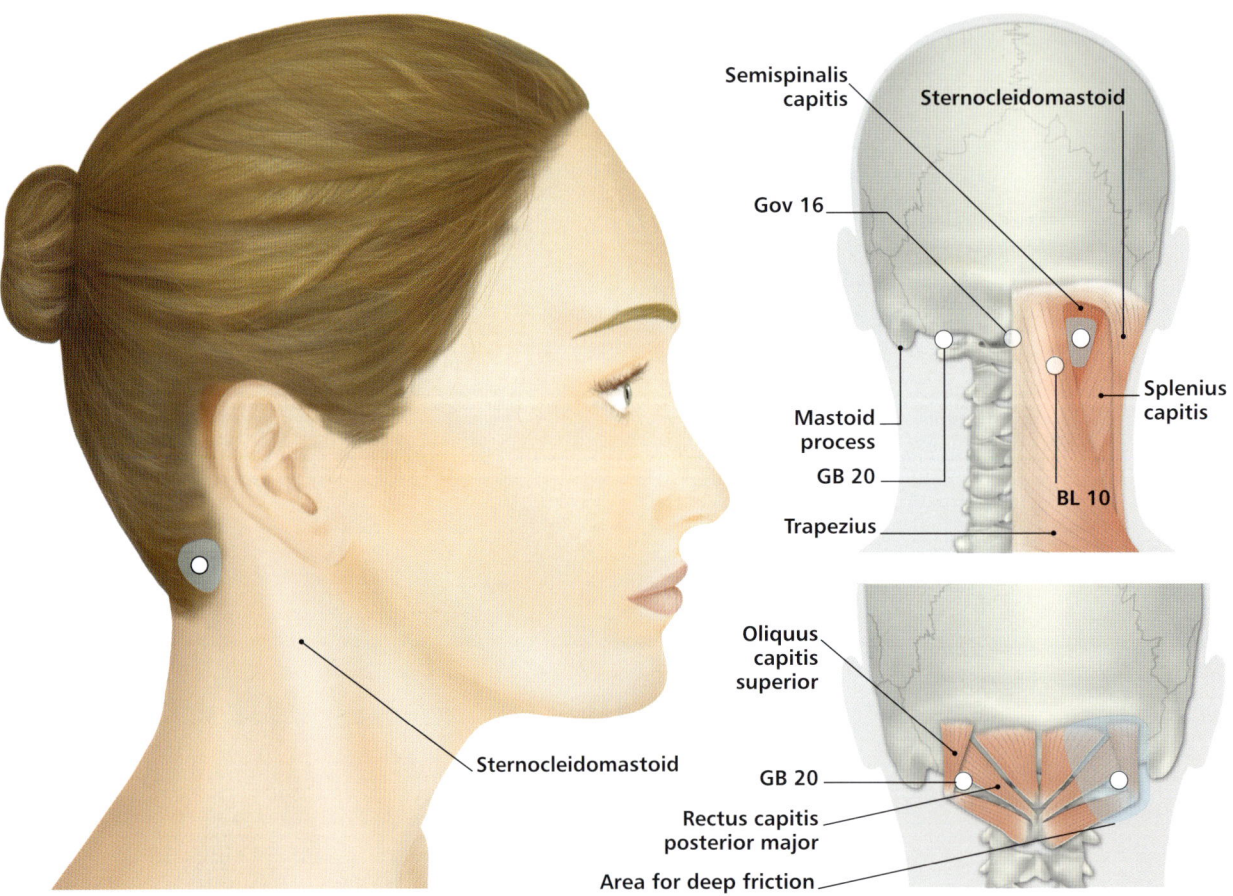

Location
Situated below the occipital bone in the depression between the start of the sternocleidomastoid process and the trapezius muscle.

Needle
Needle up to 1.2 cun using an oblique insertion directed towards the opposite corner of the mouth.

> Be aware that very occasionally needling at this point can bring about shock and fainting due to sympathetic nerve stimulation.

Moxa and pressure
Direct moxa is difficult at this point due to hair being present. A moxa stick may be used at this point and along the Gall Bladder channel towards the shoulder. There are several different acupressure techniques that may be applied at this influential point; it may be stretched (along with the occipital base), stimulated in the case of attempting to improve blood flow to the head or sedated to aid headaches and wind dizziness. Magnets are also very effective between GB 20 and GB 21 to help in cervical spine pain and dizziness.

Indications
GB 20 has a marked effect on the head and brain and is an important point in reducing pain and calming the mind. Symptoms and conditions that this important acupoint is used for are headache, migraine, eye inflammation, dizziness, vertigo, stiff neck, hypotension (postural), tinnitus, impaired hearing, Ménière's syndrome, facial paralysis, TMJ syndrome, vertigo, nose bleeds, poor memory, mental restlessness, irritability and mood swings.

Special properties
Many traditional manipulative therapies use GB 20 as a reflected point of the superior and lateral aspect of the sacrum and, as such, may be used in the treatment of sacral, sacro-iliac and lower lumbar conditions.

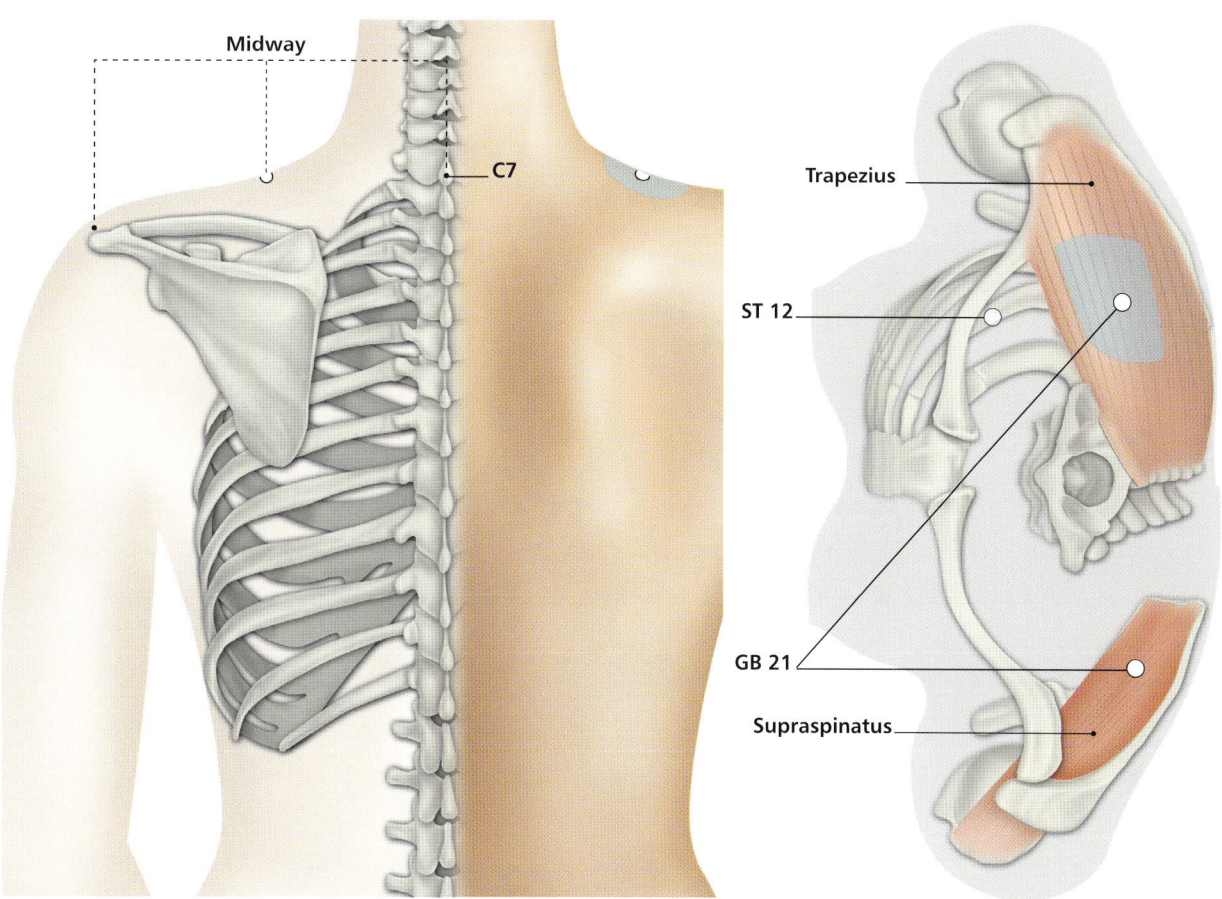

Location

Situated at the midpoint between the depression below the spinous process of C7 and the acromion.

Needle

Up to 1.5 cun using a posterior oblique insertion into the trapezius muscle fibres. It may also be inserted up to 0.8 cun using a perpendicular approach.

Do not needle any deeper as there is a risk of pneumothorax through the lung apex – ALSO do not treat during pregnancy, or in patients with low blood pressure or severe energy depletion.

Moxa and pressure

Direct moxa may be difficult to administer especially if the patient is lying down but a moxa stick is extremely useful at this point in energy depletion. This acupoint may be acutely painful due to the underlying adjacency of the brachial plexus and because the trapezius muscle is often in spasm. For these reasons it is not wise to massage this point too vigourously. Sedation acupressure can work wonders in head and neck conditions and to help clear the mind and relax the tissues.

Indications

This wonderful polychrest of a point has many different uses and actions. It is excellent in helping pain in the head and neck, calming and clearing the mind, relaxing the throat, treating constipation, helping with gynaecological conditions as well as localised trapezius spasm. Symptoms and conditions include headache, migraine, sinusitis, facial paralysis, TMJ syndrome, tinnitus, deafness, amnesia and insomnia. It is one of the great points in treating disorders of the neck and shoulders such as stiff and painful neck, sore shoulders, frozen shoulder, trapezius spasm and difficulty with lifting the arm. Due to the channel's connection with the uterus, it is very effective in treating amenorrhea, abnormal uterine bleeding, prolonged labour, mastitis and difficult lactation. Finally, it helps with dizziness, vertigo, hemiplegia and many other neurological symptoms.

Special properties

GB 21 is associated with easing pain and spasms during the final stages of labour. It is also one the greatest points in helping people who cannot express themselves or who suffer from shyness and diffidence.

GB 24 *Ri Yue* (Sun and Moon)

日月 ★★★

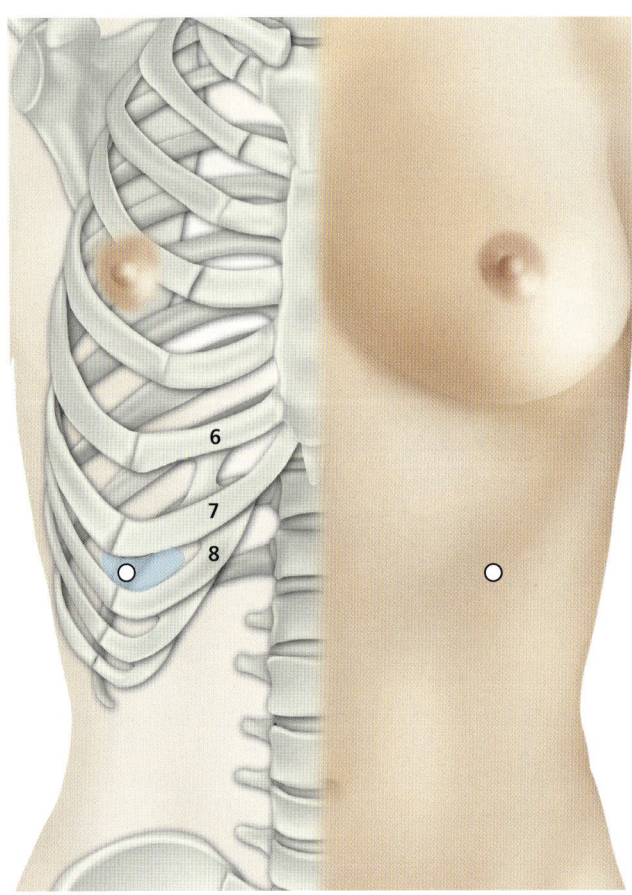

Location
Situated below the breast in the 7th intercostal space, 4 cun lateral to the ventral midline.

Needle
Insert to a depth of up to 0.8 cun using an oblique direction along the intercostal space.

Moxa and pressure
This point will take heavy moxa, direct or moxa stick in cases of liver and gall bladder energy depletion. Gentle massage may be performed to help 'stuckness' of chi in the gall bladder – be aware that this is an extremely tender point.

Indications
GB 24 is used mostly for disorders of the liver and gall bladder and to treat sore ribs in the region. Symptoms and conditions include nausea, epigastric pain, heartburn, gastric ulcers, abdominal distension, mastitis, rib pain and intercostal shingles. It has also been used in treating some psychosomatic disorders such as depression, sadness, indecision and lack of fibre or metal.

Special properties
GB 24 is the Alarm (Mu) point of the gall bladder organ and is used to indicate gall bladder disorders.

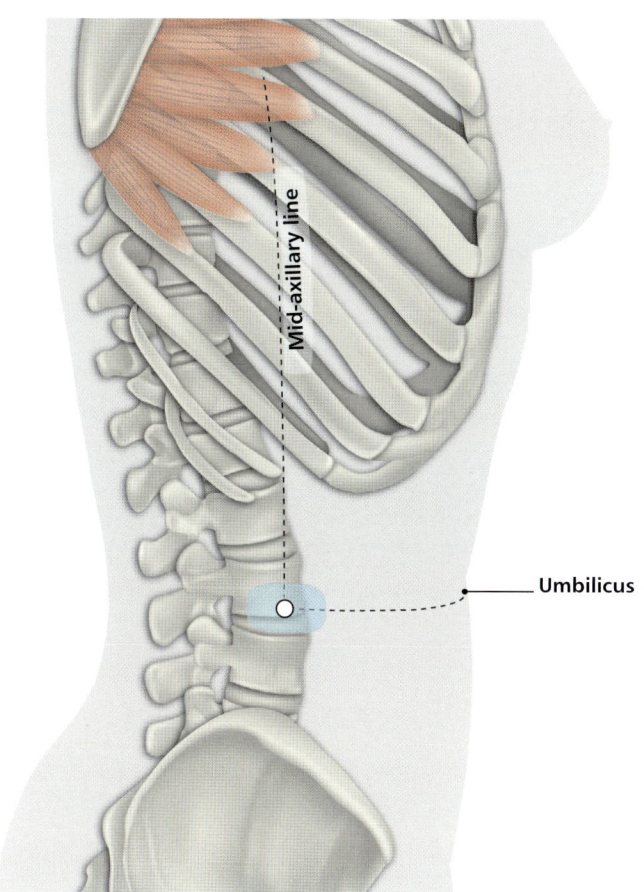

Mid-axillary line

Umbilicus

Location

Situated on the lateral aspect of the abdomen, level with the umbilicus, below the end of the eleventh rib on the mid-axillary line.

Needle

Up to 1 cun using a perpendicular approach.

> Do not needle any deeper in case the peritoneum is ruptured.

Moxa and pressure

Moxa, with the patient in side-lying, is very useful to create heat and energy to the lower abdomen. It is specifically used to ease coldness in the loin region. This is also a useful self-help acupressure point in doing the same thing, see 'special properties'.

Indications

GB 26 is one of the unsung heroes in acupuncture in that it is surprisingly versatile. It may be used for energising, strengthening and warming the lower heater that includes the abdomen and uterus. It is therefore used in the following symptoms and conditions: pain, distension and flaccidity of the abdomen, coldness in the loins, amenorrhoea, leucorrhoea and irregular menstruation.

Special properties

GB 26 is the most powerful acupoint on the Dai Mai (Girdle) channel, which is one of the extraordinary vessels that is controlled by the Key point of GB 41. It is therefore used in all cases of lower abdominal and uterine congestion. This point is also used as a self-help point in weight loss programmes because it helps to strengthen the abdomen. Magnets may also be useful in this endeavour.

GB 29 *Ju Liao* (Stationary Crevice)

居髎 ★★★★

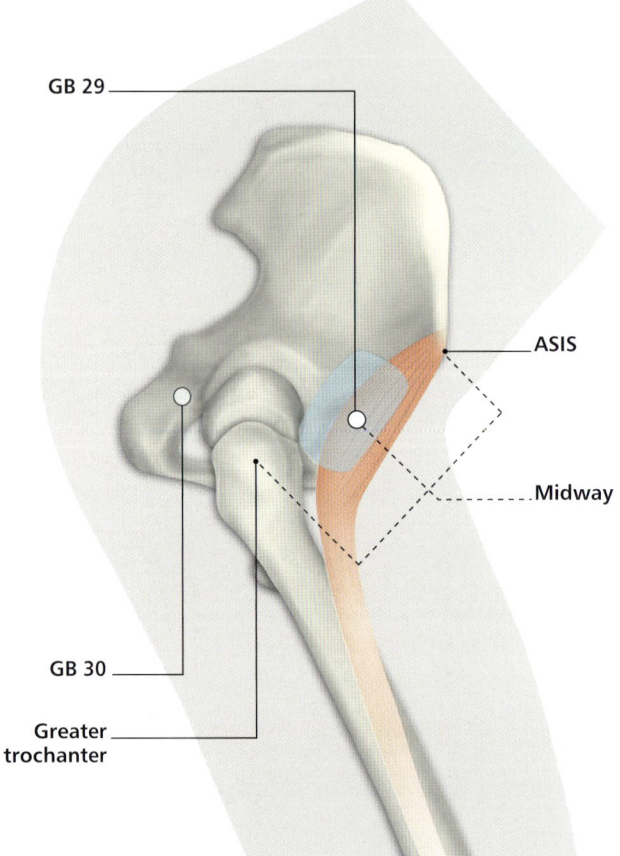

Location

Situated superior to the hip joint at the centre of the large depression formed when the hip joint is flexed. It is midway between the anterior superior iliac spine (ASIS) and the greater trochanter.

Needle

This is a very deep acupoint and therefore requires needling up to 2.5 cun with a perpendicular approach.

Moxa and pressure

This point answers well to heavy moxa in cases of chronic pain and stiffness of the hip joint. A heated needle is also extremely effective. Deep stimulating or passive pressure may help anterior hip pain. This may be performed by the finger pad, thumb pad or even the elbow.

Indications

GB 29 works on many hip disorders – pain and inflammation, osteoarthritis, capsulitis of the lateral and anterior aspect of the joint and lumbo-sacral pain and stiffness. It also helps with improving blood and lymphatic circulation to the leg.

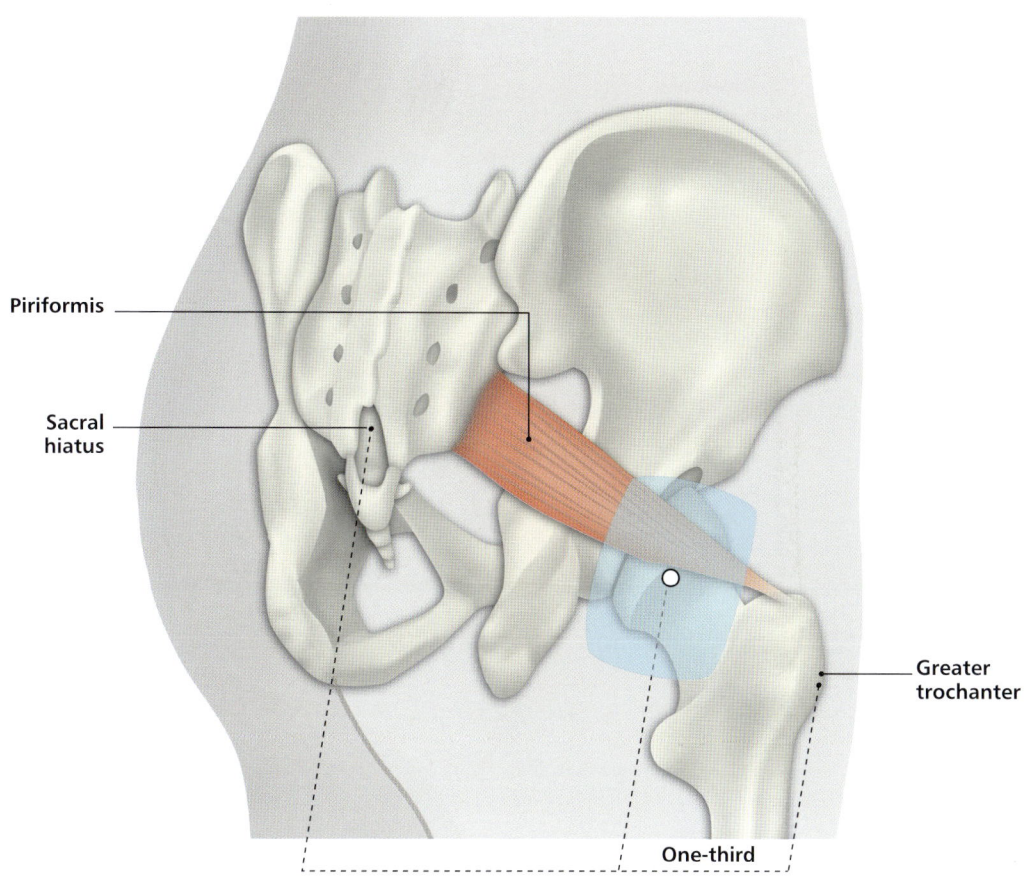

Piriformis

Sacral
hiatus

Greater
trochanter

One-third

Location

Situated in the large depression behind the
hip joint, one-third of the distance between the
greater trochanter and the sacral hiatus. The
point is located with the thigh flexed. The ideal
patient position is side-lying so that GB 29 and
GB 30 may be treated at the same time.

Needle

This acupoint is deep within the tissues so
requires a 3 cun depth using a perpendicular or
slightly oblique insertion.

Moxa and pressure

For moxa and pressure use GB 39. Acupressure
is also indicated in sciatica.

Indications

GB 30 is a wonderful acupoint in the treatment
of hip and lower spine conditions. Symptoms
and conditions include sciatica, hip pain and
stiffness, osteoarthritis, atrophy and weakness
in the lower limb, hemiplegia and lymphatic
and blood stagnation.

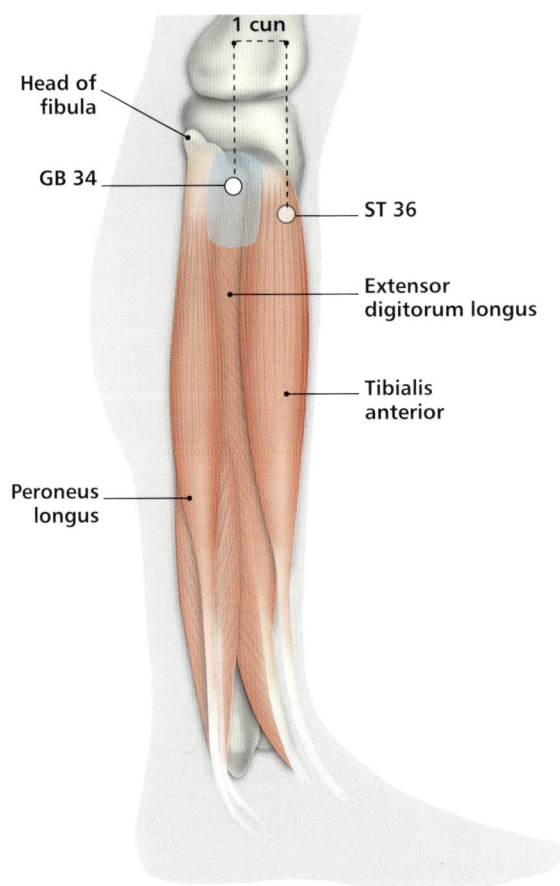

Location
Situated in the depression anterior and inferior to the head of fibula. It is 1 cun lateral and superior to ST 36.

Needle
Up to 1.5 cun using a perpendicular approach.

Moxa and pressure
Heavy moxa is indicated in general energy depletion, especially of the muscular system. Acupressure may be applied in several ways. Stimulating massage should be applied as a prelude to the main thrust of treatment in cases of chronic tendon and muscle imbalance. Deep massage (such as connective tissue massage – CTM) may be performed down the length of the Gall Bladder meridian so as to aid circulatory stagnation in such conditions as hemiplegia. Sedative acupressure using a light to deep touch is used in localised lateral knee and superior tibio-fibular pain and stiffness.

Indications
Along with its close partner ST 36, GB 34 is used when there is general depletion of energy in the body. It is also said to be the Gathering (Hui) point of sinews (tendons) and should be thought of in all acute and chronic conditions of that soft tissue type. It also helps support the liver and gall bladder organs as well as being used in spasticity and flaccidity conditions (such as hemiplegia). Symptoms and conditions include hypertension, headaches (hemi-cranial), irritability and anger, jaundice and cholecystitis, abdominal distension and pain, diarrhoea, premenstrual tension and mastitis. GB 34 is also extremely useful in all muscular and tendon conditions – acute or chronic and helping musculo-skeletal conditions along its channel. These include TMJ, shoulder, cervical spine, lumbar spine, hip, knee and ankle.

Special properties
Because of its propensity to aid musculo-skeletal conditions and also to aid in general energy depletion, GB 34 is perfectly suited to pre-match or pre-event 'tuning' prior to an important athletic event. Athletes should be encouraged to used bilateral GB 34 points as a self-help procedure.

GB 37 *Guang Ming* (Illumination or Bright Light)

光明 ★★★

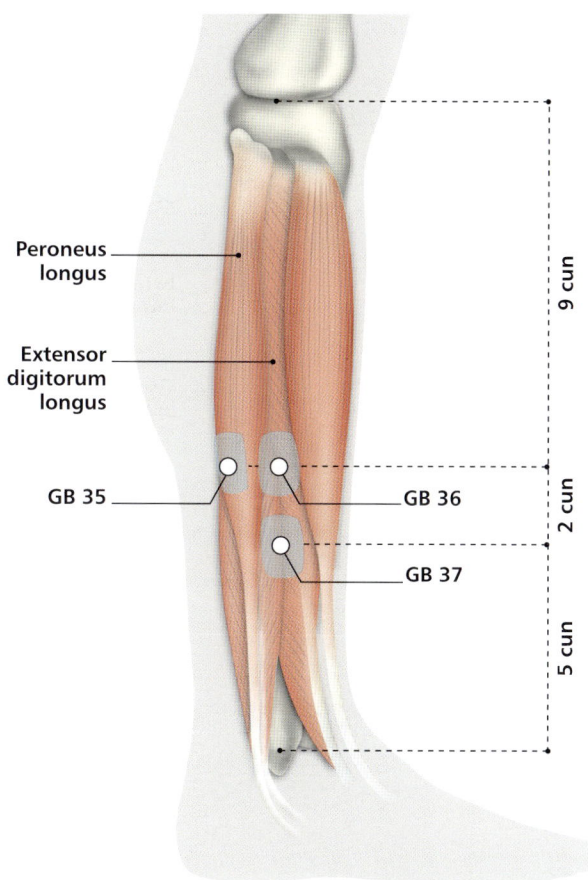

Peroneus longus

Extensor digitorum longus

GB 35

GB 36

GB 37

9 cun

2 cun

5 cun

Location

Situated in the depression between the peroneus longus and brevis and the extensor digitorum longus muscles, at the anterior border of the fibula, 5 cun proximal to the lateral malleolus.

Needle

Up to 1.5 cun using a perpendicular insertion.

Moxa and pressure

Moxa is not contraindicated but rarely used. Acupressure may be useful as a distal point in eye conditions, also in conjunction with other local points around the mid aspect of the fibula; it can be used in shoulder pain and stiffness.

Indications

GB 37 is the Connecting (Luo) point to LR 5, thus it is used in gall bladder and liver organic imbalance. Symptoms and conditions include gall bladder colic, tension and pain in the chest and breast region and the early stages of mastitis, headache, teeth grinding, irritability and depression.

Special properties

GB 37 is a wonderful distal point in the treatment of eye conditions. These include; iritis, pain, itching, grittiness, inflammation, excessive lacrimation, night blindness and failing vision.

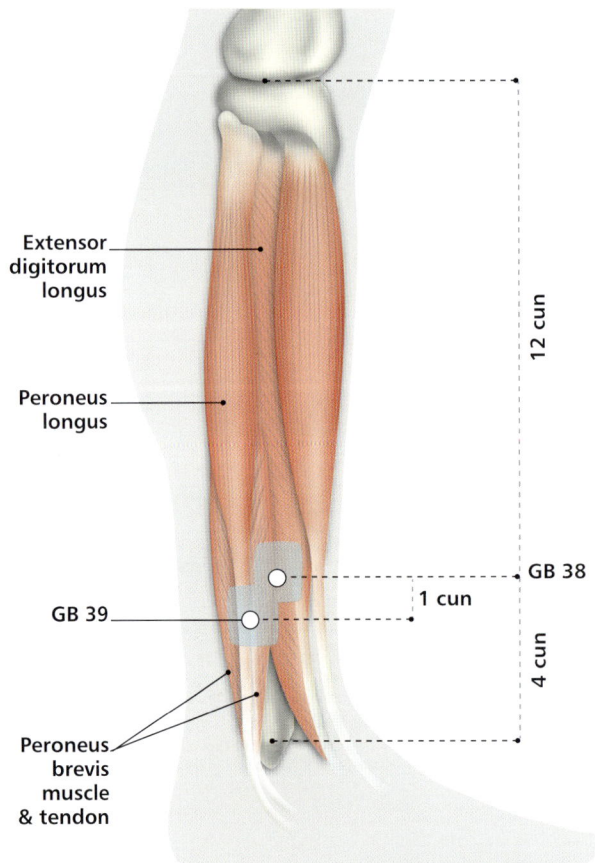

Location
Situated 3 cun proximal to the prominence of the lateral malleolus on the anterior aspect of the fibula.

Needle
Up to 1 cun using a perpendicular insertion.

Moxa and pressure
Moxa is very effective on this point in chronic conditions affecting tendons and muscles, e.g. rheumatoid arthritis. Acupressure may be used in conjunction with other Gall Bladder and some localized Stomach meridian points to help acute and chronic tendo-muscular and soft tissue conditions.

Indications
GB 39 is specifically used to aid conditions associated with tendo-muscular conditions. Symptoms and conditions include spinal conditions, particularly the cervical spine, osteoporosis, osteoarthritis, rheumatoid arthritis, ankylosis, pain, stiffness and swelling of the joints, lower limb symptoms of hemiplegia. GB 39 has a limited effect on channel symptoms. In TCM it is called the Gathering (Hui) point for the Marrow.

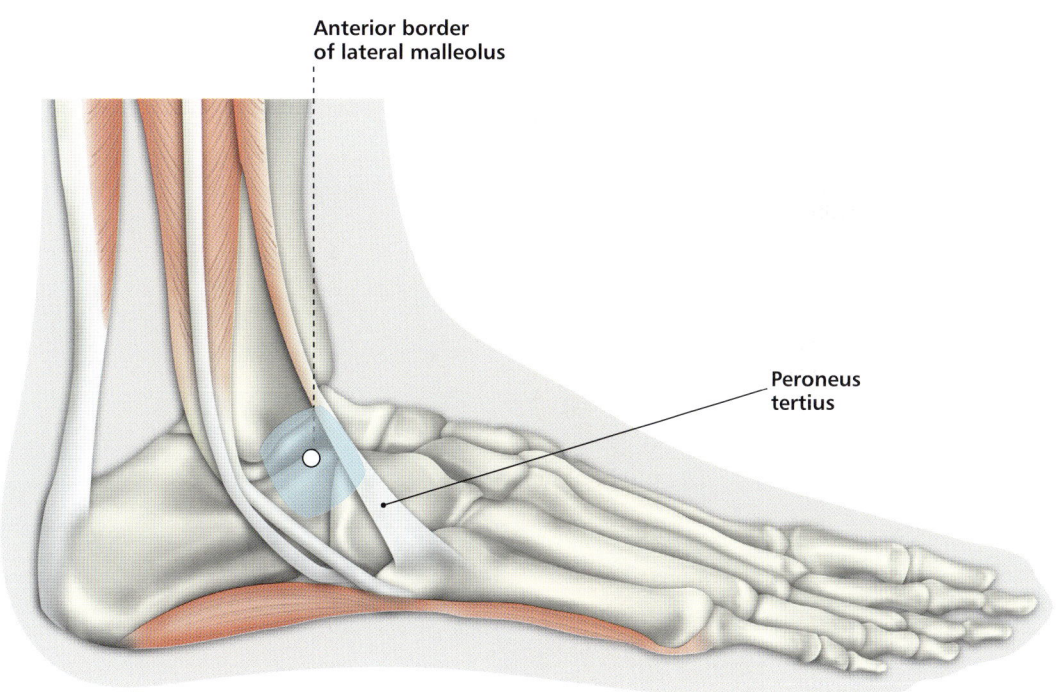

Anterior border
of lateral malleolus

Peroneus
tertius

Location

Situated anterior and distal to the lateral malleolus, in a depression lateral to the tendon of the extensor digitorum longus muscle.

Needle

Up to 0.8 cun using a perpendicular insertion.

Deeper needling could jeopardize the saphenous vein or the peroneal nerve.

Moxa and pressure

Use mild moxabustion only to aid channel energy insufficiency and also to help with chronic and repeated lateral ligament tears of the ankle joint.

Indications

GB 40 is the Source (Yuan) point of the Gall Bladder channel and therefore has a special relationship with the gall bladder. It is a very good point in the treatment of diseases and conditions of the gall bladder including hypochondrial distension and pain, cholecystitis, heartburn and shoulder discomfort. It is also an excellent point in eye conditions. Further, it has a good reputation in the treatment of certain psychosomatic conditions such as depression, weakness of the mind and irritability. Finally, it is a very suitable point for localized treatment of acute and chronic lateral ankle sprains.

GB 41 *Zu Lin Qi* (Foot Governor of Tears)

足臨泣 ★★★★★

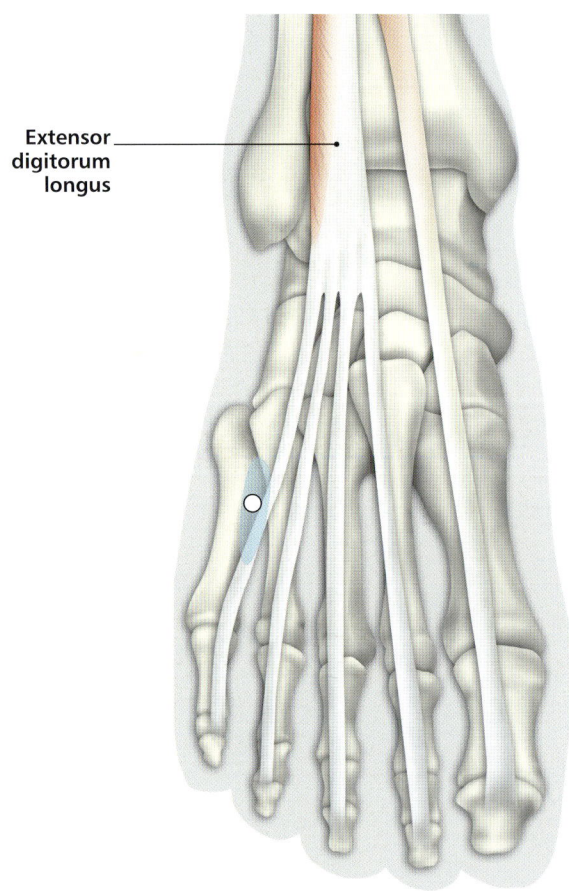

Extensor digitorum longus

Location
Situated on the dorsum of the foot, in the proximal angle between the 4th and 5th metatarsal bones, in the depression lateral to the tendon of the extensor digitorum longus to the little toe.

Needle
Up to 0.5 cun with a perpendicular insertion. Be careful to move the tendon slightly medially so as to affect the point.

Moxa and pressure
This point answers extremely well to stimulating moxa both directly and with a moxa stick in all cases of channel sluggishness. In particular it is very effective in helping hemiplegia. Pressure can be effective but be aware that the point is acutely sore to the touch.

Indications
GB 41 is the most energetically 'powerful' and useful channel point on the foot. It is the Wood (Horary) point and is therefore used predominantly in all Gall Bladder meridian imbalances. Symptoms and conditions include conditions of the eyes and ears, hemi-cranial headaches and migraine, paralysis and loss of sensation following this, pain in the abdominal and lumbar regions, dysmenorrhoea and regulating menstruation. It is also one of the acupoints that may be used for pain during childbirth.

Special properties
GB 41 is the Key (Opening) point of the Dai Mai (Girdle Vessel). It is therefore instrumental in aiding all symptoms associated with the Dai Mai, e.g. lower abdominal and uterine discomfort. GB 41 is usually linked with TE 5, which is the Key point of the Yangwei Mai (Regulating channel). These two may be treated in unison with needle, pressure or magnets and make a very powerful duo in the treatment of many diverse conditions.

Liver Meridian (LR)

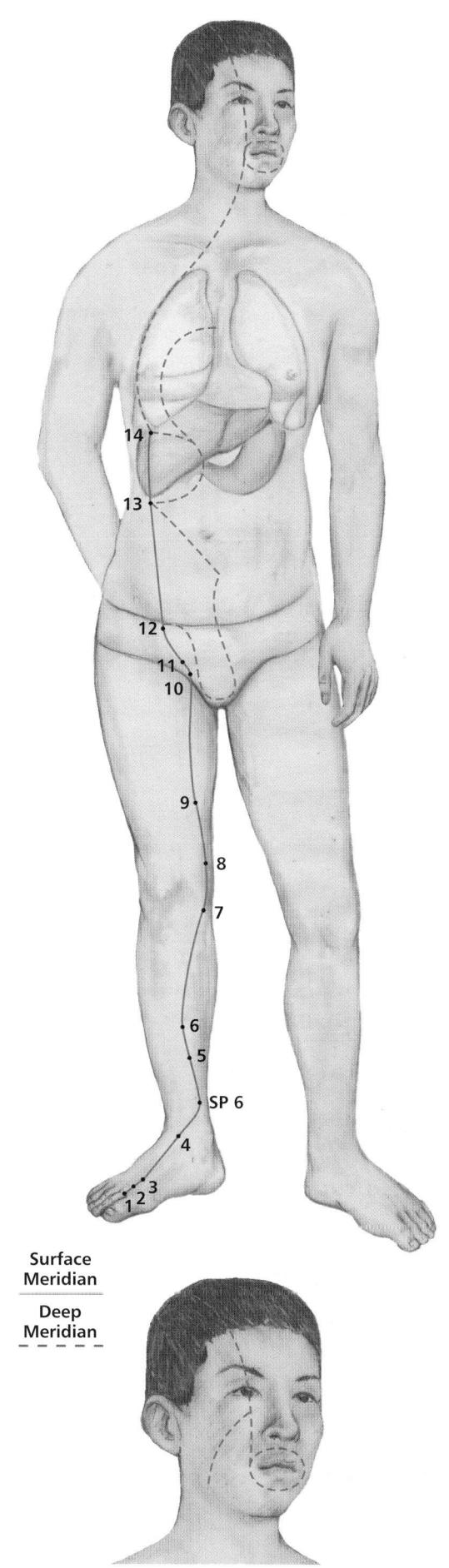

Surface Meridian

Deep Meridian

The Liver meridian represents the Yin aspect of the Wood element. There are only fourteen (14) points on the surface channel from great toe to the chest. The meridian commences at the lateral aspect of the great toe and travels up the medial aspect of the leg to the very medial aspect of the knee and up to the groin. Here the channel diverges into a deep channel that supplies the genitalia before linking back to the surface channel again at LR 13 and LR 14 below the breast where the surface channel ends. A further deeper channel supplies the diaphragm and lungs before ascending to the top of the head via the mouth and eyes. We shall discuss LR 2, LR 3, LR 5, LR 8, LR 13 and LR 14.

LR 2 *Xing Jian* (Moving Between)

行間 ★★★

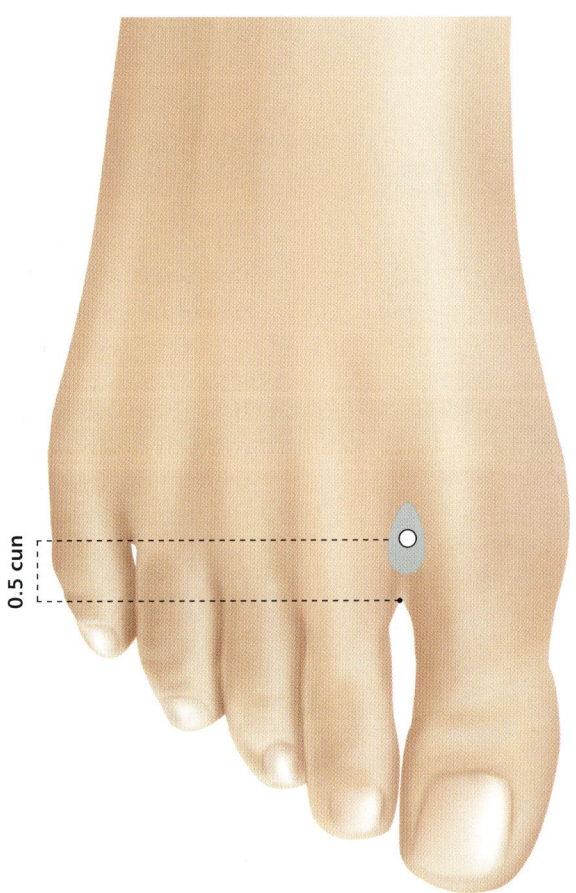

0.5 cun

Location
Situated on the dorsal aspect of the foot, in the web between the 1st and 2nd metatarsophalangeal joints.

Needle
This point is needled either up to 0.5 cun with a perpendicular insertion or, more commonly, up to 1 cun with an oblique insertion directed towards the heel.

Moxa and pressure
Moxa may be used in energy depletion in the liver or following a stroke. Acupressure is very useful on this point as it works well in clearing heat and inflammation from the head and eyes; do not use tonifying techniques.

Indications
LR 2 is the Fire (Tonification) point of the Liver channel and is mainly used in easing pain and inflammation along the channel. Symptoms and conditions include migraine, headache, eye inflammation, dizziness, hypertension, facial paralysis, groin strain, genital conditions, irregular menstruation, insomnia and irritability. LR 2 is also indicated in many conditions affecting the bladder, especially cystitis, urinary retention and incontinence.

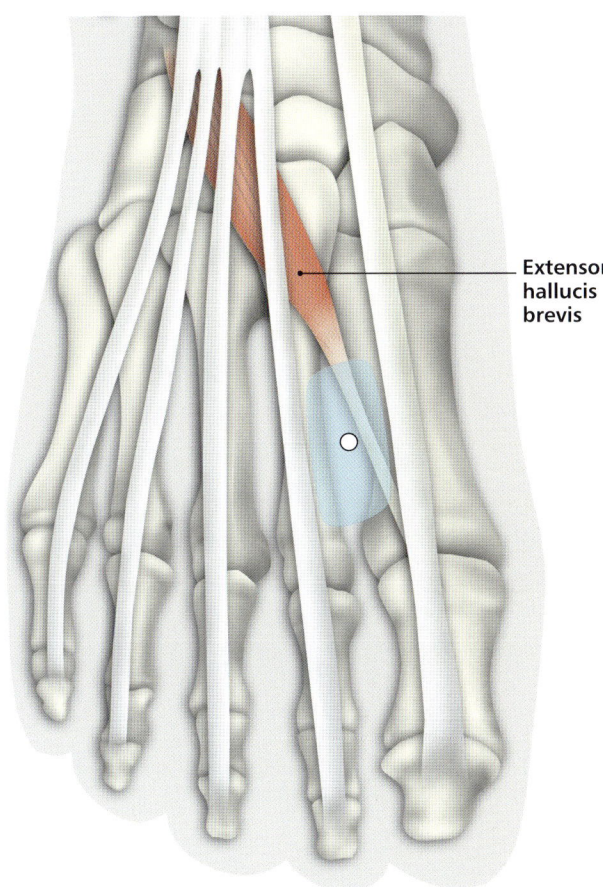

Extensor
hallucis
brevis

Location
Situated on the dorsum of the foot, in the depression distal to the proximal corner between the 1st and 2nd metatarsal bones.

Needle
Up to 1 cun using a perpendicular insertion.

Moxa and pressure
Moxa is indicated in channel energy depletion and in situations of muscular congestion. Acupressure is extremely effective on this point and ranges from stationary pressure for local conditions and eye anomalies to tonifying massage in energy depletion. (See 'special properties'.)

Indications
LR 3 is probably the second most used acupoint on the body next to LI 4. In anatomical terms these two points are located in the same position – one on the hand and the other on the foot. Its actions and indications are as follows:

- Either in isolation or in combination with LI 4 (known as the Four Gates), LR 3 is extensively used in anaesthesia and pain relief for almost anywhere in the body – it is especially useful in muscular pain and spasm.
- It has an excellent calming effect on the mind and is used to treat anger, irritability, frustration, mental restlessness, insomnia, nightmares, sighing and some of the physical symptoms associated with these symptoms.
- Due to the fact that the internal Liver channel supplies the eyes, mouth and head, LR 3 is a prime point in treatment of headaches, migraine, cranial nerve involvement, spasm, cramp, seizures and vertigo. The point has a great affinity for the eyes and is used extensively in all eye conditions.
- It is also indicated in many neurological conditions such as hemiplegia, symptoms of multiple sclerosis, paralysis, atrophy and facial paralysis.
- Using its property of being the Source (Yuan) point of the Liver channel, it has a direct link with the liver and, as such, is used in many liver and gall bladder conditions.
- It is also indicated in many gynaecological and respiratory conditions including tightness of the chest, throat inflammation, premenstrual symptoms, mastitis, infertility and vaginal discharge.
- It is a powerful point in the treatment of many musculo-skeletal conditions especially in athletes who over exert themselves and suffer from sprains and strains.
- It is one of the more powerful points in helping reduce hypertension.

Special properties
LR 3 is the first aid point in the treatment of cramp – anywhere in the body (including the diaphragm). Acupressure is preferable to needle, but the point just needs to be held with a moderate pressure for up to half a minute for cramp to be released; do NOT stimulate the point!

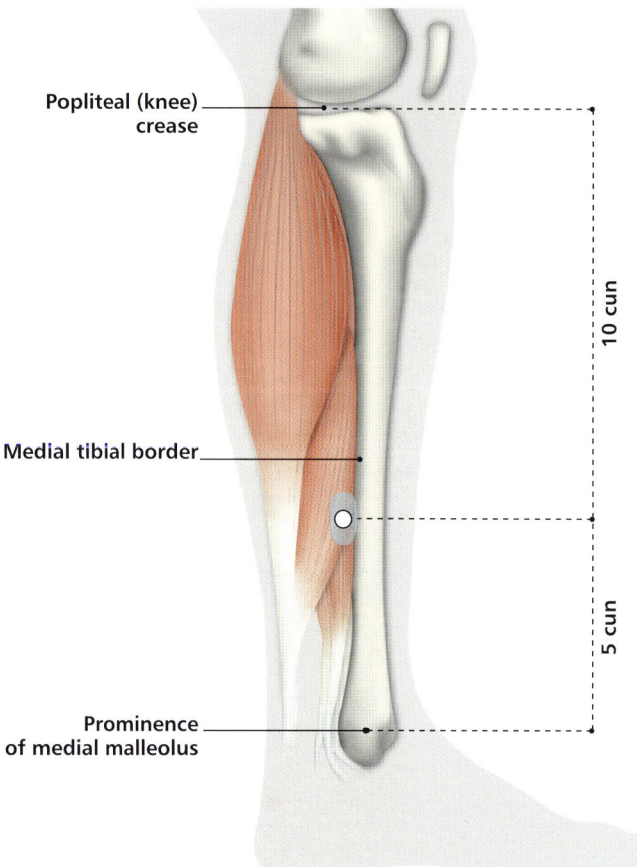

Popliteal (knee) crease

10 cun

Medial tibial border

5 cun

Prominence of medial malleolus

Location
Situated 5 cun superior to the medial malleolus just posterior to the medial tibial border.

Needle
Either up to 1 cun using a perpendicular approach or 1.5 cun depth if the approach is oblique.

> Do not needle any deeper for fear of affecting the crural or saphenous nerve.

Moxa and pressure
Direct and indirect moxa is indicated in channel depletion but also in any underlying local muscle condition such as shin splints. Acupressure is very effective on this point in the local treatment of shin splints in unison with other Liver, Spleen and Kidney acupoints on the posterior aspect of the tibia. The best way is, with oil, to perform some connective tissue massage deeply up the tibialis posterior. Please note that I believe that true shin splints is a condition affecting mostly the tibialis posterior and not the tibialis anterior which is known as anterior tibial compartment syndrome. For other pressure indications, see 'special properties'.

Indications
Although LR 5 may be used in many channel conditions such as eye, liver, gall bladder, chest and abdominal ones, it is in its effect on the uterus, pelvis and genitals that it excels. Symptoms and conditions include; pain, itching and inflammation of the genitalia or urethra, vaginal discharge, irregular menstruation, dysmenorrhoea, insufficient dilatation during labour, uterine prolapse, inguinal or scrotal hernia, prostatitis and impotence.

Special properties
In reflextherapy terms, LR 5 is one of the reflected points of the shoulder, in particular the medial aspect of the gleno-humeral joint. It is therefore very effective in pain, stiffness and frozen shoulder. This may be achieved with needle or better still with acupressure with the middle finger pad on LR 5 and the other middle finger pad on the region of the shoulder pain. Magnets on these two points are also effective. It is no surprise therefore that LR 5 is also one of the Key points of the Throat chakra which also controls the shoulders.

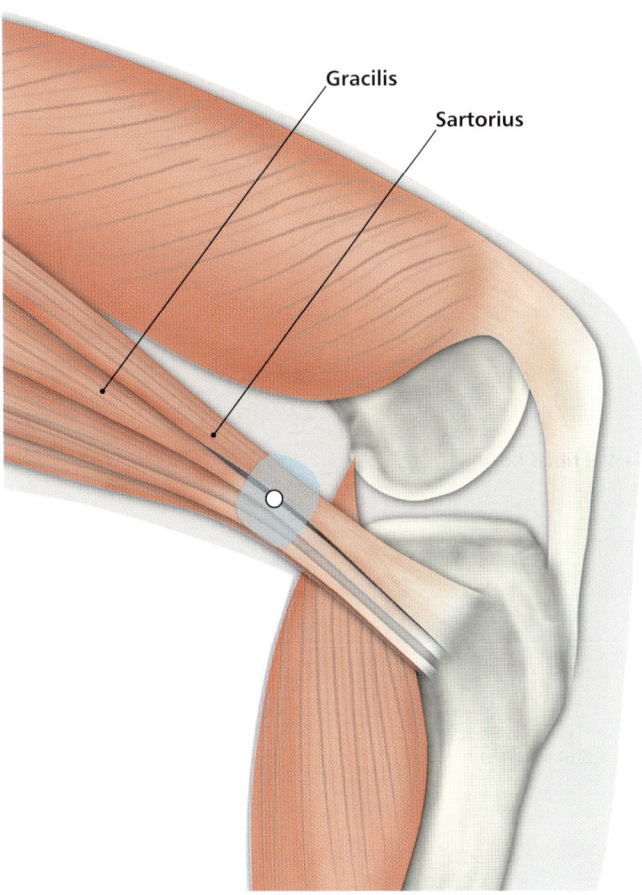

Gracilis

Sartorius

Location

Situated at the medial end of the popliteal crease, dorsal to the medial condyle of the tibia, in the depression at the anterior border of the semimembranosus and the semitendinosus muscles. The knee should be slightly flexed both in palpation and treatment.

Needle

Up to 1.5 cun with a perpendicular insertion.

> Deeper needling may pierce the great saphenous vein.

Moxa and pressure

Moxa with light stimulation only preferably using a moxa stick.

> Do not use moxa if there are any varicosities in the area.

Frictions may be applied across the two tendons or the point may be used with stationary acupressure in energy balancing with LI 11 on the lateral border of the elbow using parallel acupressure between the knee and elbow.

Indications

LR 8 is the Water (Tonification) point on the Liver channel. It therefore benefits the kidneys, bladder and urogenital system amongst others. Symptoms and conditions include itching and inflammation of the genital region, cystitis, urethritis, vaginal discharge, dysmenorrhoea, endometriosis, impotence and pain along the leg portion of the meridian.

Special properties

LR 8 is the Key (Opening) acupoint of both the Base chakra at Con 1/Gov 1 (major) and the Clavicular chakra at KI 27 (minor). It is therefore essential with either needle or pressure when utilizing these energy systems.

LR 13 *Zhang Men* (Completion Gate)

章門 ★★★★

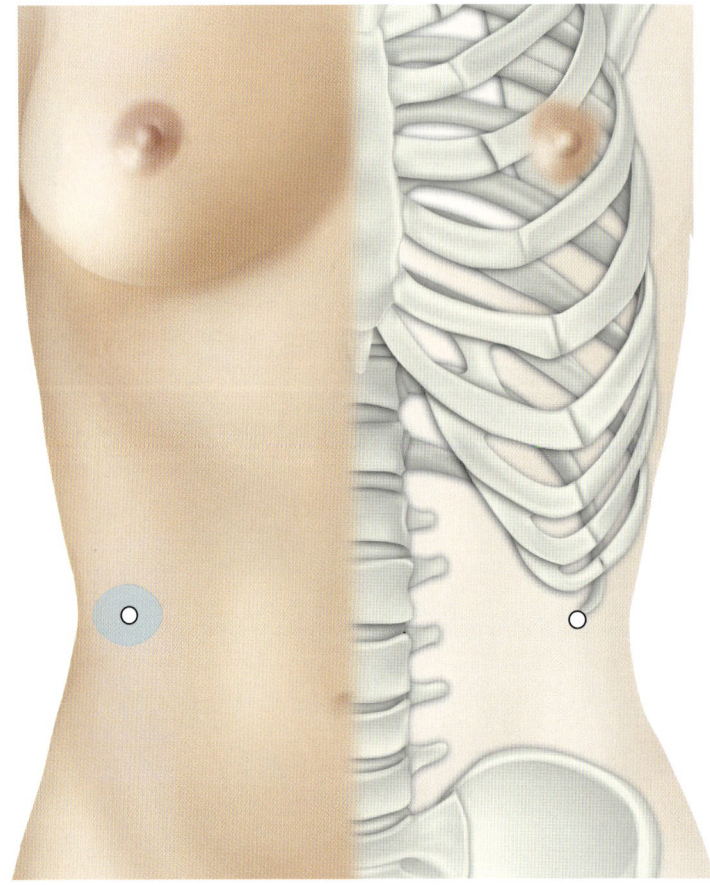

Location

Situated on the inferior border of the free end of the eleventh rib.

Needle

Up to 1.0 cun if using a perpendicular approach or up to 1.5 cun if using a transverse approach by needling along the line of the rib.

> Do not needle any deeper as there is a danger of puncturing the liver on the right or spleen on the left.

Moxa and pressure

This point will respond well to stimulating moxa in order to boost liver and spleen chi. Pressure is used in analysis (see 'special properties') but is very tender if used in treatment mode. Self-help acupressure may be helpful as patients do not massage with such vigour!

Indications

LR 13 is predominantly used in improving chi to the liver and spleen although it may be used for many other conditions, such as acute and chronic gastroenteritis, chronic diarrhoea, acute and chronic cholecystitis, abdominal distension, nausea and vomiting, chronic tiredness (especially to aid the recovery of patients with chronic fatigue syndrome), pain and inflammation in the ribs and thorax.

Special properties

LR 13 is the Alarm (Mu) point of the spleen and indicates when this organ is in a state of distress and requires treatment.

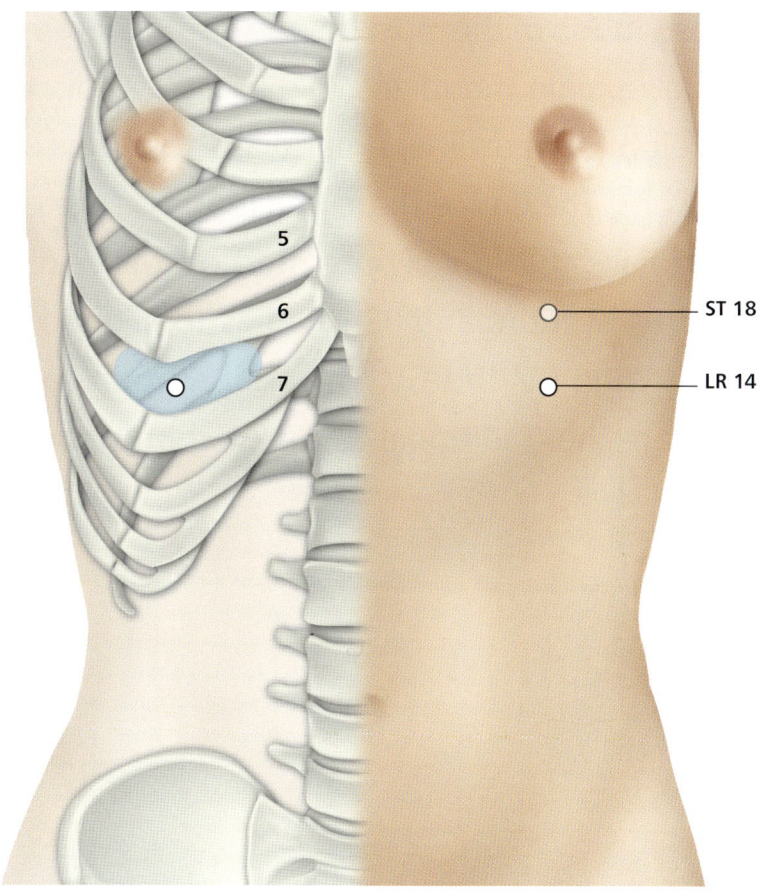

Location
Situated below the nipple in the sixth intercostal space, 4 cun lateral to the midline.

Needle
Up to 0.8 cun using an oblique insertion directed laterally along the intercostal space.

> Do not needle any deeper as there is a considerable risk of puncturing the lung tissue.

Moxa and pressure
Only use very light moxa, if at all. Acupressure on the point and massage around the area is excellent in helping relieve lymphatic stagnation due to chronic mastitis or following breast surgery.

> Never use massage directly on inflamed lymph nodes or in any cases of active cancerous tissue.

Indications
This much used acupoint is important in the treatment of many liver, spleen, stomach and gynaecological conditions. Symptoms and conditions include breast pain, mastitis, premenstrual syndrome, tightness and pain in the chest, irritability, abdominal pain and distension, diaphragmatic spasm, hepatitis, gallstones, stomach ache, gastritis, nausea and vomiting.

Special properties
LR 14 is the Alarm (Mu) point of the liver and is used in both analysis and treatment in acute hepatitis.

That concludes description of the most powerful and therapy useful acupoints that lie on the twelve main meridians. We shall now discuss the two most important of the eight extraordinary meridians that have no single organic or system associations. The Conception (Ren Mai) and the Governor (Du Mai) are unilateral meridians that are represented on the midlines of the body. I shall use the initials of 'Con' and 'Gov' so as to avoid confusion between the more popularly used CV and GV. The abbreviations of Ren and Du may be used but these are the traditional forms of abbreviation.

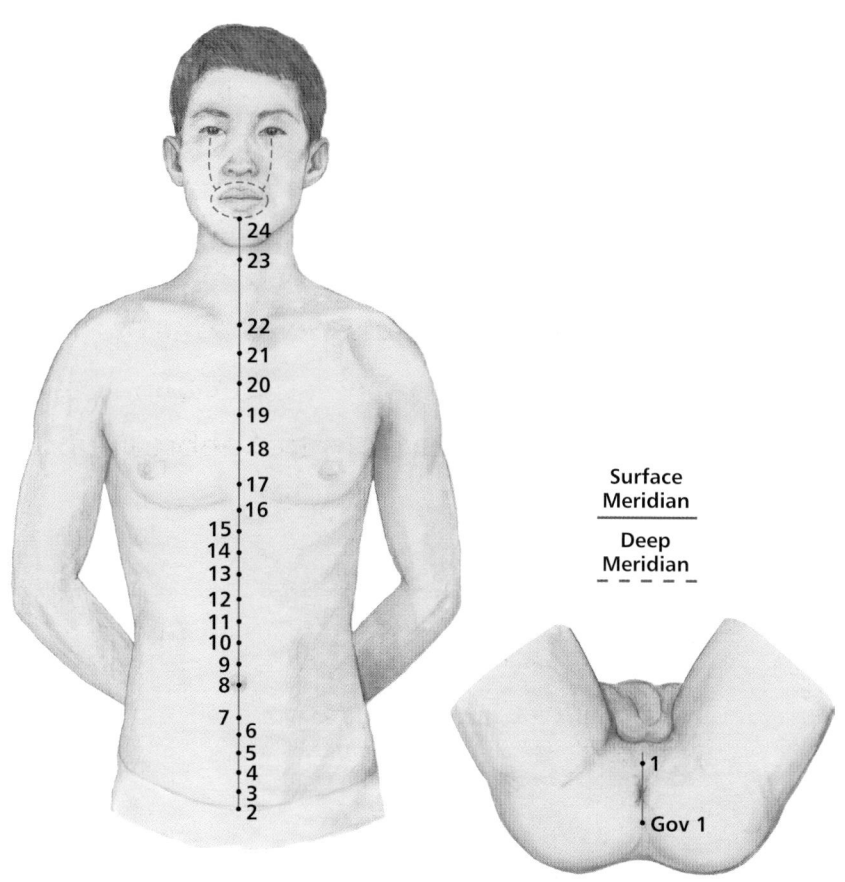

The Conception channel is sometimes called the Intake channel. There are twenty-four (24) acupoints on the surface pathway of this channel that commences at the perineum and ends at the lower lip, having travelled directly up the ventral midline. From the end point at Con 24, a deep channel supplies the mouth, outer aspect of the nose and the eyes. It is considered to be a Yin channel so its main thrust is in the treatment of chronic conditions. Its Key (Opening) point is LU 7. Although each point along its surface meridian is important, some are much more powerful and versatile than others and it will be these that are discussed. They are: Con 1, Con 3, Con 4, Con 6, Con 8, Con 12, Con 14, Con 17 and Con 22.

Con 1 *Hui Yin* (Meeting of Yin)

會陰 ★★★★★

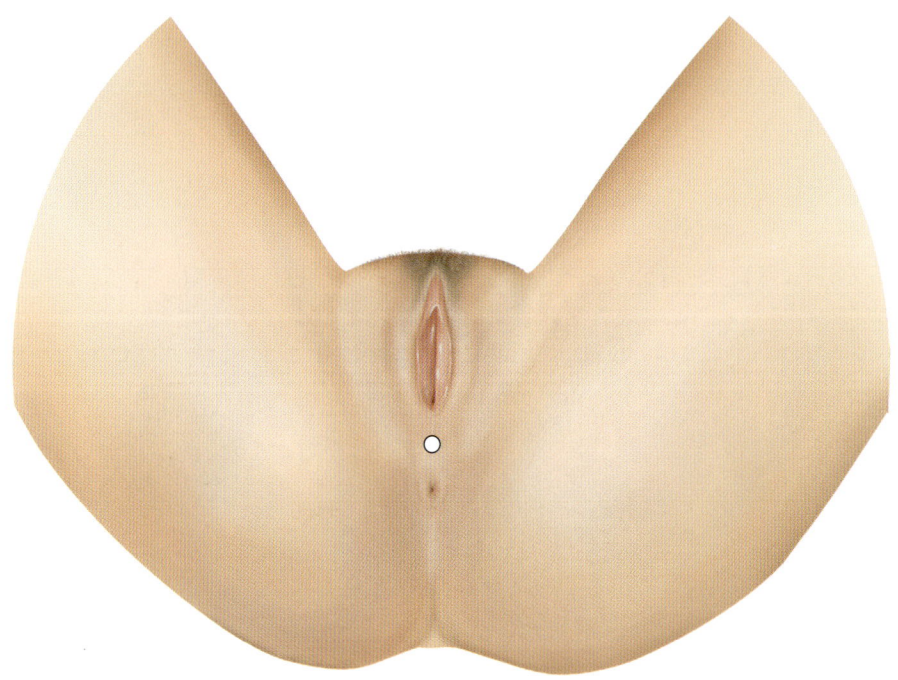

Location
Situated at the centre of the perineum, midway between the anus and the posterior border of the genitals.

Needle
Traditional texts tell us that this point is forbidden to needle, probably due its intimate location. As each acupoint has an energy area of influence that surrounds it, it is possible to needle Con 2 (on the superior border of the symphysis pubis) instead, although Con 1 is more powerful. You must be an experienced practitioner to use this point and have a chaperone in the room. Depth is up to 1 cun using a perpendicular insertion.

Moxa and pressure
Moxa is forbidden on this point and direct pressure is also very rarely used except in cases of it being a first aid point in drowning – where it should be tonified. Use Con 2 with pressure techniques if you are at all uncomfortable.

Indications
Con 1 may be used in treating both local and general conditions. Local symptoms and conditions include fertility disorders, diminished libido, uterine bleeding, prolapsed uterus, haemorrhoids, scrotal pain and inflammation, incontinence, vaginal dryness and leucorrhoea. By using this point either with stimulating needle, self-help acupressure or with faradism (electro-stimulation), it may help to strengthen the pelvic floor muscles. Con 1 is also used to ease stress, help with tiredness, depression, poor circulation and low blood pressure. Self-help acupressure is very useful in all these symptoms. It is also used to help with anxiety and some psychic and psychosomatic disorders.

Special properties
Con 1 is said to be the Base (Muladhara) chakra and is considered in many traditional philosophies to represent the earthing or grounding point of the body. It is specifically used in meditation, yoga and other Eastern arts. It is also the 'opposite' point to Gov 20 (Crown chakra) and a useful exercise in aiding energy balancing or homoeostasis is to place the hands on these two points to allow an energy balance. Magnets are also effective on these two points. If though, as stated before, you are uncomfortable in treating this point, Con 2 may be used as a very good substitute and is especially useful in balancing the chakra energies.

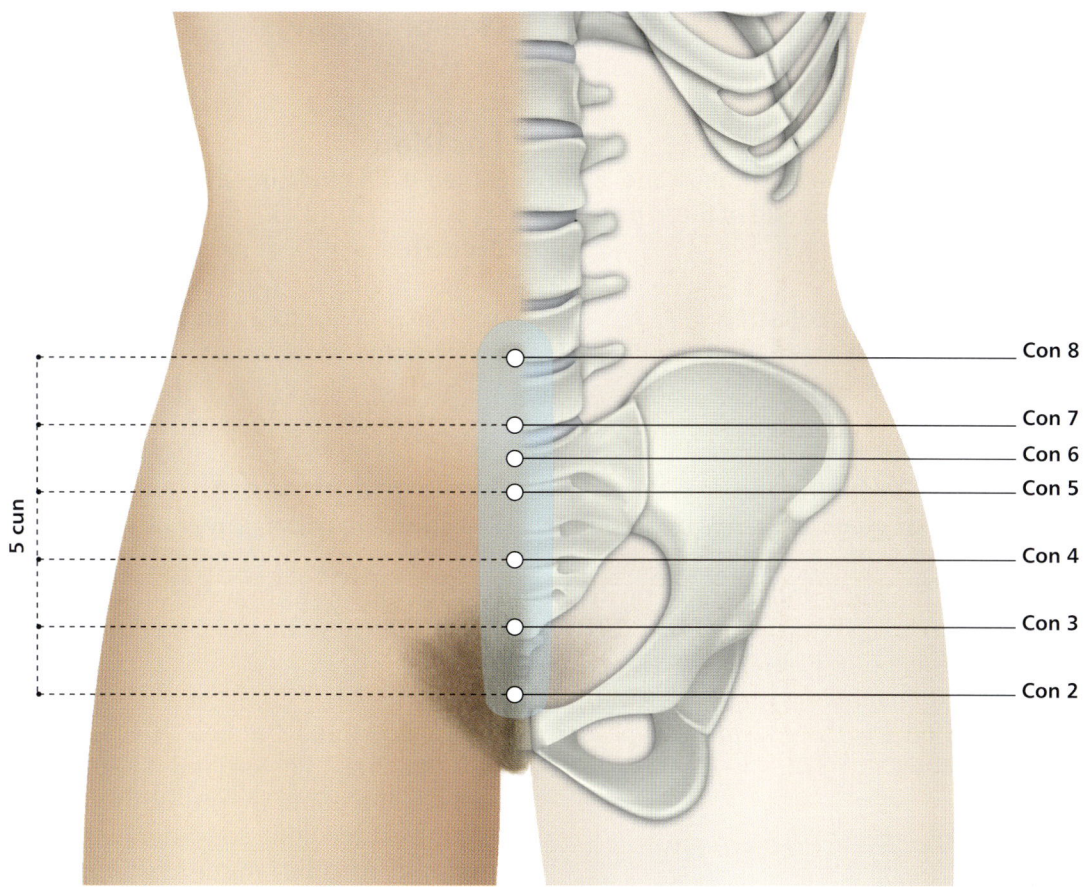

5 cun

Con 8
Con 7
Con 6
Con 5
Con 4
Con 3
Con 2

Location
Situated 4 cun below the umbilicus and 1 cun superior to the upper border of the symphysis pubis.

Needle
Up to 1.5 cun with a perpendicular insertion.

Do not needle in pregnancy.

Moxa and pressure
Direct moxa is not recommended due to presence of pubic hair but this point answers very well to a moxa stick to encourage energy flow to the bladder and uterus. Acupressure is effective as either practitioner led or self-help in helping some of the symptoms listed below.

Indications
This is a powerful point in the treatment of bladder, sexual dysfunction and gynaecological disorders. Symptoms and conditions include dysuria, frequent urination or retention, cystitis, urethritis, prostatitis, impotence, leucorrhoea, prolapsed uterus, irregular menstruation and dysmenorrhoea.

Special properties
Con 3 is the Alarm (Mu) point of the bladder as well as being an intersection point of the Spleen, Kidney, Liver and Conception channels. Apart from being used to treat all the symptoms mentioned above, it is used to indicate acute conditions of the bladder.

Con 4 *Guan Yuan* ★★★★

(Original Gate or Barrier of Vital Energy)

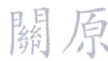

Location
Situated 3 cun below the umbilicus and 2 cun above Con 2 at the superior end of the symphysis pubis.

Needle, moxa and pressure
This point responds to exactly the same needle, moxa and pressure as Con 3.

Indications
The same as Con 3 with the addition that Con 4 may be treated for general energy depletion as well as localised conditions. It is used mostly in conjunction with Con 3 and is more powerful in the treatment of gynaecological conditions. As per Con 3, this point is an intersection point of the three yin channels with the Conception meridian but Con 4 is the Alarm (Mu) point of the small intestine.

Do not needle in pregnancy.

Con 6 *Qi Hai* ★★★★★

(Sea of Energy)

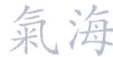

Location
Situated 1.5 cun directly below the umbilicus.

Needle
Either up to 1.5 cun using a perpendicular approach or up to 2 cun by slanting the needle towards the umbilicus.

Do not needle in pregnancy.

Moxa and pressure
Traditionally, the lower Conception points may use moxa cones on slices of ginger as this tonifies the yang chi more than straightforward moxa. For pressure, see 'special properties'.

Indications
Con 6 is named the Sea of Energy (Chi) and, as such, may be tonified to increase general energy depletion in the body. It is therefore recommended that conditions such as chronic tiredness, chronic fatigue syndrome, exhaustion and weakened immunity are treated with this point as a priority. It is also extensively used to treat many abdominal, urological and gynaecological conditions including abdominal distension and pain, bloating and irritable bowel syndrome, constipation, dysmenorrhoea, amenorrhoea, uterine collapse, frequent urination and sexual dysfunction (both sexes) and impotence amongst others.

Special properties
Con 6 is the anterior aspect of the Sacral chakra (Gov 3 is the posterior aspect). It is extensively used in yoga and meditation as the focal point in 'hara' breathing. It is linked with the Throat chakra at Con 22 and these two points may be used in energy balancing of these two chakras by needle, pressure or magnets. It is its use with acupressure and bodywork though, which is paramount.

Con 8 *Shen Que* (Spirit Gateway or Palace of Providence)

Location
Situated at the centre of the umbilicus.

Needle

Con 8 is forbidden to needle.

Moxa and pressure
This point is traditionally treated with just moxa by pouring salt into the umbilicus and burning moxa punk either directly over the salt or using ginger over the salt to burn the cones. A moxa box may also be used over the area. Do not over-stimulate this point in cases of depletion or where it is not warranted. Pressure is also said to be forbidden, but I have used it for many years with extremely good results. The most effective technique is to place the whole hand gently over the umbilicus with the other hand directly underneath the back at approximately L3–4 to perform energy balancing.

Indications
In many forms of tribal and traditional cultures, the umbilicus (navel) was considered the point where the spirit enters and leaves the body. It may, therefore, be utilised in the treatment of chronically sick patients and those who are dying. I have used this point extensively with patients in hospices. Although it is a unique point, it is not extensively used, hence its apparently low star rating.

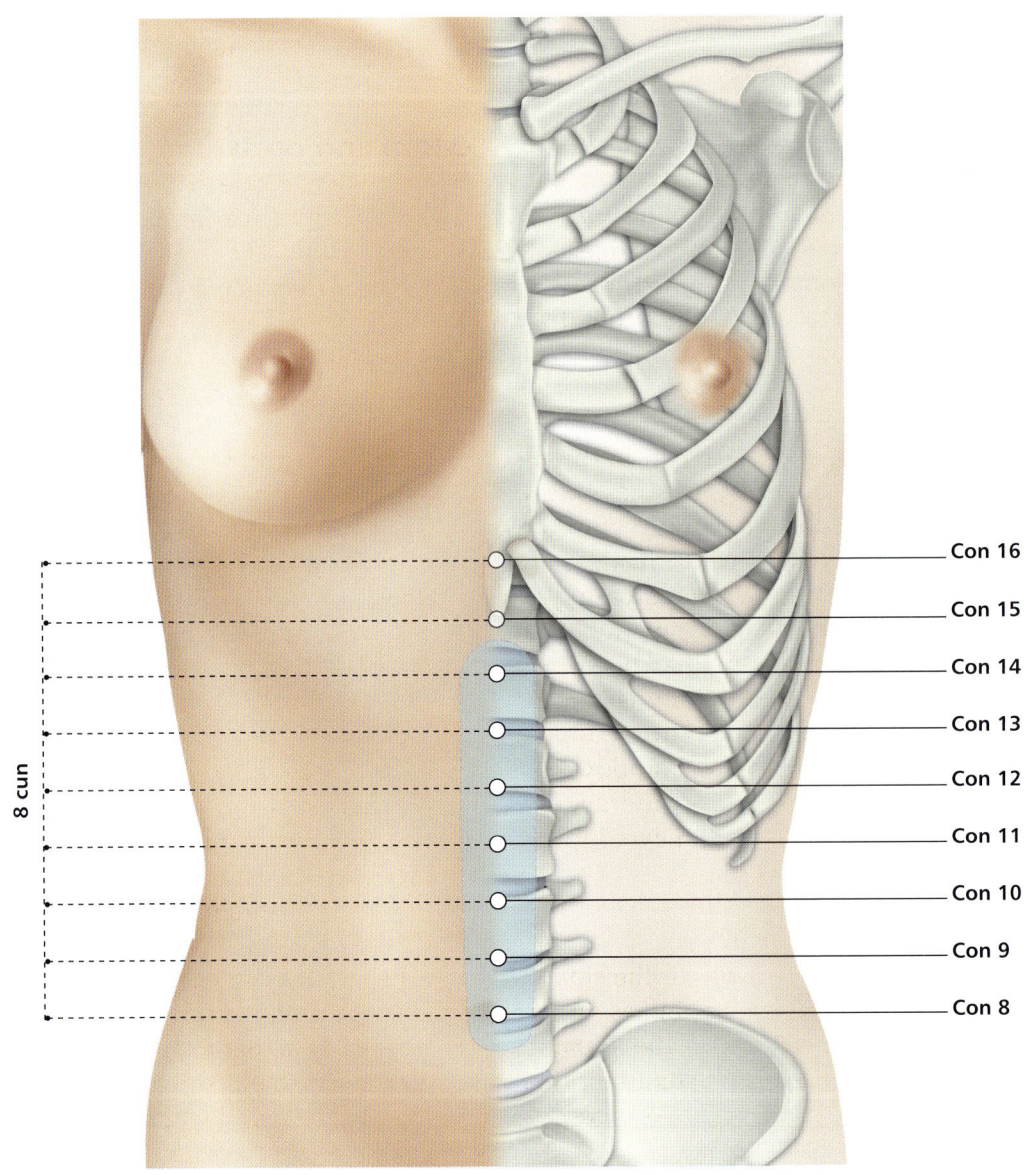

Con 16

Con 15

Con 14

Con 13

Con 12

Con 11

Con 10

Con 9

Con 8

8 cun

Con 12 *Zhong Wan* ★★★★★

(Stomach Centre)

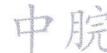

Location
Situated 4 cun directly above the umbilicus, halfway between the umbilicus and the xiphisternal junction.

Needle
Up to 1.5 cun using a perpendicular insertion.

> Do not needle this point in thin and emaciated patients.

Moxa and pressure
This point answers very well to heavy moxa either with cones (you may use ginger with the moxa) or with a moxa stick. Acupressure is extensively used and is particularly helpful as self-help in stomach conditions.

Indications
This acupoint is primarily used to harmonise the stomach and spleen organs and may be used with the following conditions and symptoms: acute and chronic gastroenteritis, gastric ulcers, stomach pain, loss of taste, bloating and heaviness in the stomach, diaphragmatic tension, hiatus hernia, constipation and diarrhoea, acute or chronic cholecystitis and hiccoughs. It is also used in general energy depletion syndromes and where there are problems with body fluids as in dry mouth, urine conditions and dry skin. It is a very important point to relieve digestive conditions caused by stress.

Special properties
Con 12 is the Alarm (Mu) point for the stomach and is used as a diagnostic point as well as in treatment. It is also where the Stomach, Triple Energizer and Small Intestine meridians intersect with the Conception – hence its powerful actions.

Con 14 *Ju Que* ★★★★★

(Great Palace)

Location
Situated 6 cun superior to the umbilicus, 1 cun below the tip of the xiphoid process.

Needle
Up to 1.5 cun with a perpendicular insertion.

> Do not needle in thin and emaciated patients. Do not needle with the needle angled upwards.

Moxa and pressure
Mild moxa only due to the proximity of the celiac plexus. Do not use any heavy or stimulating pressure because of the celiac plexus and the xiphoid process being nearby.

Indications
This excellent acupoint treats many heart conditions as well as being a major point in calming the mind and helping with stress. Symptoms and conditions include palpitations and arrhythmia, dyspnoea, pain and constriction of the chest, coronary heart disease, angina pectoris, anxiety, epilepsy, diaphragmatic spasm and tension, insomnia, psychic and psychosomatic disorders.

Special properties
- Con 14 is the Alarm (Mu) point of the heart and as well as treating heart and chest conditions, it is used as a diagnostic point as to possible treatment.
- Con 14 is the anterior aspect of the Solar Plexus chakra (Gov 10 being the posterior aspect). This is a very powerful acupoint in esoteric medicine as it represents the highest point of our lower energies and the lower part of our upper energies. In most people the Solar Plexus chakra is either over-stimulated by the sheer pace of life, or congested by eating denatured or additive-filled foods. Stimulation can cause nervous disorders that affect the stomach, gall bladder, liver and spleen/pancreas.

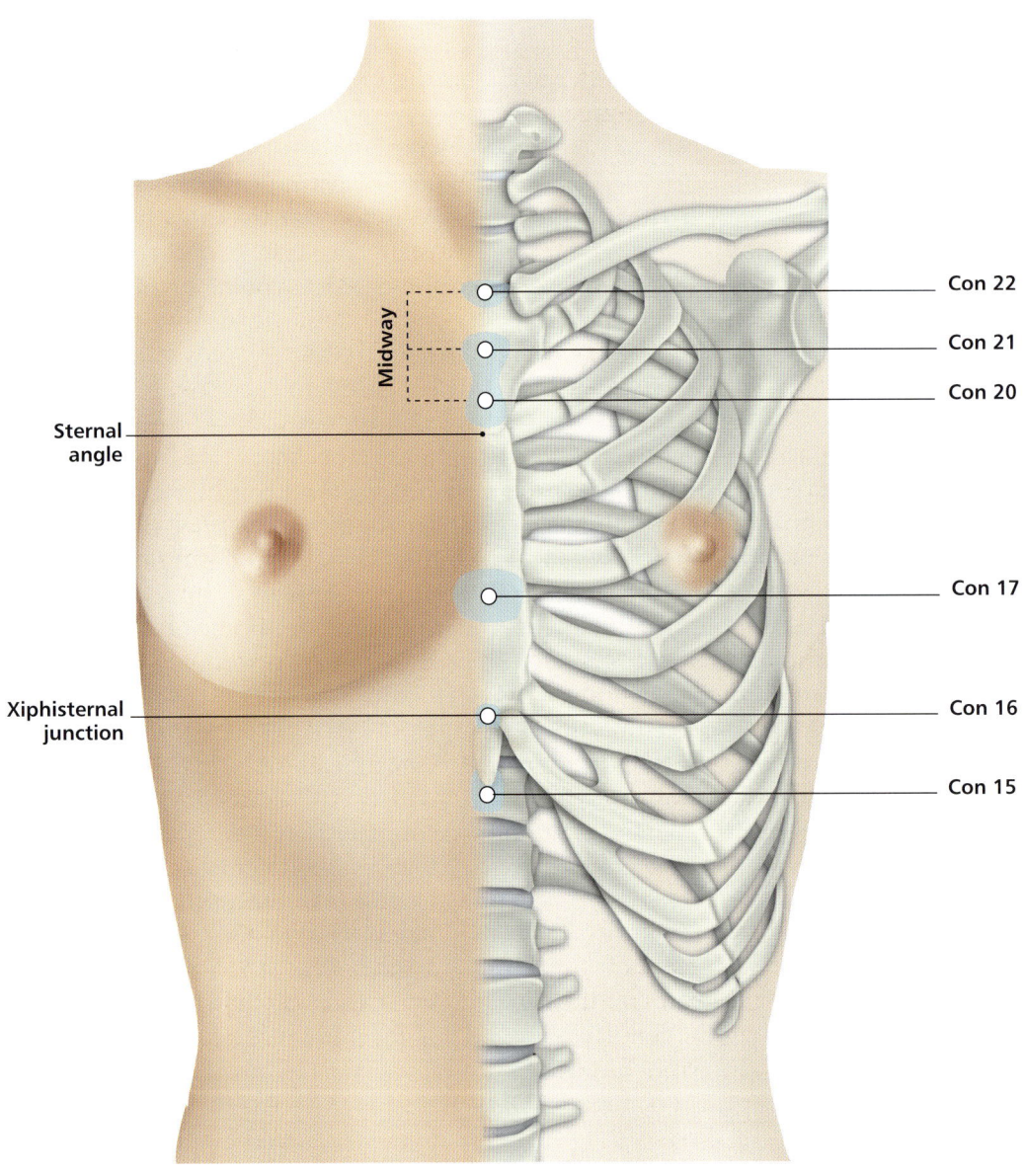

Midway

Con 22

Con 21

Con 20

Sternal angle

Con 17

Xiphisternal junction

Con 16

Con 15

Con 17 *Dan Zhong* ⭐⭐⭐⭐⭐

(Chest Centre)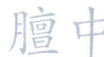

Location
Situated at the centre of the chest level with the 4th intercostal space, between the nipples.

Needle
Although some traditional texts inform us that it is forbidden to needle, presumably as it is possible to puncture the sternum and pierce the heart, but in reality it is a highly effective point. Needle up to 0.8 cun using a transverse insertion downwards.

> Do not needle this point with a perpendicular approach.

Moxa and pressure
Moxa may be performed but there is very little need for it. For pressure, see 'special properties'.

Indications
Con 17 is used to treat two main sets of symptoms (which are sometimes linked). Firstly, it is used to treat many heart conditions such as chest constriction, pain and heaviness in the region, palpitation and arrhythmia, congestive heart symptoms, wheezing and coughing. Secondly it is a major player in calming the mind and spirit and is extensively used in anxiety, panic attacks, grief, sadness, sighing, insomnia and hysteria. It is also used as a 'local' point in breast conditions such as insufficient lactation.

Special properties
- Con 17 is the Alarm (Mu) point of the Pericardium and is used as a point of analysis for pericardial and heart conditions.
- It is an intersection point of the Spleen, Kidney, Small Intestine and Triple Energizer with the Conception channel. It is, therefore, highly effective in many widespread syndromes. It is colloquially called the centre point of the body.
- Con 17 is the anterior aspect of the Heart (Anahata) chakra (the posterior aspect is Gov 10) and is utilised extensively in calming the mind and spirit in very many emotional and psychosomatic conditions. It is a brilliant point used with gentle acupressure in meditation and is probably the best point on the body for calming the mind and body.

Con 22 *Tian Tu* ⭐⭐⭐⭐⭐

(Heavenly Prominence)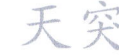

Location
Situated on the midline just superior to the suprasternal notch.

Needle
As this acupoint is almost 'hidden' beneath the manubrium, firstly needle 0.3 cun perpendicular, then direct it downwards along the posterior border of the manubrium to 1 cun.

> Do not needle any deeper as there is a great danger of piercing the thyroid gland or the numerous blood vessels and nerve plexii in the region.

Moxa and pressure
Use only mild moxa directly or with a moxa stick. Stimulating point massage is effective for localised thyroid imbalance but generally use gentle acupressure, see 'special properties'.

Indications
This point is extensively used for local energy imbalance. Symptoms and conditions include diseases of the respiratory tract such as bronchial asthma, throat congestion and constant sore throats, sudden loss of voice (as in Clergyman's throat), wheezing, hoarseness, pain and swelling of the throat, goitre and thyroid gland imbalance. It is also used in some cases of heartburn, nausea and heartburn.

Special properties
Con 22 is the anterior aspect of the Throat (Vishuddha) chakra (the posterior aspect is at Gov 14). It is coupled with the Sacral chakra at Con 6 and is extensively used in esoteric and Ayurvedic medicine in emotional and physical conditions where the patient is unable to excrete or express themselves. It is therefore used as one of the points in shyness, grief, the bottling up of emotions and worries, frozen shoulder, constipation, anger and frustration.

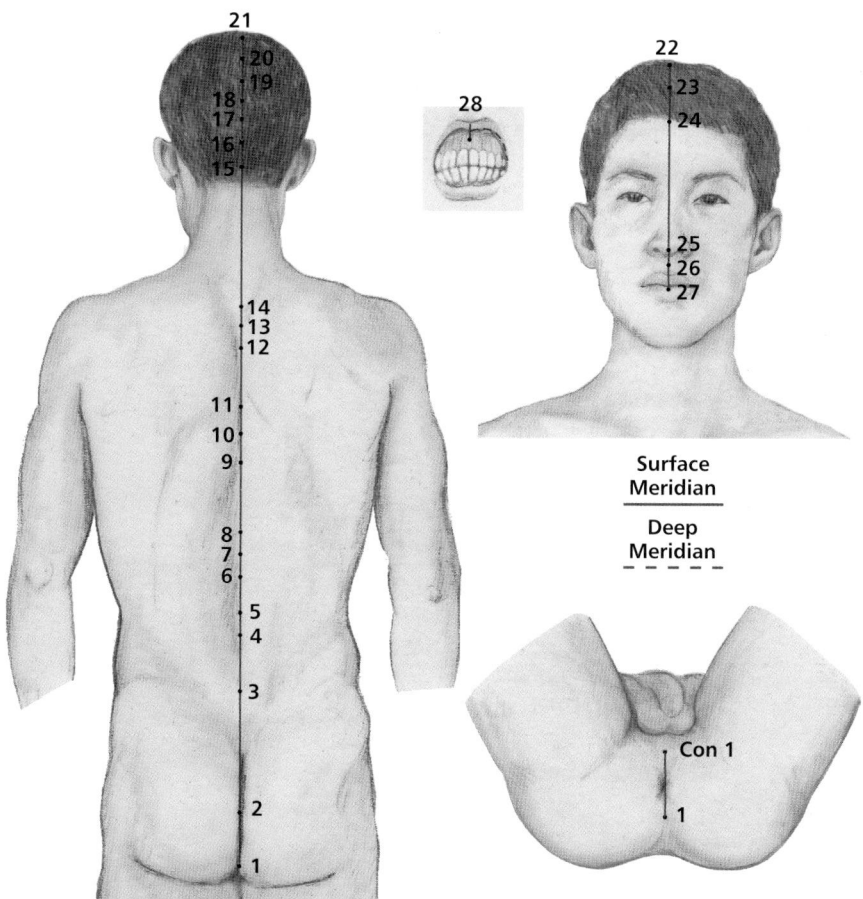

Surface Meridian

Deep Meridian

Con 1

The Governor channel is sometimes called the Steering or Governing channel. There are twenty-eight (28) acupoints along its surface pathway beginning at the distal aspect of the coccyx (being joined to the Conception at the perineum by a deep channel). The meridian then ascends directly up the midline of the spine, continues over the head and ends in the underside of the upper lip. It is considered to be Yang in nature and is generally used to treat musculo-skeletal and spinal conditions although internal organic conditions are treated at the many levels of this channel. The Key point is SI 3 (on the ulnar aspect of the ring finger). The posterior aspects of many of the major chakras are situated along its course and these powerful points are used with needle, pressure or magnets in the treatment of many spinal and spinal-related disorders. We shall discuss the following points: Gov 1, Gov 2, Gov 3, Gov 4, Gov 5–Gov 13, Gov 14, Gov 16, Gov 20, Gov 24, Gov 25 and Gov 26.

Gov 1 *Chang Qiang* (Always Strong)

長強 ★★★★★

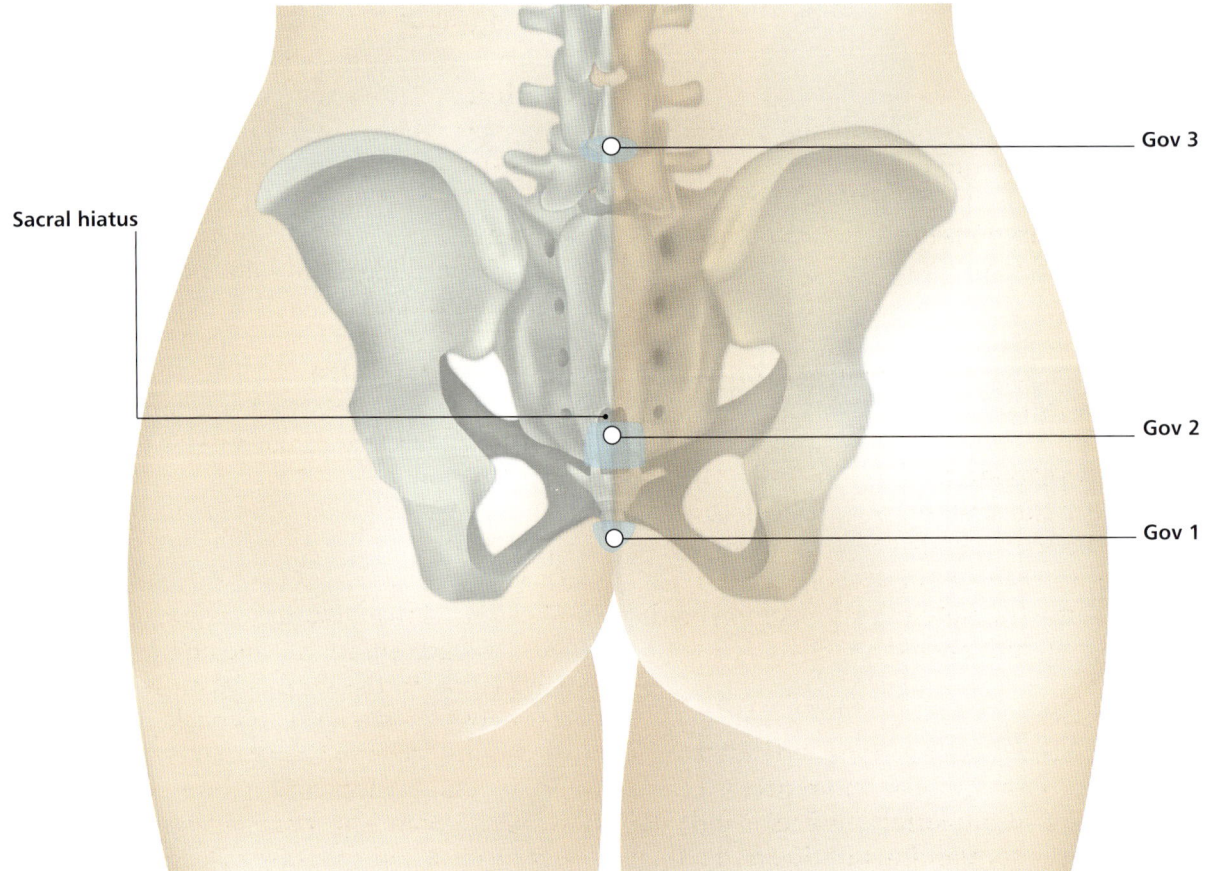

Gov 3

Sacral hiatus

Gov 2

Gov 1

Location

Situated midway between the tip of the coccyx and the anus.

Needle

Up to 1 cun using a perpendicular approach. Because of its anatomical position, please note that it is sometimes either very difficult or not in the patient's best interest to needle this point; if you are at all uncomfortable with needle or pressure, use Gov 2 instead.

Moxa and pressure

Direct moxa is not forbidden but for obvious reasons it is not recommended. For pressure techniques, see 'special properties'.

Indications

In traditional forms of acupuncture, the point is used for localised conditions such as: haemorrhoids, prolapsed rectum, constipation, anal bleeding, lumbar pain, painful urination and kidney chi congestion.

Special properties

Gov 1 is considered to be the posterior aspect of the Base (Muladhara) chakra and is linked with the Crown chakra at Gov 20. In some ways it could be the most important acupoint of the body as it should be used in every chronic condition of the spine, kidneys, bladder, any 'bone' condition and any hereditary imbalance. It is said to be the body's main 'earthing' or grounding point and a strong Base chakra will keep us on the ground with regards to our mental attitudes. It is also the main ancestral point of the body and, as such, is used along with other points to help with many congenital deformities. It is obviously used as a focal point in qigong and tai chi exercises and is much used in meditation and yoga. It is a super point in clearing the mind as well as stabilising a person's emotions. It is extensively used in balancing and treating the chakra energies with acupressure and in cranio-sacral therapy. If you are at all uncomfortable using this point, then use Gov 2 instead as it has all the clinical attributes of Gov 1.

Gov 2 *Yao Shu* ★★★★★

(Lumbar Point)　腰俞

Location
Situated on the midline between the sacrum and coccyx. Some texts indicate that it is located in the sacral hiatus at its inferior end but classical charts (and commonsense) indicate that it is where I have stated.

Needle
Up to 1 cun using a perpendicular or oblique upwards insertion.

Moxa and pressure
Although it is still anatomically difficult to moxa this point directly. Persistence brings rewards. Indirect moxa using a stick is very effective in general energy depletion and haemorrhoids. Pressure techniques are as Gov 1.

Indications
Gov 2 possesses the same actions and indications as its partner Gov 1 but is more accessible to needle, moxa and pressure. Some texts indicate that this is just a local point, but due to its huge influence as a major chakra point, it warrants a high star rating.

Gov 3 *Yao Yyang Guan* ★★★★★

(Yang Barrier)　腰陽關

Location
Situated in the midline below the spinous process of L4.

Needle
Up to 1.5 cun using a perpendicular or upwards oblique insertion.

Moxa and pressure
Heavy moxa is indicated in lumbar spine sluggishness and large bowel symptoms such as constipation.

Indications
This is an effective point in treating lower lumbar and lower internal organ imbalance. Conditions and symptoms include pain and/or inflammation in the lumbo-sacral region, pain and/or loss of strength in the legs, dysuria, urinary tract infections, irregular menstruation, infertility, impotence, constipation and irritable bowel syndrome. This point is also indicated in lower cervical and shoulder discomfort.

Special properties
Gov 3 is the posterior aspect of the Sacral chakra (the anterior aspect is at Con 6). It is therefore indicated in acute conditions in gynaecological conditions as well as oedema of the legs. It is partnered with the posterior Throat chakra at Gov 14 and this is an excellent duo in the treatment of lower cervical conditions.

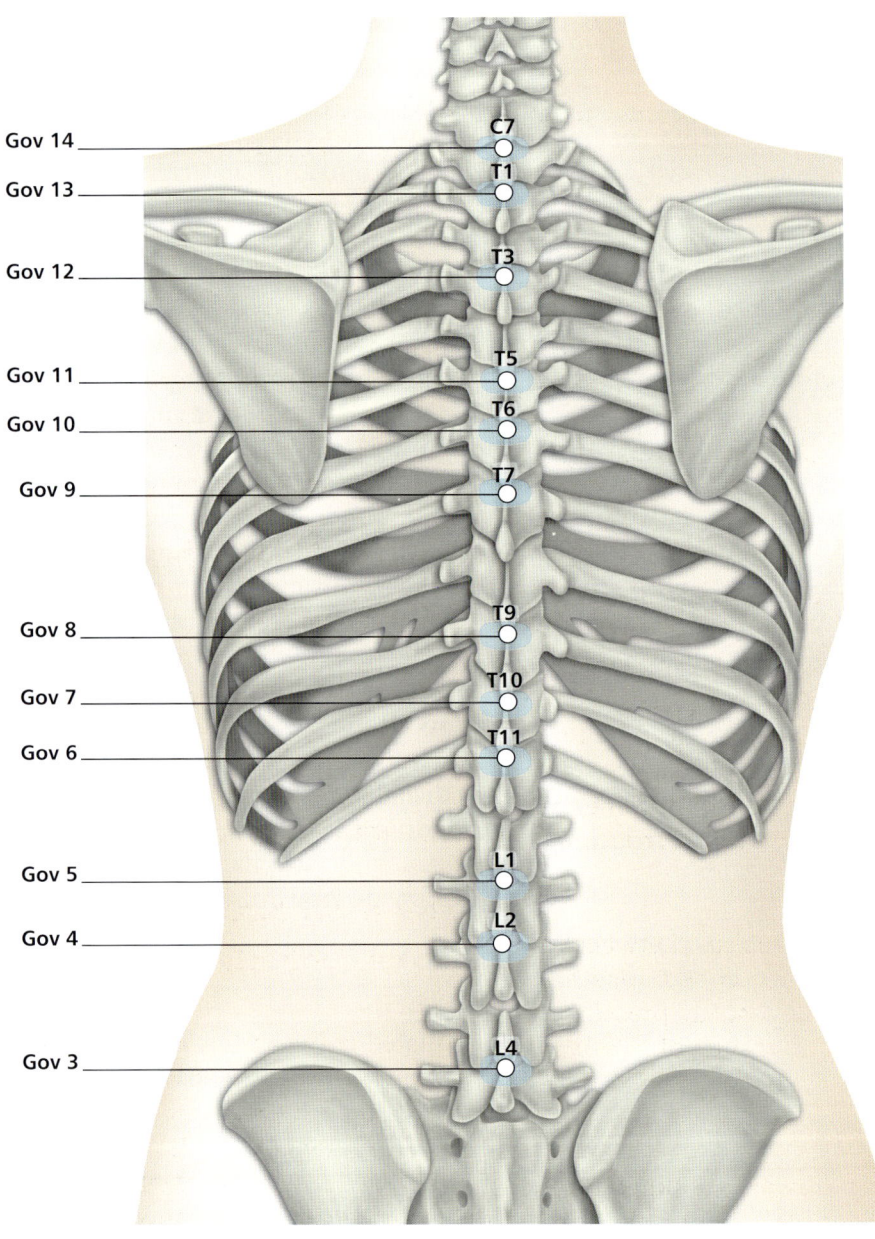

Gov 14 — C7
Gov 13 — T1
Gov 12 — T3
Gov 11 — T5
Gov 10 — T6
Gov 9 — T7
Gov 8 — T9
Gov 7 — T10
Gov 6 — T11
Gov 5 — L1
Gov 4 — L2
Gov 3 — L4

Gov 4 Ming Men
(Door of Life)

Location
Situated in the depression below the spinous process of L2. It is level with BL 23 and also on the same girdle line as the umbilicus.

Needle
Up to 1 cun using an upwards oblique insertion.

Moxa and pressure
Heavy direct or indirect moxa is indicated in energy depletion syndromes. A moxa box is ideally used here due to the flatness of the anatomy. This point is also ideal for stimulating massage and pressure either in unison or combined with bilateral BL 23 points. It makes an excellent self-help region to stimulate kidney and general energy.

Indications
Gov 4 is an excellent acupoint in general energy depletion conditions, with kidney energy being paramount. Symptoms and conditions include chronic and acute lumbar pain, sciatica, spinal stiffness, lumbago, male sexual dysfunction (e.g. impotence), tinnitus, poor memory, chronic tiredness and chronic fatigue syndrome, rectal prolapse and many chronic gynaecological conditions.

The Governor channel points between Gov 5 and Gov 13 will be described together as each has similar needle, moxa, pressure and indication. Each has a star rating of ⭐⭐⭐ with the exception of Gov 9 which is ⭐⭐⭐⭐.

Needle
Up to 1 cun using an upwards oblique insertion going with the angle of the spinous process.

Moxa and pressure
Moxa is indicated at each of the points in cases of energy depletion with the exception of Gov 6 where it is forbidden. Pressure is sometimes difficult to do as the points are 'buried' by bony prominences. Flat of hand acupressure is often practiced in many esoteric and traditional practices such as reiki.

Gov 5 *Xuan Shu*
(Suspended Pivot)

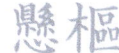

Situated between the spinous process of L1–L2. It is used in localised spinal conditions, enteritis and diarrhoea and for strengthening the spleen.

Gov 6 *Ji Zhong*
(Spine Centre)

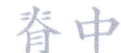

Situated between the spinous processes of T11–T12. It is used in localised spinal pain and conditions, jaundice, diarrhoea, abdominal distension and enteritis. Similarly to Gov 5, this point strengthens the spleen. Although it represents the posterior aspect of the Solar Plexus chakra, it is only used in that capacity in energy balancing with the Heart chakra.

Gov 7 *Zhong Shu*
(Central Pivot)

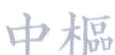

Situated between the spinous processes of T10–T11. Indications are similar to adjacent Governor points with the exception that it aids the gall bladder. It also promotes urination and helps with loss of appetite.

Gov 8 *Jin Suo*
(Sinew Contraction)

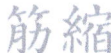

Situated between the spinous processes of T9–T10. Indications are similar to other Governor acupoints. Gov 8 is associated with BL 18 and the liver and, as such, is used in muscular conditions such as cramp as well as some psychological disturbances, dizziness, fever, spasm and hepatitis.

Gov 9 *Zhi Yang*
(Arrival of Yang)

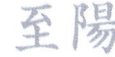

Situated between the spinous processes of T7–T8. It is associated with the diaphragm, liver and gall bladder so is used to treat diaphragmatic spasm, gall bladder colic, hepatitis, jaundice, abdominal tension and acute mastitis.

Gov 10 *Ling Tai*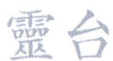
(Spirit Tower)

Situated between the spinous processes of T6–T7. According to many ancient texts, this point is forbidden to needle but I have yet to find out why! It is used for alleviating coughing and breathing difficulties as well as pain in the spine and is particularly helpful in treating adolescent kyphosis and some forms of scoliosis. Gov 10 helps with spinal deformities that are predisposed by emotional imbalance. It is particularly effective in the treatment of idiopathic juvenile scoliosis.

Gov 11 *Shen Dao*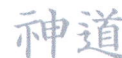
(Path of Providence)

Situated between the spinous processes of T5–T6. Indications include dyspnoea, cough, asthma, depression and sadness, palpitations and neurasthenia.

Gov 12 Shen Zhu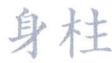
(Body Pillar)

Situated between the spinous processes of T3–T4. Indications include bronchial and chest conditions as well as some psychic and psychosomatic disorders. It is also indicated in epilepsy, cramps, fever, colds and localised spinal pain.

Gov 13 *Tao Dao*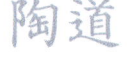
(Way of Happiness)

Situated between the spinous processes of T1–T2. As well as being useful as local spinal pain point, it is also used in upper respiratory chest infections, colds and influenza.

Gov 14 *Da Zhui*
(Great Vertebra)

Location
Situated between the spinous processes of C7–T1.

Needle
Up to 1 cun in an upwards oblique direction.

Moxa and pressure
In the traditional texts, moxa is indicated as one moxa per year of age. With the patient in prone lying this point answers very well to stimulating direct or indirect moxa as well as the moxa box. Cupping is also very effective. Acupressure is indicated at this point either in stimulation mode where local muscles are tight and indurated, or in sedation mode when energy balancing is required. (See 'special properties'.)

Indications
This acupoint is one of the most heavily used in many different types of conditions, especially musculo-skeletal ones. It lies at the centre of a parallelogram of forces with one axis being the spine and the other being the horizontal line between the shoulders. The area is therefore prone to much physical tension, and it is tension and stress where this point is mostly used. This very powerful point is the intersection of five different meridians (some by deep channels) so is influential in many energy imbalances. Symptoms and conditions include:
- Pain and stiffness of the neck and upper back, trapezius spasm, fibromyalgia and kyphosis.
- Colds, fever, cough and sore throat, asthma, wheezing and upper respiratory chest conditions.
- Palpitations, tachycardia, tightness in the chest, insomnia, mental restlessness and depression, poor memory, poor concentration and tinnitus.
- Headache and migraine, hypertension, dizziness and eye conditions.

Special properties
Gov 14 is considered to be the posterior aspect of the Throat (Vishuddha) chakra and is used in combination with the anterior aspect at Con 22. This combination with needle, pressure, healing or magnets is used for all the symptoms mentioned plus constipation, inability to express emotions, shyness and diffidence amongst others.

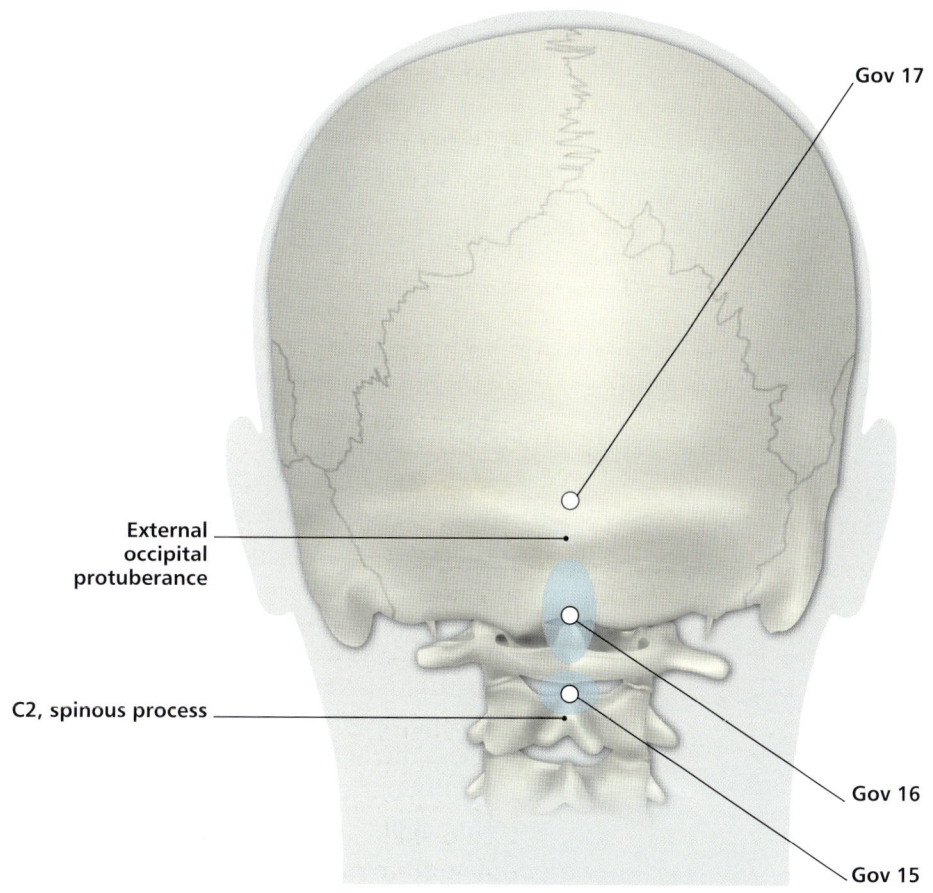

Location

Situated directly below the external occipital protuberance, in the depression between the attachments of the trapezius muscle.

Needle

Up to 1 cun with a perpendicular insertion directed slightly downwards.

> Do not apply strong manipulation – some patients may faint with this! Do not needle any deeper as there is a considerable risk of touching the spinal cord.

Moxa and pressure

Some texts insist that this point is forbidden to moxa, but I think it is perfectly permissible to treat it by using a moxa stick. Acupressure using many different techniques is widely used on this point. Be careful not to stimulate this point too much – sedative pressure has much more effect. Gov 16 is localised in therapies such as craniosacral therapy, cranial osteopathy, shiatsu, reiki, yoga and many other philosophies. Be careful not to stretch the occiput too much in some neurological conditions.

Indications

Gov 16 is indicated to bring clarity to the brain and to open the senses as well as many other syndromes. Symptoms and conditions include hemiplegia, aphasia, dizziness, headache, migraine, vertigo, blurred vision, epistaxis, tinnitus, dyspnoea and vomiting, mental confusion, restlessness, agitation, insomnia and anxiety.

Special properties

Gov 16 is the posterior counterpart of the Brow (Ajna) chakra. With its anterior counterpart Yin Tang they form the best two acupoints in the body to create calmness in the mind and for treating all stress-related conditions.

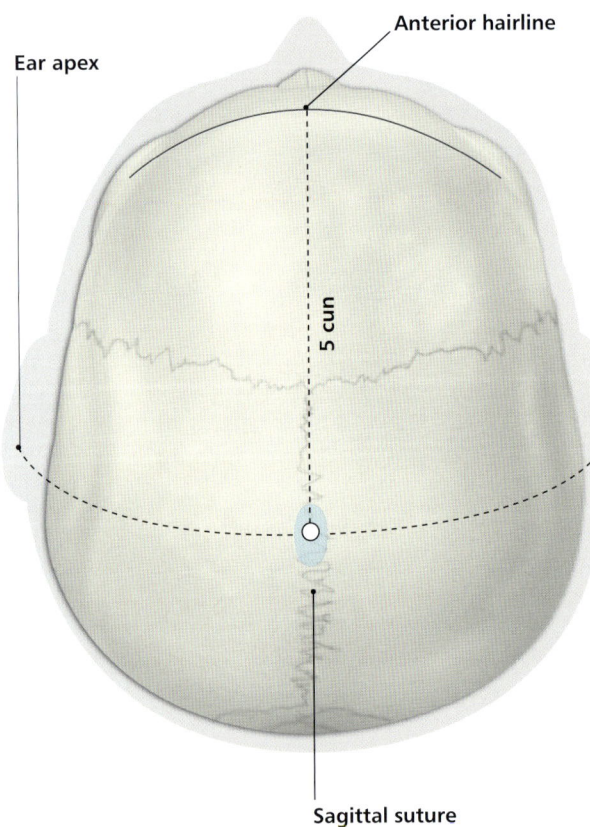

Ear apex
Anterior hairline
5 cun
Sagittal suture

Moxa and pressure

Moxa is an excellent treatment at this point either with a moxa stick or directly. If using direct moxa, the hair must be parted and the point marked with a pen prior to treatment. Moxa up to 20 times using direct moxa in cases of haemorrhoids and anal conditions.

> Do not perform any stimulating acupressure on this point as it may cause fainting. For further pressure techniques, see 'special properties'.

Indications

Gov 20 is considered to be the most Yang point on the body (opposite to both Con 1 and KI 1). It has many functions including; clearing the head and mind, calming, many emotional imbalances, as well as helping conditions on the opposite end of the Governor channel including haemorrhoids. Symptoms and conditions include apoplexy, dizziness, headache, migraine, numbness, anxiety, vertigo, palpitations, excess heat and hypertension, tinnitus, blurred vision, sadness, stage fright and mental agitation. It also helps with haemorrhoids, rectal and uterine prolapse and diarrhoea.

Location

Situated on the dorsal midline, 5 cun posterior to the anterior hairline, at the midpoint of the line connecting the apex of the two ears. An easy way to find this important point is that it is exactly halfway between Gov 16 and Yin Tang.

Needle

Use 0.5 cun subcutaneously or up to 1 cun by threading the needle in a transverse manner along the channel.

> Do not needle in patients under 12 years old as the fontanelle may not have closed. Do not tonify with any degree of exuberance as the patient may feel faint and 'spaced out'.

Special properties

In classical and traditional medicine this point is considered to be the Crown (Sahasrara) chakra. It is colloquially called the Thousand Petalled Lotus and is where a person is connected with their spiritual selves via their auras that house the subtle bodies. It is therefore extensively used (and abused) in many forms of yoga, meditation, Eastern arts and chakra healing. As stated before, be very careful not to over treat this point as the patient may soon become spaced out and feel 'other worldly'. The best way to do acupressure on this point is to place both hands either side of the head with the middle fingers resting on the point opposing each other. Gently stretch the hands apart to affect the point.

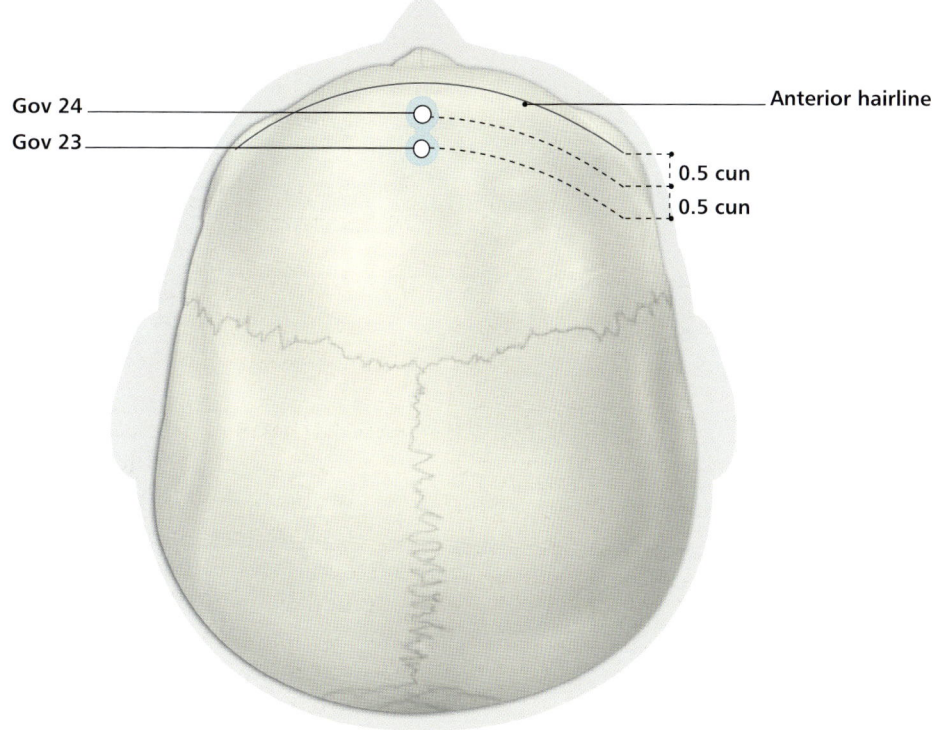

Location
Situated on the midline 0.5 cun within the anterior hairline.

Needle
Only use subcutaneous needling on this point.

> Do not tonify or stimulate the needle.

Moxa and pressure
Moxa is rarely called for on this point but not forbidden. Do not use stimulating acupressure but gentle sedating touch and hand pressure are excellent in self-help strategies, with other points, in many stress conditions.

Indications
Gov 24 pacifies the spirit, calms the mind and helps in neurasthenia. Symptoms and conditions include some psychic and psychosomatic disorders, insomnia, apoplexy, headache and migraine, epistaxis, blocked or runny nose, hemiplegia, fear and anxiety. This point is widely used in reflextherapy and cranio-sacral therapy.

Gov 25 *Su Liao* (White Crevice or Bone of the Nose)

素髎 ★★★

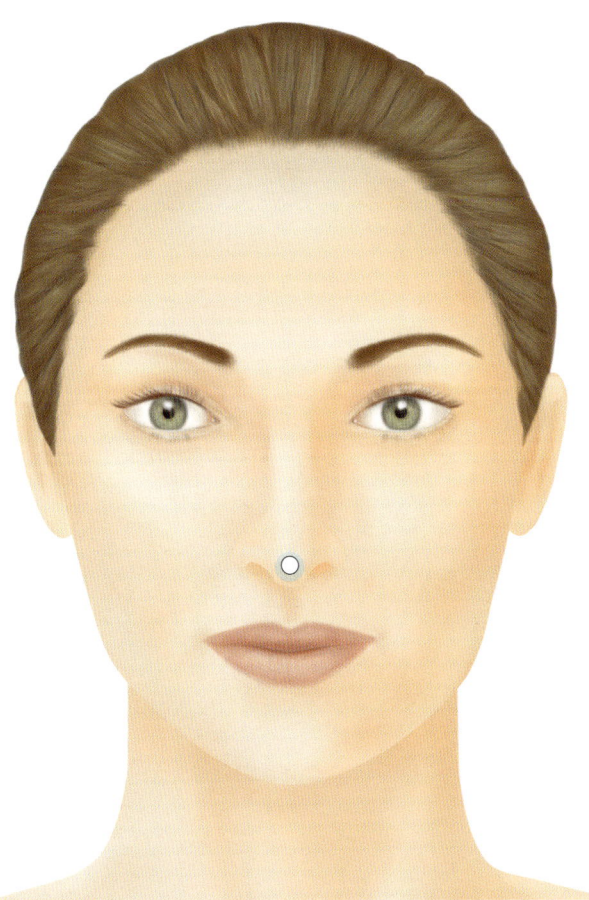

Location
Situated at the midpoint at the tip of the nose.

Needle
Up to 0.5 cun only using a perpendicular insertion.

> It is a very tender point and will make the eyes water!

Moxa and pressure
Acupressure is seldom called for except in emergencies, (see 'special properties').

> Moxa is forbidden.

Indications
This surprisingly useful point is an excellent one in clearing the mind, detoxification and helping with some nasal disorders. Symptoms and conditions include rhinitis, sinusitis, blocked nose, epistaxis and loss of smell, dyspnoea, excessive lacrimation, inflammation and swelling of the eyes.

Special properties
It is colloquially called the Command Point for the Consciousness and is an excellent first aid point in treating shock, fainting and coma. The point must be stimulated with a finger nail for maximum affect. Gov 25 is also used as one of many 'trigger' points in helping cessation of smoking or aiding other addictions. It works as well as the more popular auricular points.

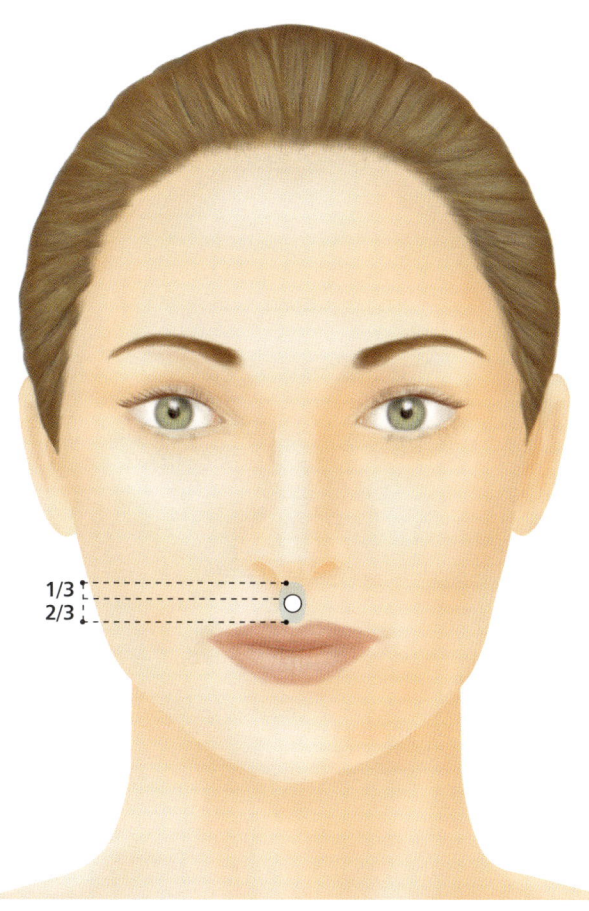

Location

Situated on the anterior midline at the dividing line between the upper and middle thirds of the philtrum (external top lip).

Needle

Up to 0.5 cun with an upward oblique insertion.

Moxa and pressure

Although moxa is not forbidden, it is very unpleasant and rather unnecessary to have moxa smoke so close to the nostril and eyes. Acupressure acts in one of two ways; stimulating pressure revives from drowsiness and unconsciousness (as in Gov 25) and sedative acupressure calms and clears the mind and is a super point to teach patients in self-help.

Indications

As stated above, Gov 26 is used in both revival and calming. It is also indicated in localised mouth and nasal conditions such as runny and blocked nose, sinusitis, deviation of the mouth, thirst, halitosis and it is a very useful point in treating some psychic and psychosomatic conditions. This point is said to be one of the best 'first aid' points for excessive sneezing.

That concludes description of the most popular acupoints on the main fourteen meridians. We shall now describe some commonly used acupoints that mostly lie outside the effect of meridian flow.

Before acupuncture point standardization in the 1990s, these were named Extra 1, Extra 2, etc. They were re-categorized as being Miscellaneous Points (M), also known as Extraordinary, Additional or New Points, that exist in various areas of the body under the following classifications:

M-HN	Head and Neck
M-B	Back
M-CA	Chest and Abdomen
M-AH	Arm and Hand
M-LF	Leg and Foot

Some of the acupoints are singular whilst others are groups of points. I have chosen nine of the most commonly used and effective of these acupoints to serve as additions to your repertoire. Many other influential acupoints and major reflex points exist on the body but do not come under the remit of this publication.

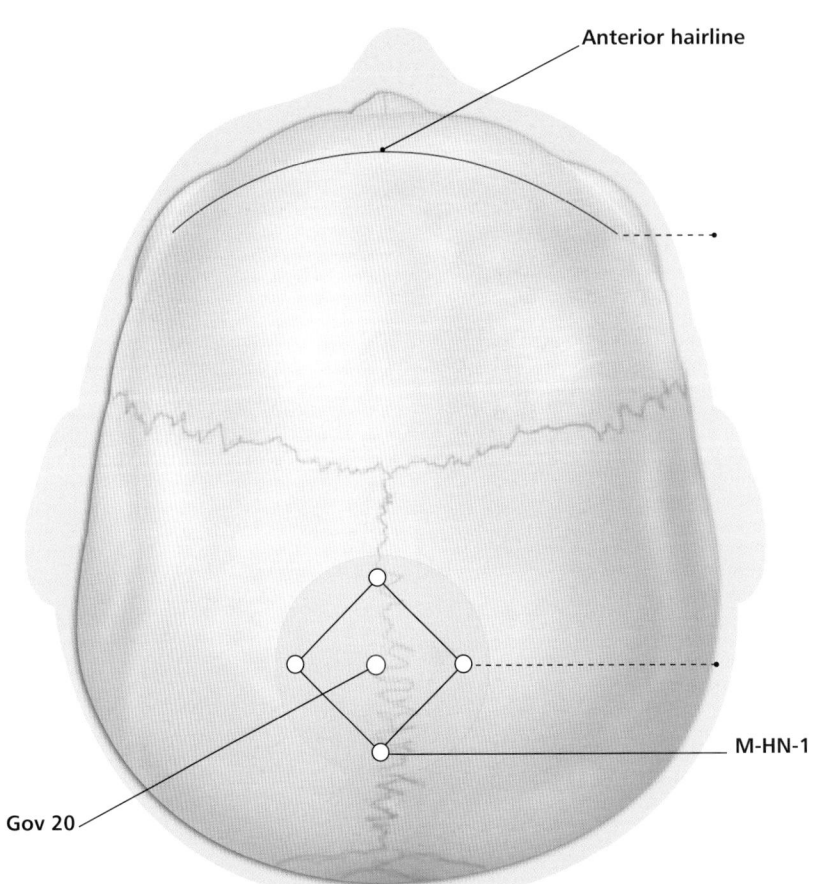

Anterior hairline

M-HN-1

Gov 20

Location
Consists of four points either side of the vertex, 1 cun lateral, anterior and posterior to Gov 20.

Needle
Use subcutaneous needling only directed towards Gov 20. Tiny copper needles are very effective on these points but only in people with little hair!

Moxa and pressure
Moxa is seldom used due to presence of hair. These points answer well to sedatory acupressure in conjunction with Gov 20. Two useful techniques would be to gently stretch the points (it is just possible to do all four at the same time) or to place the whole hand over the area with the middle of the palm (PC 8) centred on Gov 20. Acupressure and chakra balancing can then be performed between this area and other areas in need of treatment.

Indications
In conjunction with Gov 20 these points help clear the mind, brain, eyes and nose. Symptoms and conditions include headache, dizziness, migraine, vertigo, hemiplegia, epilepsy, depression, insomnia, poor memory, disorders of the eyes and nose, and some psychosomatic disorders.

印堂 ★★★★★

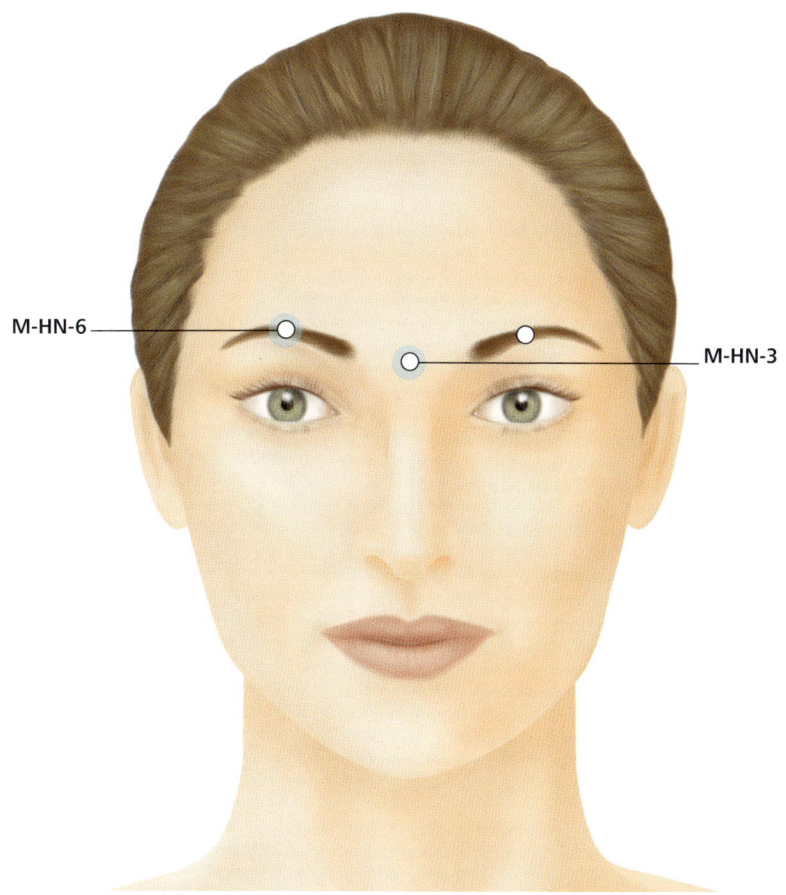

M-HN-6

M-HN-3

Location
Situated midway between the eyebrows on the anterior midline at the glabella.

Needle
Up to 0.5 cun subcutaneously with a perpendicular insertion or up to 1 cun using an oblique insertion with the needle directed towards the eye.

Moxa and pressure
Moxa is hardly ever indicated or warranted on this point and in some cultures is frowned upon. Acupressure is extensively used, especially in sedation techniques in calming the mind. (See 'special properties'.)

Indications
Yin Tang is extensively used in clearing the mind, easing pain, treating conditions of the ears, nose and eyes and as a very powerful point in hormonal imbalance. Although it lies on the Governor channel, it has never been classified as a Governor acupoint and yet it is one of the most powerful points on the body! It is sometimes called Gov 24.5 due to this apparent discrepancy by our forefathers. Symptoms and conditions include; anxiety, insomnia, depression, frontal headache, tiredness and many disorders of the eyes, nose and ears.

Special properties
Yin Tang is the anterior aspect of the Brow (Ajna) chakra and, as such, may be used in isolation or with other points in the treatment of many endocrine imbalances due to its effect on the hypothalamus and pituitary glands. It is also a master point in people who are susceptible to adverse or perverse radiation and is extensively used in yoga, meditation and many Eastern arts.

M-HN-5 *Tai Yang* (The Sun or Supreme Yang)

太陽 ★★★★★

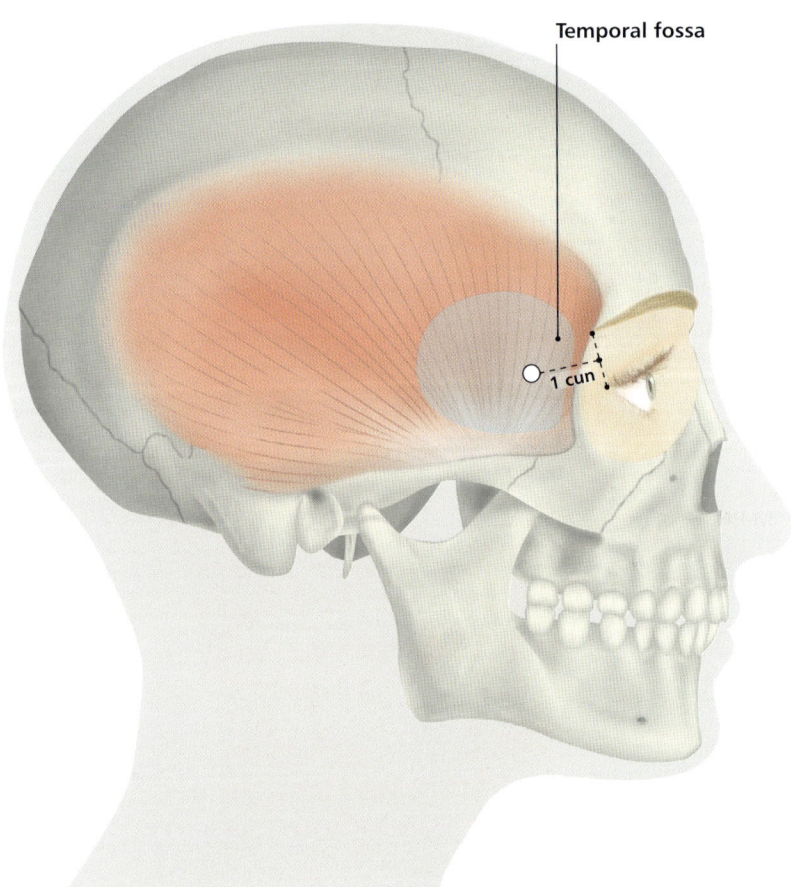

Temporal fossa

1 cun

Location
Situated in the depression of the temporal fossa, 1 cun posterior to the midpoint between the outer canthus of the eye and the eyebrow.

Needle
Use up to 0.8 cun with perpendicular approach or up to 1 cun using oblique insertion.

> Do not needle any deeper as there are many vital nerves and veins below.

Moxa and pressure
Moxa is not indicated at this point. Do not use stimulating acupressure as it will cause headaches and overheating. Sedatory acupressure works magnificently in temporal headaches and eye conditions plus some endocrine imbalance.

Indications
This is a very useful point in the treatment of all forms of headache, especially temporal. It is also very effective in trigeminal neuralgia, eye pain and inflammation, facial paralysis, tired and gritty eyes and general energy debility.

Special properties
Cranial osteopaths and cranio-sacral therapists will know this point well as it lies within the fissure line of the spheno-basilar-synchondrosis, which is where the sphenoid bone may be affected.

M-HN-8 *Bi Tong* (Nose Passage)

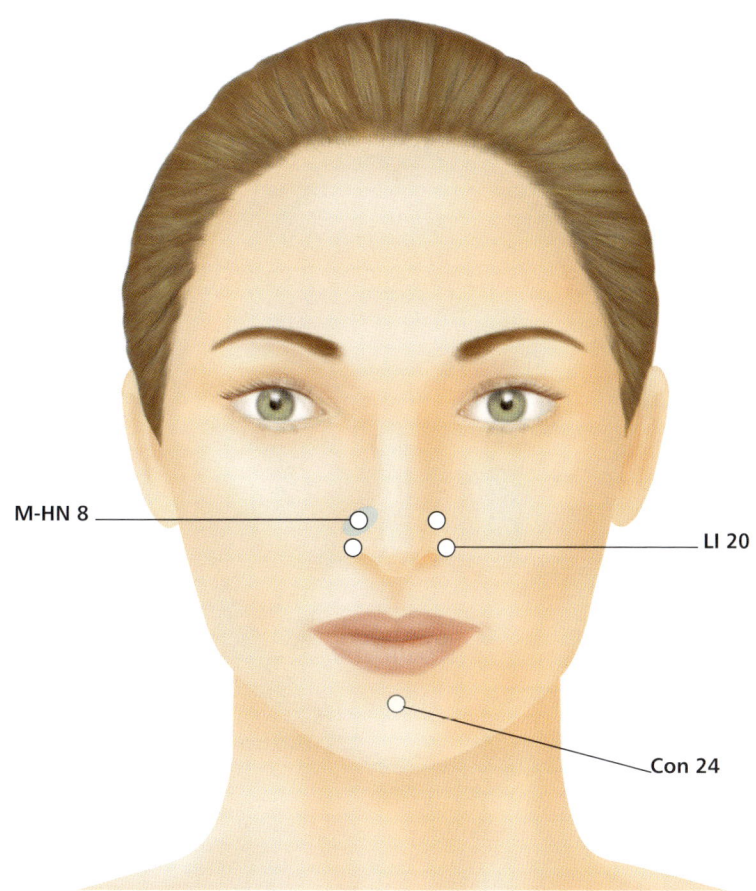

M-HN 8   LI 20

Con 24

Location
Situated in the depression below the nasal bone, at the superior end of the nasolabial sulcus.

Needle
Up to 0.5 cun only using a transverse insertion towards the bridge of the nose. It may also be joined up with LI 20.

Moxa and pressure
Acupressure performed by the patient is extremely helpful in clearing the nasal passages and in rhinitis.

Moxa is contraindicated.

Indications
This point works very well with LI 20 and is indicated in rhinitis, sinusitis, nasal congestion and polyps, discharge and catarrh.

M-B-2 *Hua Tuo Jia Ji* (Paravertebral or Ah Shi Points) 華佗夾脊 ⭐⭐⭐⭐⭐

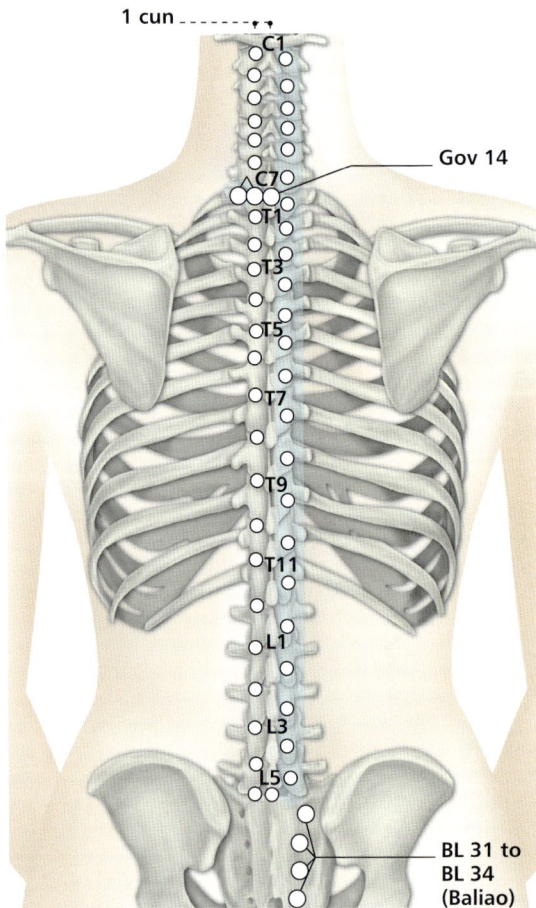

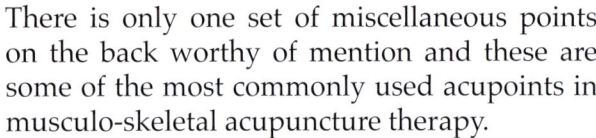

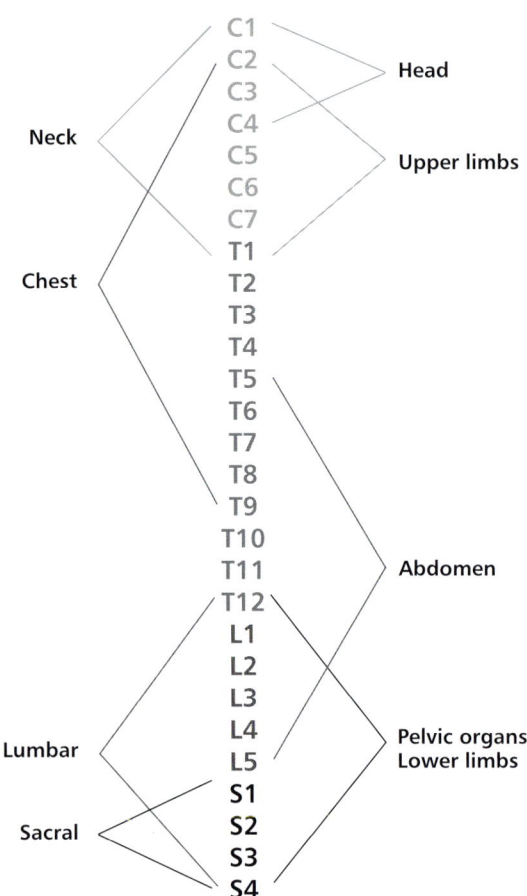

There is only one set of miscellaneous points on the back worthy of mention and these are some of the most commonly used acupoints in musculo-skeletal acupuncture therapy.

Location

Situated in the paraspinal groove, approximately 0.5 cun lateral to the posterior midline and situated over the facet joints of each vertebra from C1 to L5. Some authorities indicate these points lie over the emergence of the spinal nerves and others say that they are further away from the spine. In a way, they are considered to be reflex points and are used in analysis as well as treatment; they are often called 'ouch' points. Treatment is carried out with needle or pressure wherever there is a tender point, indicating local or distal energy imbalance.

Needle

Up to 1 cun in a perpendicular or slightly medially oblique direction.

Moxa and pressure

Moxa is indicated alongside the treatment of Governor channel and Inner Bladder channel points either with a moxa stick or moxa box. Cupping is also very effective on these points. Acupressure is usually performed along many of the vertical lines together either with the finger pads, thumbs or with many different forms of massage.

Indications

As stated before, this set of points may be used diagnostically as well as in treatment. They are generally used in spinal conditions such as spondylosis and spondylitis, pain, chronic inflammation, ankylosing spondylitis, hemiplegia, fibrositis and lumbago. They are also useful in producing relaxation. As individual acupoints they have internal links to various systems – these are shown in the above diagram.

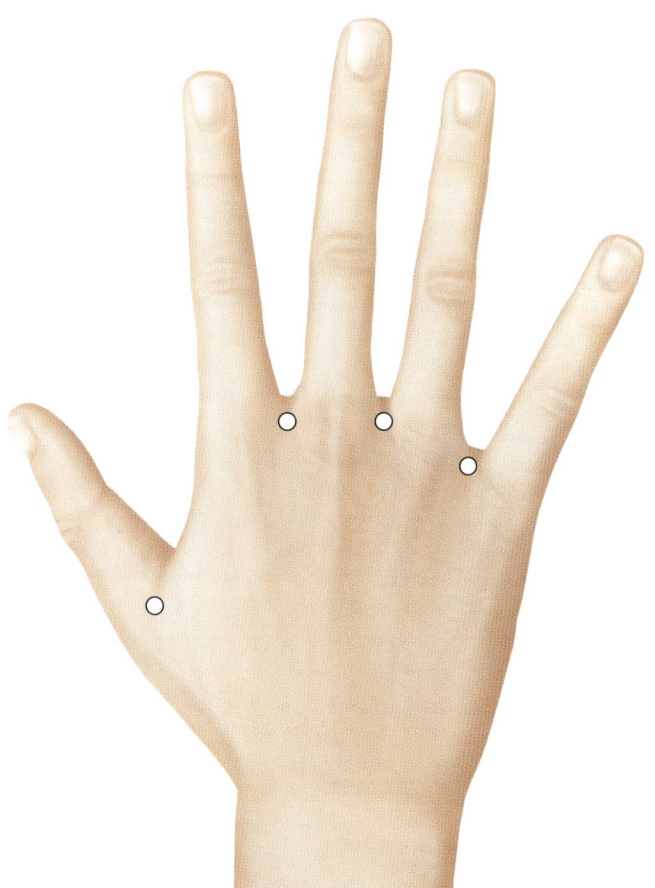

There are several miscellaneous acupoints and reflex points on the hands but Ba Xie represents the most useful in an everyday clinical setting.

Location
Eight points (four on each hand) situated between the metacarpo-phalangeal joints approximately 0.5 cun proximal to the web margins.

Needle
Up to 1 cun with an oblique insertion towards the middle of the palm.

Moxa and pressure
Direct or indirect moxa can be extremely effective in chronic arthritis of the hands. Acupressure, too, is indicated in this condition and can be an excellent self-help tool.

Indications
These points are excellent as ancillary ones to treat many different hand conditions including; rheumatoid and osteo-arthritis, swelling and oedema, stiffness and contractures as well as post trauma (accident or surgery) treatment.

Miscellaneous Points of the Arm and Hand (AH)

M-LF-5 *Xi Yan* (Eyes of the Knee)

膝眼 ★★★★

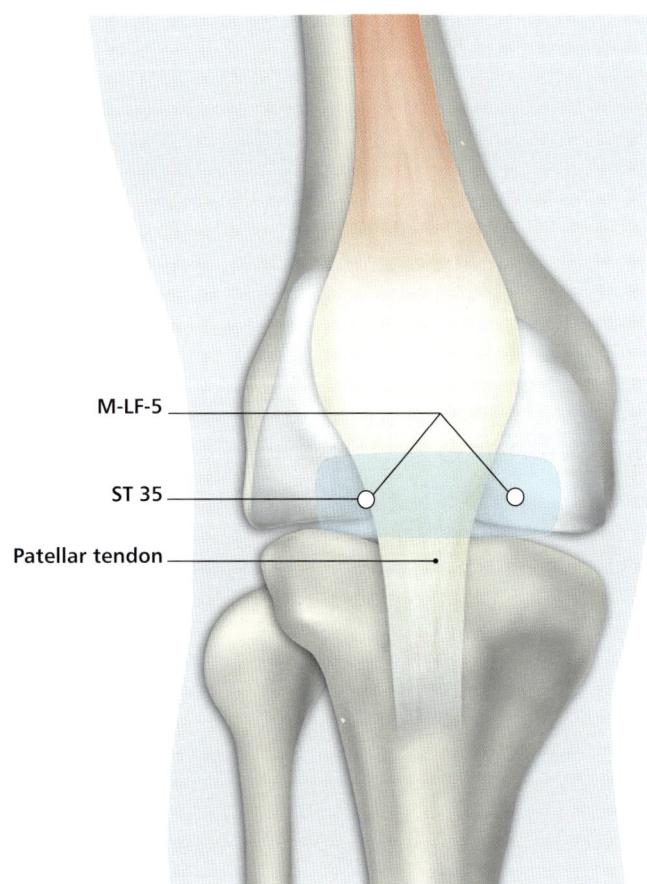

M-LF-5

ST 35

Patellar tendon

Location
Two points situated just below the patella, one in the medial and one in the lateral depression formed by the quadriceps tendon when the knee is flexed. The lateral point is ST 35 (Wai Xi Yan).

Needle
With the patient's knee flexed to 90 degrees (if possible) and supported by firm cushions, use an oblique insertion of up to 3 cun using a long needle.

Moxa and pressure
Use moxa punk on the end of a copper (fire) needle in any case of chronic pain and stiffness of the knee. Acupressure is also very effective if the patient does not wish to have needles. The tips of the two middle fingers need to pressed against each point and held for up to five minutes.

Indications
These two excellent points are used in all chronic conditions of the knee including osteoarthritis, stiffness, swelling and oedema and post surgery rehabilitation.

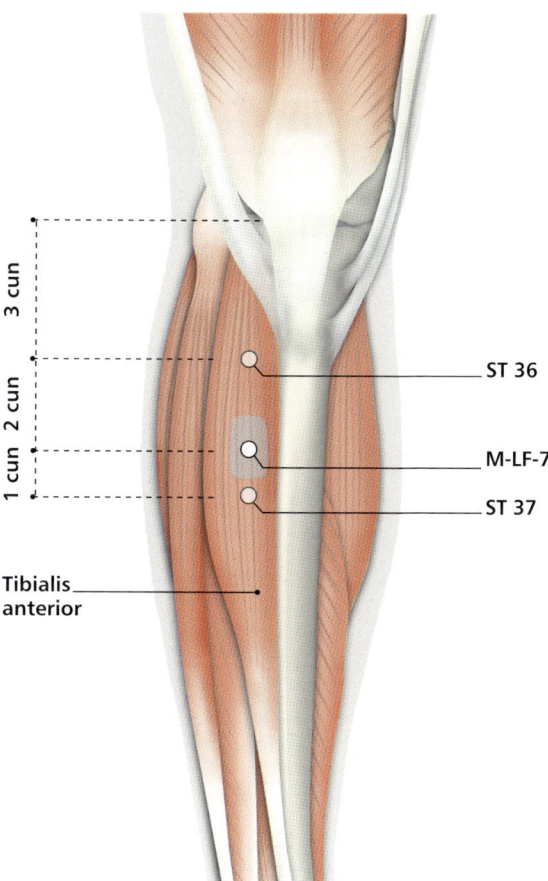

3 cun

2 cun

1 cun

ST 36

M-LF-7

ST 37

Tibialis
anterior

Location
Situated approximately 2 cun directly below ST 36 on the Stomach channel of the right leg only.

Needle
Up to 1.5 cun using a perpendicular insertion.

Moxa and pressure
Moxa is not as effective as needle or pressure on this point, but is not ruled out. Acupressure serves as both analytical and treatment for acute appendix and lower abdominal discomfort.

Indications
This point is extensively used for the diagnosis and treatment of acute and chronic appendicitis as well as lower abdominal discomfort, bloating and indigestion. It is also a useful point to help in the treatment of ileo-caecal valve syndrome.

M-LF-10 *Ba Feng* (Eight Winds)

八風

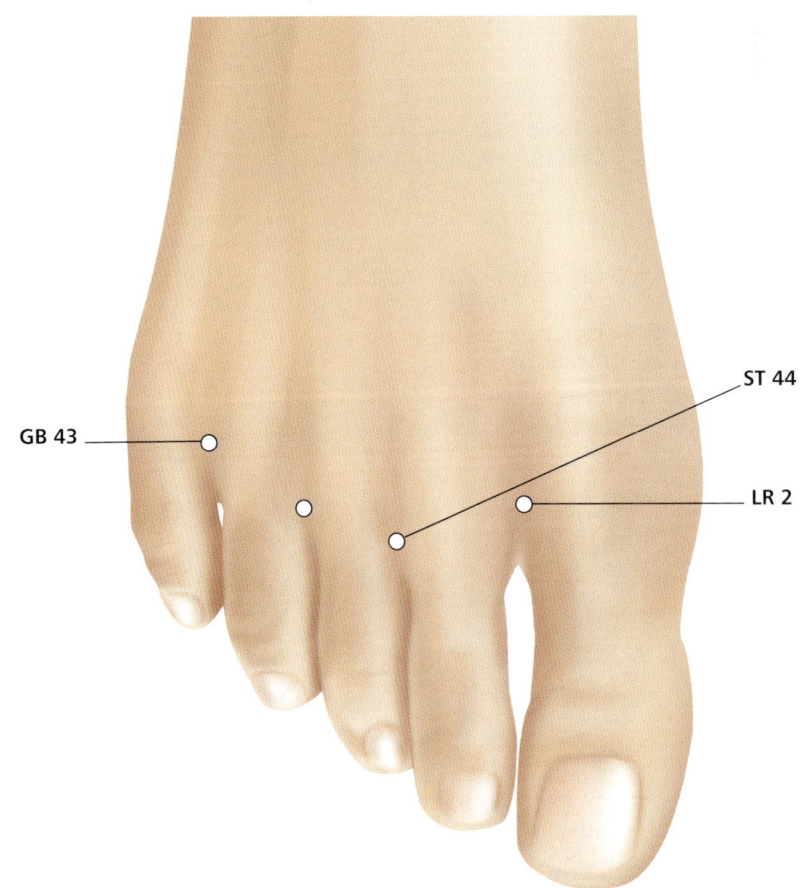

Location
Eight points (four on each foot) on the dorsal surface of the foot situated in the webs between each toe, distal to the metatarso-phalangeal joints, approximately 0.5 cun proximal to the web margins. These points are the equivalent to the Ba Xie points on the hands and include GB 43, ST 44 and LR 2 in their ranks.

Needle
Use an oblique insertion of 1 cun directed towards the heel.

Moxa and pressure
Direct or indirect moxa can be very effective in chronic conditions of the toes and feet. Acupressure is equally effective with patients who cannot tolerate needles.

Indications
These are excellent points that may be used in local foot conditions as well as general imbalance. Conditions and symptoms include pain, stiffness and swelling of the toes (ideal in some cases of rheumatoid arthritis). They are also indicated in headache, tinnitus, eye inflammation and hypertension.

Resources

Cheng, Xinhong.: 1999. *Chinese Acupuncture and Moxibustion*. Foreign Languages Press, Beijing.

Clemente, C.: 1985. *Gray's Anatomy of the Human Body, thirtieth edition*. Lippincott, Williams & Wilkins, Baltimore.

Cross, J.R. 2000. *Acupressure: Clinical Applications in Musculo-skeletal Conditions*. Butterworth Heinemann, Oxford, England

Cross, J.R. 2001. *Acupressure and Reflextherapy in the Treatment of Medical Conditions*. Butterworth Heinemann, Oxford, England

Cross, J.R. 2006. *Healing with the Chakra Energy System: Acupressure, Bodywork and Reflexology for Total Health*. North Atlantic Books, Berkeley, California

Cross, J.R. 2008. *Acupuncture and the Chakra Energy System: Treating the Cause of Disease*. North Atlantic Books, Berkeley, California

Deadman, P., Baker, K., Al-Khafaji, Mazin.: 2007. *A Manual of Acupuncture, second edition*. Journal of Chinese Medicine Publications, Brighton.

Ding, Li, Professor.: 1991. *Acupuncture, Meridian Theory and Acupuncture Points*. English translation by You Benlin and Wang Zhaorong, Nanjing College of Traditional Chinese Medicine and Nanjing International Acupuncture Training Centre. Foreign Languages Press, Beijing.

Ebner, M.: 1962. *Connective Tissue Massage: Theory and Therapeutic Applications*. Churchill Livingstone, Edinburgh

Ellis, A., Wiseman, N., Boss, K..: 1989. *Grasping the Wind*. Paradigm Publications, Brookline, Massachusetts.

Ellis, A., Wiseman, N., Boss, K.: 1991. *Fundamentals of Chinese Acupuncture, revised edition*. Paradigm Publications, Brookline, Massachusetts.

Ellis, N.: 1994. *Acupuncture in Clinical Practice: A Guide for Health Professionals*. Chapman and Hall, London

Hecker, Hans-Ulrich, Steveling, Angelika, Peuker, Elmar, Kastner, Jorg, Liebchen, Kay.: 2001. *Color Atlas of Acupuncture: Body Points, Ear Points, Trigger Points*. Thieme Medical Publishers, Germany.

Hoppenfeld, S.: 1976. *Physical Examination of the Spine and Extremities*. Appleton-Century-Crofts, a Publishing Division of Prentice-Hall, USA.

Jarmey, C.: 1999. *Shiatsu: a Complete Guide*. Harper Collins, London.

Jarmey, C.: 2004. *The Atlas of Musculo-skeletal Anatomy*. Lotus Publishing / North Atlantic Books, Chichester / Berkeley.

Jarmey, C.: 2006. *The Foundations of Shiatsu*. Lotus Publishing / North Atlantic Books, Chichester / Berkeley.

Jarmey, C. & Bouratinos, I.: 2008. *A Practical Guide to Acu-points*. Lotus Publishing / North Atlantic Books, Chichester / Berkeley.

Kendall, F. P., McCreary, E. K. & Provance, P. G.: 1993. *Muscles: Testing and Function, 4th edition*. Lippincott, Williams & Wilkins, Baltimore.

Lade, A.: 1989. *Acupuncture Points: Images and Functions*. Eastland Press, Seattle, Washington.

Lian, Yu-Lin, Chen, Chun-Yan, Hammes, M., Kolster, B. C. *The Pictorial Atlas of Acupuncture: an Illustrated Manual of Acupuncture Points*. Edited by Hans P. Ogal and Wolfram Stor. Translation from German by Colin Grant. Konemann Publishers.

Longmore, M., Wilkinson, I., Torok, E.: 2001. *Oxford Handbook of Clinical Medicine, fifth edition*. Oxford University Press.

Maciocia, Giovanni.: 1989. *The Foundations of Chinese Medicine: a Comprehensive Text for Acupuncturists and Herbalists, first edition*. Churchill Livingstone, Edinburgh.

McCracken, T.: 2005. *Black's Concise Atlas of Human Anatomy*. A & C Black, London.

Netter, F. H.: 1995. *Atlas of Human Anatomy*. Ciba-Geigy Corporation, Summit, New Jersey.

Platzer, W.: 2003. *Color Atlas and Textbook of Human Anatomy, Vol. 1: Locomotor System*. Thieme Medical Publishers, Germany.

Putz, R., Pabst, R., Weiglein, A. H.: 2001. *Sobotta Atlas of Human Anatomy, thirteenth edition*. Lippincott, Williams & Wilkins, Baltimore.

Rohen, Johannes W., Yokochi, Chihiro, Lutjen-Drecoll, Elke.: 2002. *Color Atlas of Anatomy: a Photographic Study of the Human Body, fifth edition*. Lippincott, Williams & Wilkins, Baltimore.

Schuenke, M., Schulte, E., & Shumacher, U.: 2005. *General Anatomy and Musculo-skeletal System*. Thieme Medical Publishers, Germany.

Shanghai College of Traditional Medicine.: 1981. *Acupuncture: a Comprehensive Text*. Translated and edited by John O'Connor and Dan Bensky. Eastland Press, Seattle, Washington.

Wang, Deshen.: 1993. *Manual of International Standardization of Acupuncture (Zhenjiu) Point Names*. The Higher Education Press of China.

Zhong, Yi Xue, Chu, Ji.: 1995. *Fundamentals of Chinese Medicine, revised edition*. Translated and amended by Nigel Wiseman and Andrew Ellis. Paradigm Publications, Brookline, Massachusetts.

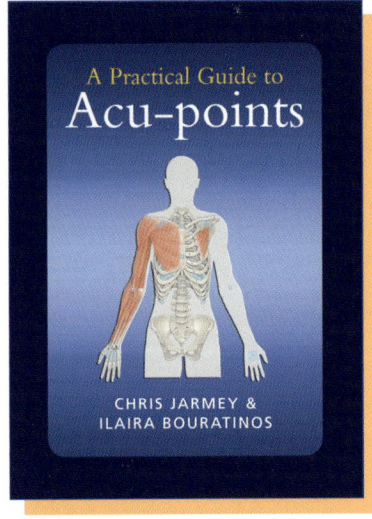

A Practical Guide to Acu-points

**Chris Jarmey
Ilaira Bouratinos**

978 0 9543188 4 0; **£24.99**; 360 pages; 275 mm x 212 mm; 440 colour illustrations; paperback

Written with Ilaira Bouratinos, this book is an exceptionally well-illustrated guide to the location and properties of acu-points, and uniquely provides additional information for bodyworkers such as shiatsu and tuina therapists. The point is given as a precise anatomical location and illustrated with a dot, along with alternative locations where relevant, but this book delineates the larger area where the point can be activated by pressure, gua sha and other means. Also the optimum position for treatment via acupuncture, acupressure and other treatment strategies is given. The distribution of sensation resulting from point stimulation is also documented, and differentiated between pressure and needle application where appropriate.

Chris Jarmey, M.C.S.P., D.S., M.R.S.S., qualified as a Chartered Physiotherapist in 1979, and taught anatomy, shiatsu, qigong, and bodywork therapy throughout Europe. He authored several best-selling books, including Acupressure for Common Ailments and Shiatsu: the Complete Guide. The founder of the European Shiatsu School, Chris tragically died in November 2008: the books he wrote for Lotus and for other publishers are a fitting legacy, and will help students with their studies for years to come.

Ilaira Bouratinos, Dip.Ac., D.S., is Principal of both the European Institute of Oriental Medicine, and the Greek branch of the European Shiatsu School. Ilaira received her diploma in acupuncture from the London School of Acupuncture and Traditional Chinese Medicine in the early 1990's.

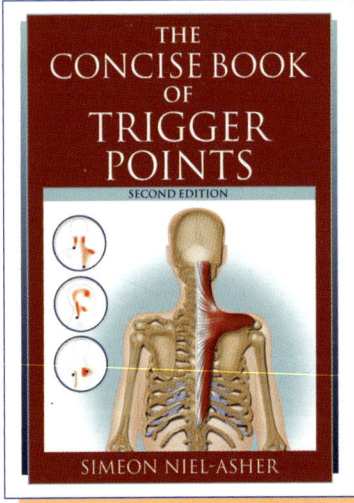

The Concise Book of Trigger Points, Second Edition

Simeon Niel-Asher

978 1 905367 12 2; **£17.99**; 224 pages; 275 mm x 212 mm; 260 colour / black and white illustrations; paperback

The new edition of the bestselling The Concise Book of Trigger Points includes a self-help section, and up-to-date research on trigger points. Written for the student and early practitioner, the book provides a sound background to the physiology of trigger points, and the general methods of treatment. The following six chapters are organized by muscle groups, with each major skeletal muscle identified, and physiological implications of the trigger points and techniques for treatment discussed.

Simeon Niel-Asher, B. Phil., B.Sc., (Ost.), qualified as an osteopath in 1992. He is involved in treating, research, writing, and teaching throughout Europe, the Middle East, and the USA.